Illustrated Diagnosis of
SYSTEMIC DISEASES

Illustrated Diagnosis of
SYSTEMIC DISEASES

R. DOUGLAS COLLINS, M.D.

Attending Physician in Internal Medicine and Neurology at the Berwick Hospital, Berwick, Pennsylvania; Consultant in Internal Medicine and Neurology to the Bloomsburg Hospital, Bloomsburg, Pennsylvania, and the Locust Mountain Hospital, Shenandoah, Pennsylvania; Consultant Neurologist to the White Haven State Hospital, White Haven, Pennsylvania; Diplomate of the American Board of Internal Medicine

Color Illustrations by
JOSEPH ALEMANY, B.A.

166 Cases Illustrated in Color

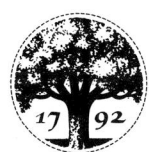

J. B. Lippincott Company
Philadelphia   Toronto

COPYRIGHT © 1972 BY J. B. LIPPINCOTT COMPANY

This book is fully protected by copyright and, with the exception of brief excerpts for review, no part of it may be reproduced in any form by print, photoprint, microfilm, or any other means without written permission from the publisher.

ISBN-0-397-50281-8

Library of Congress Catalog Card Number 71-157908

Printed in the United States of America

3 5 6 4 2

To Pauline, my wife

Preface

Understanding and recalling the many facets of systemic diseases can tax the minds of even the most astute clinicians. With the ever-increasing subspecialization of medicine, these diseases, which may involve many organ systems, are frequently forgotten in the differential diagnosis. Each specialist is well-acquainted with the local diseases of his particular specialty. For example, the urologist would scarcely forget renal calculus or hypernephroma in the differential diagnosis of hematuria. But he might fail to consider lupus erythematosus or Wegener's granulomatosis in this differential.

Thus the purpose of this book is easily defined: first, to draw together the most significant facts about each systemic disease into one composite picture, and second, to present a systematic approach to the differential diagnosis.

To fulfill the first of these objectives, I have used a technique I first applied in *Illustrated Manual of Neurologic Diagnosis* to produce, in the present book, Profiles of Systemic Disease (Part One).

A full-color anatomic illustration of the human body becomes the background on which are portrayed over 150 important systemic diseases. The organs involved in each disease are shaded, speckled in black, or merely marked. As disease of each organ gives rise to certain symptoms, many of the symptoms of each systemic disease are symbolized by this technique. Where there is skin or eye involvement an additional drawing of each is included, but I have deliberately left these out where they are not typically involved. A clinical synopsis of a typical case accompanies the illustration as well as clinical notes and a brief description of the pathology, providing a composite summary and a basis for easy recall of the most significant clinicopathologic facts of each disease. These cases, which are summaries of actual cases, present the pertinent symptoms and signs as the physician actually sees them.

The second of the above objectives is accomplished by the Introduction and by the tables in Part Two. The presenting symptoms and signs of a case of possible systemic disease will usually indicate the organ systems involved. Knowing which organs are involved is the key to the differential diagnosis of what the systemic disease is. Most systemic diseases characteristically involve certain tissues or organs of the body. The reason is that, as Virchow pointed out, the vulnerability of the tissue of each organ system to each etiologic agent is variable. The approach to the diagnosis and the organization of the tables are formulated on this principle.

The reader will quickly note that the text of this book is brief, increasing the omnipresent risk of being misleading. Much information regarding systemic diseases has been deliberately omitted, but since the avowed purpose is to emphasize those features having broad clinical application, I make no apology for this brevity. The backbone of the material is generally accepted knowledge, and this is valuable for the student, the general physician, or the specialist.

R. Douglas Collins

Acknowledgments

To acknowledge everyone who helped make this book possible would take several pages. Obviously my patients deserve immeasurable credit because, next to God, they are my most important teachers! For the first time in my career I have a brilliant, efficient, and cooperative office staff, and therefore I have had more time to spend on this book.

Rose Anne Volpicelli Minier and Bonnie Beck typed the manuscript. Joseph Alemany produced the vital color illustrations.

Finally, I am deeply grateful to Brooks Stewart, Stuart Freeman, Mildred Purnell, and all the other personnel at J. B. Lippincott Company for their continued assistance throughout all the stages of preparation.

R.D.C.

Contents

Introduction: The Diagnosis of Systemic Diseases 1

PART ONE: PROFILE OF SYSTEMIC DISEASE

1 Allergic Diseases 5

   Serum Sickness 6

2 Blood Diseases 9

   Aplastic Anemia 10
   Mediterranean Anemia 12
   Sickle Cell Anemia 14
   Henoch-Schönlein Purpura 16
   Idiopathic Thrombocytopenic Purpura 18
   Thrombotic Thrombocytopenic Purpura 20
   Hemophilia 22

3 Collagen Diseases 23

   Rheumatoid Arthritis 24
   Dermatomyositis 26
   Periarteritis Nodosa 28
   Scleroderma 30
   Ankylosing Spondylitis 32
   Still's Disease (Juvenile Rheumatoid Arthritis) 34
   Wegener's Granulomatosis 35
   Lupus Erythematosus, Case 1 36
   Lupus Erythematosus, Case 2 38
   Lupus Erythematosus, Case 3 40

4 Congenital Diseases 41

   Arachnodactyly 42
   Fibrocystic Disease 44
   Gargoylism 45
   Mongolism 46
   Neurofibromatosis 48
   Osteopetrosis 50
   Polycystic Disease 51
   Peutz-Jegher's Syndrome 52
   Sturge-Weber Syndrome 54
   Tuberosclerosis 56
   Porphyria Cutanea Tarda 58
   Porphyria Erythropoietica 60
   Porphyria, Intermittent Abdominal Type 62

5 Deficiency Diseases 63

   Pernicious Anemia 64
   Beriberi 66
   Plummer-Vinson Syndrome 67
   Kwashiorkor 68
   Pellagra 70
   Scurvy 72
   Vitamin A Deficiency 74
   Hypervitaminosis A 76
   Rickets 78

6 Endocrine Diseases 79

   Addison's Disease 80
   Acromegaly 82
   Adrenogenital Syndrome 83
   Aldosteronism 84
   Cretinism 86
   Cushing's Syndrome 88
   Primary Hyperparathyroidism 90
   Hyperthyroidism 91
   Hypoparathyroidism 92
   Hypopituitarism 94
   Hypothyroidism 96
   Klinefelter's Syndrome 98
   Islet Cell Adenoma 100
   Lawrence-Moon-Biedl Syndrome 101
   Menopause 102
   Pheochromocytoma 104
   Zollinger-Ellison Syndrome 105
   Pseudohypoparathyroidism 106
   Turner's Syndrome (Gonadal Dysgenesis) 108

7 Infectious Diseases 111

Viral Diseases 113

   Chickenpox (Varicella) 114
   Yellow Fever 116
   Infectious Mononucleosis 117
   Lymphogranuloma Venereum 118
   Mumps 119
   Measles (Rubeola) 120
   Rubella 122
   Smallpox 124
   Poliomyelitis 126

Rickettsiae 127

   Rocky Mountain Spotted Fever 128
   Epidemic Typhus 130
   Scrub Typhus 132
   Q-Fever 134

Bacteria 135

   Diphtheria 136
   Subacute Bacterial Endocarditis 138
   Acute Rheumatic Fever 140
   Scarlet Fever 142
   Streptobacillary Fever 144
   Typhoid Fever 146
   Brucellosis 148
   Gonorrhea 149
   Listeriosis 150
   Meningococcemia 152
   Plague 154
   Miliary Tuberculosis 155
   Pulmonary Tuberculosis 156
   Tularemia 158

xii   Contents

Spirochetes 159
   Relapsing Fever 160
   Spirillary Rat-Bite Fever 162
   Weil's Disease... 164
   Congenital Syphilis 166
   Syphilis, Case 1 168
   Syphilis, Case 2 170

Mycoses.. 171
   North American Blastomycosis 172
   Coccidioidomycosis 174
   Cryptococcosis 175
   Disseminated Histoplasmosis 176
   Mucormycosis... 178
   Nocardiosis... 179
   Sporotrichosis... 180

Parasites 181
   Chagas' Disease 182
   Amebiasis... 184
   Cysticercosis 185
   Echinococcosis 186
   Filariasis (Bancroftian) 187
   Kala-azar 188
   Malaria 189
   Schistosomiasis (S. Mansoni) 190
   Toxoplasmosis 192
   African Trypanosomiasis 194
   Trichinosis 196

8 Metabolic Diseases 197
   Alkaptonuria and Ochronosis.................... 198
   Primary Systemic Amyloidosis 200
   Renal Tubular Acidosis 202
   Secondary Amyloidosis 203
   Diabetes Mellitus, Case 1......................... 204
   Diabetes Mellitus, Case 2......................... 205
   Diabetes Mellitus, Case 3......................... 206
   Diabetes Mellitus, Case 4......................... 208
   Glycogen Storage Disease (Von Gierke's Disease,
      Etc.) 209
   Essential Hypercholesterolemia................. 210
   Essential Hypertriglyceridemia 212
   Galactosemia 214
   Gout 216
   Idiopathic Hemochromatosis 218
   Lignac-Fanconi Syndrome (Cystinosis) 220
   Phenylpyruvic Oligophrenia 222
   Wilson's Disease....................................... 224

9 Neoplasms... 227
   Carcinoid Syndrome................................. 228
   Metastatic Carcinoma, Case 1................... 230
   Metastatic Carcinoma, Case 2................... 231
   Metastatic Carcinoma, Case 3................... 232
   Hodgkin's Disease 233
   Acute Lymphatic Leukemia....................... 234
   Chronic Lymphatic Leukemia 236
   Chronic Myelogenous Leukemia 237
   Macroglobulinemia 238
   Myelofibrosis with Myeloid Metaplasia 240

   Multiple Myeloma 241
   Polycythemia Vera.................................... 242

10 Organ Failure 245
   Chronic Pulmonary Emphysema................ 246
   Chronic Congestive Heart Failure 247
   Chronic Hepatic Failure............................ 248
   Chronic Renal Failure............................... 250
   Malabsorption Syndrome 252
   Chronic Pancreatitis 254

11 The Reticuloendothelioses 257
   Gaucher's Disease 258
   Histiocytosis X: Hand-Schüller-Christian
      Disease 260
   Histiocytosis X: Letterer-Siwe Disease 262
   Niemann-Pick Disease 264

12 Toxic Diseases 267
   Alcoholism 268
   Hypokalemia... 269
   Digitalis Intoxication 270
   Phenothiazine Intoxication 271
   Dilantin Intoxication 272
   Arsenic Poisoning 274
   Carbon Tetrachloride Poisoning 276
   Lead Poisoning... 278
   Benzene Poisoning 280

13 Diseases of Unknown Etiology................ 281
   Acrodynia 282
   Atherosclerosis... 284
   Ulcerative Colitis...................................... 286
   Essential Hypertension 288
   Myotonia Atrophica 290
   Reiter's Syndrome 292
   Sarcoidosis... 294
   Whipple's Disease 296

PART TWO: TABLES

   I. Clinical Key to Organ System Involvement... 301
  II. Prominent Physical Signs of Systemic
     Disease 309
 III. Organ Involvement as a Key to the Diagnosis
     of Systemic Disease 311
 IV. Systemic Disease With the Organs That
     Show Significant Functional or Pathologic
     Changes.. 319
  V. Local Disease as a Symptom of Systemic
     Disease 322
 VI. Laboratory Work-up of Systemic Diseases 327
VII. Laboratory Tests of Organ Involvement 331

Index... 333

Illustrated Diagnosis of
SYSTEMIC DISEASES

Introduction:

The Diagnosis of Systemic Diseases

The History and Physical Examination. A thorough history and physical examination are more important in diagnosing systemic diseases than in diagnosing any other group of diseases. A cold, a staphylococcal abscess, or an episode of gastroenteritis may well be diagnosed after a 5-minute examination in the office, or even over the telephone. This is not so with a systemic disease.

The *chief complaint* in diagnosing a systemic disease is developed in three ways. First it is developed in terms of time, location, intensity, and the relationship to certain events in the patient's life. Second, the chief complaint is related to the presence or absence of other symptoms or physical signs in the organ system suggested by the chief complaint. Table I (Part Two, p. 301) is organized in this fashion for easy recall of associated symptoms. For the diagnosis of local disease, the clinician might be able to stop right here. However, since systemic disease usually affects two or more organs at a time, a third step must always be taken. At this point a careful review of systems in the history and the physical is made. Does the patient complain of pain anywhere else in the body? Does the patient have any bleeding from the body orifices or skin? Are there any lumps or bumps anywhere in the body? Are there any symptoms or signs of functional changes in any of the organs, such as cough (indicating changes in the lung), tachycardia (heart), vomiting or diarrhea (gastrointestinal tract)? And so on.

In the physical examination emphasis should be placed on examination of the eye, the skin, and the nervous system. On examination of the eye one may note corneal opacities (suggestive of Hurler's disease), a Kayser-Fleischer ring (Wilson's disease), or cataracts (diabetes mellitus, galactosemia, myotonia atrophica). There are many other eye signs illustrated in Part One of this book and mentioned in Table II (Part Two, p. 309). Further discussion of this subject may be found in *Eye Signs in General Disease* by F. H. Haessler (Springfield, Ill., Charles C Thomas, 1960).

In the examination of the skin, one must note carefully the character of the lesion and the distribution. This is the key to the diagnosis of many skin lesions. The rash of scarlet fever is erythematous, the rash of measles is maculopapular, and the rash of chickenpox is vesicular. The rash of erythema multiforme is on the back of the hands, whereas the rash of erythema induratum is on the back of the calves. The illustrations in Part One of this book demonstrate the distribution and description in each case. For further discussion of this subject the reader is referred to *Difficult Diagnosis* by H. J. Roberts (Philadelphia, W. B. Saunders, 1958) and to *The Cutaneous Manifestations of Systemic Diseases* by J. G. Downing (No. 182, American Lecture Series, monograph in American Lectures in Dermatology, ed. by A. C. Curtis, Springfield, Ill., Charles C Thomas, 1954; also published in England by Blackwell and in Canada by Ryerson).

One does not have to be a neurologist to determine whether the nervous system is involved in most systemic diseases. The tremor in Wilson's disease or the wristdrop in lead poisoning are usually obvious. It does help to examine all the reflexes, power, coordination, and sensory modalities, as well as each cranial nerve. Depression is an important manifestation in many systemic diseases. The reader will find additional discussion of this subject in *Neurological Manifestations of General Diseases* by J. A. Aita (Springfield, Ill., Charles C Thomas, 1964).

Assembling and Interpreting the Data. Once the history and physical examination are complete, the symptoms and signs are listed together. Then with the help of Table I, the organ or organs involved in each case may be determined. This is the key to a differential diagnosis of systemic disease. By knowing which organs are involved one can determine the most likely systemic disease by using Table III (Part Two, p. 311). Because of the variable vulnerability of different tissues to different etiologic agents, each systemic disease characteristically involves certain organs. These are listed in Table IV (Part Two, p. 319). However, Table III lists these in reverse so that they may be applied in diagnosis. Some physicians may find the use of these tables unnecessary; others may find it more enjoyable to page through the illustrations in Part One to determine the differential diagnosis of the organ or organs involved. The data presented in these tables is not new. It is merely organized for quick reference and recall.

The busy physician who cannot take the time to analyze each case in the foregoing manner may find Table V (Part Two, p. 322) useful. Here are listed the systemic diseases that may masquerade as a local disease of each organ. This is particularly of value when a local disease seems especially resistant to therapy. It may in actuality be the first clue to a systemic disease.

Laboratory, X-ray, and Special Diagnostic Procedures. In *Illustrated Manual of Laboratory Diagnosis* this author has already discussed the use of the laboratory in clinical diagnosis. Two tables from that book have been included here with a few alterations. When the clinician is relatively certain of the diagnosis after his examination, he will find more specific tests to confirm his diagnosis in Table VI (Part Two, p. 327). All too frequently the picture is not so rosy. He needs laboratory tests to determine which organ or organs are involved. Table VII (Part Two, p. 331) will help him do just that. If the laboratory and x-ray department are of no help, then a therapeutic trial may be indicated. More often, however, a psychiatric evaluation will be rewarding. Then again, repeated examinations of the patient and additional history, as he is followed in the office at frequent intervals, may turn up the correct diagnosis.

The diagnosis of systemic disease is the most challenging of all diagnoses. As more and more of these diseases become treatable, establishing the correct diagnosis will become more and more rewarding to the doctor, his reputation, and his practice.

Part One

Profiles of Systemic Disease

1. Allergic Diseases
2. Blood Diseases
3. Collagen Diseases
4. Congenital Diseases
5. Deficiency Diseases
6. Endocrine Diseases
7. Infectious Diseases
8. Metabolic Diseases
9. Neoplasms
10. Organ Failure
11. The Reticuloendothelioses
12. Toxic Diseases
13. Diseases of Unknown Etiology

Chapter 1

Allergic Diseases

Allergic disorders typically affect only one organ system in individual cases. Thus allergies of the respiratory tract are manifested by hay fever and/or asthma, allergies of the skin by contact dermatitis and urticaria, and allergies of the intestinal tract (much less frequent) by recurrent diarrhea.

Anaphylactic shock can be considered a systemic disease because it often manifests with shock (vascular involvement), asthmatic bronchitis (respiratory involvement), and urticaria (skin involvement) simultaneously. Serum sickness, illustrated here, is a more insidious form of a systemic allergic reaction.

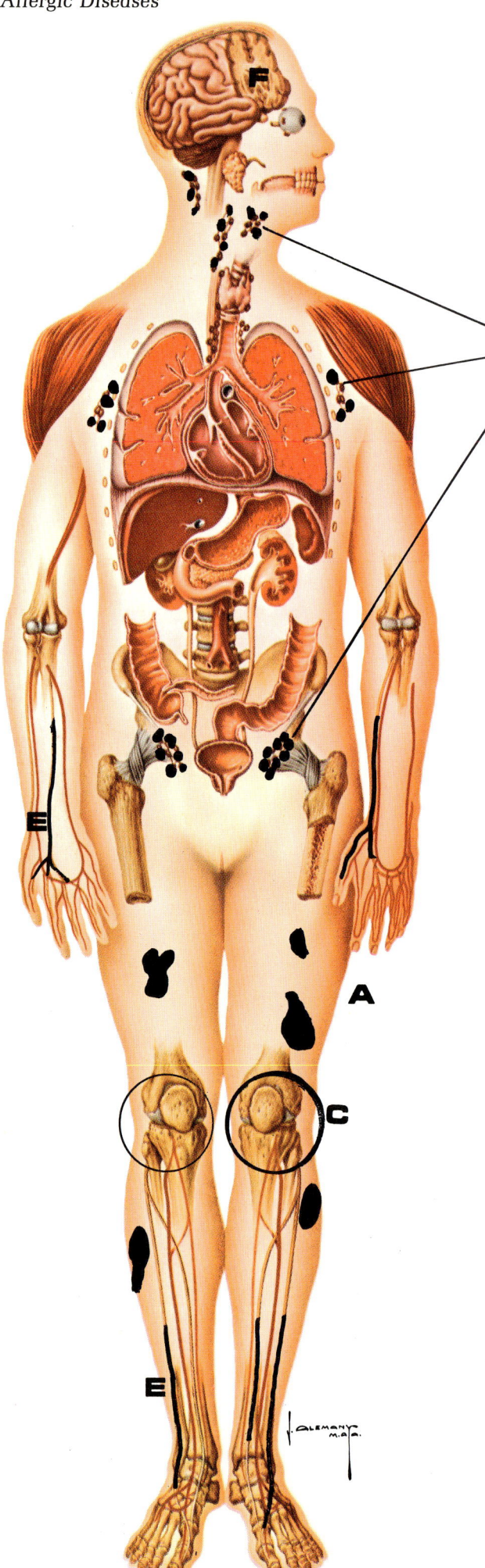

Serum Sickness

A 36-year-old white female complained of severe itching and a generalized rash. Three days later she developed fever, generalized headache, nausea and vomiting, and pain in her joints, particularly the left temporomandibular joint. She had had an injection of penicillin 1 week before for possible streptococcus pharyngitis.

Physical examination revealed generalized urticaria (A), diffuse lymphadenopathy (B), pain, swelling, and stiffness of the left temporomandibular joint and both knee joints (C).

Laboratory examination was essentially normal except for a high heterophil antibody titer which was absorbed by sheep erythrocytes. The sedimentation rate was normal.

Treatment with corticosteroids brought resolution.

Differential Diagnosis:
1. Rheumatic fever
2. Rheumatoid arthritis
3. Lupus erythematosus

4. Gonorrhea
5. Reiter's syndrome
6. Syphilitic arthritis
7. Periarteritis nodosa
8. Angioneurotic edema

Clinical Note. This reaction may occur with any foreign substance introduced into the body, particularly antisera. This condition resembles collagen disorders very much, and, in fact, periarteritis nodosa may be precipitated by penicillin, sulfonamides, and other drugs. Lupus erythematosus has been precipitated by hydralazine. The skin rash may be in many forms, but, unlike other skin disorders, it is usually associated with fever and lymphadenopathy.

Pathology. Occasionally vascular lesions are identical with those in periarteritis nodosa in the involved tissues, but generally there are few microscopic changes. Optic neuritis (D), peripheral neuritis (E), and central nervous system involvement (F) have also been observed in this condition. Actually, any organ of the body may be involved in an allergic drug reaction.

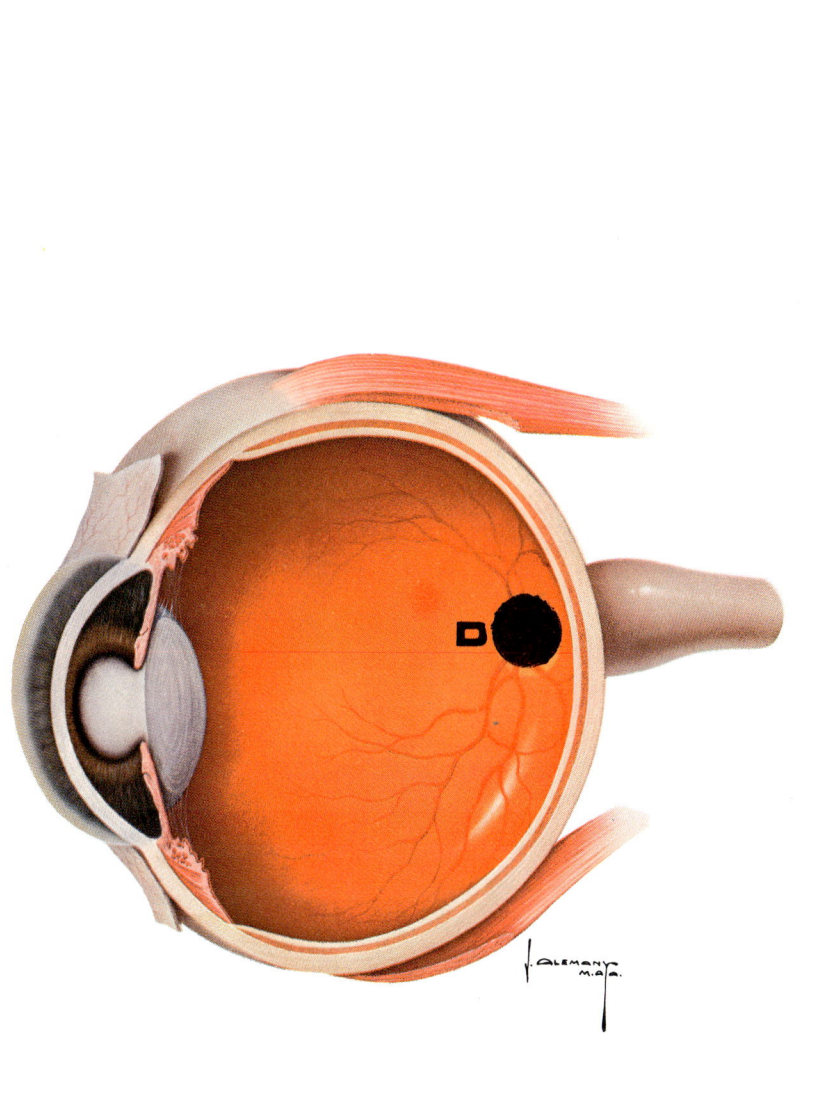
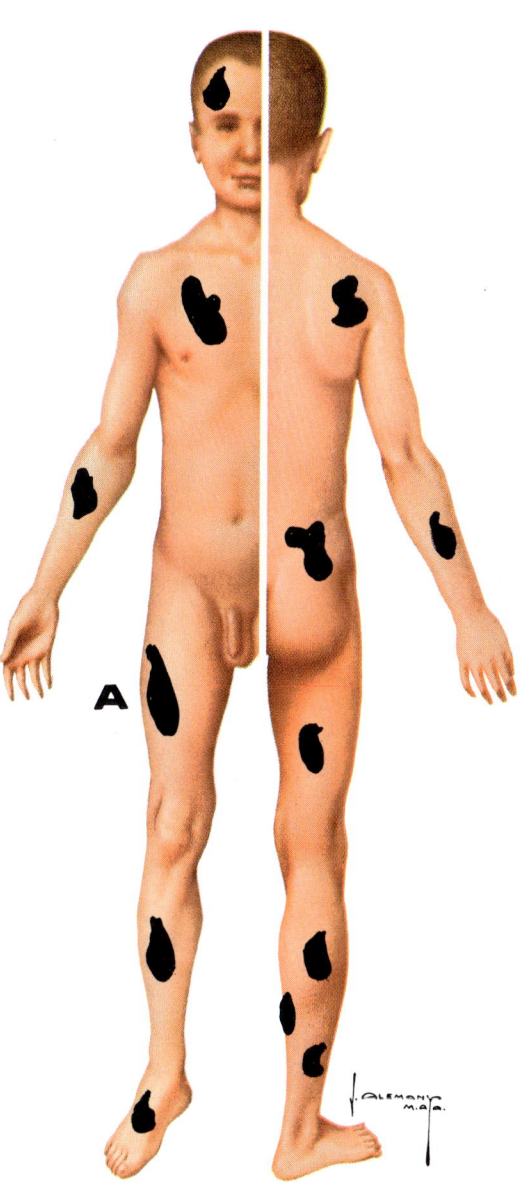

Chapter 2

Blood Diseases

Since the blood travels to all parts of the body, it is quite logical that any disease affecting the blood may involve many organs and thus be classified as a systemic disease. Furthermore, blood is formed in various organs (the bone marrow, liver, spleen, and lymph nodes), and destruction of red cells is carried on in at least 2 organs (the liver and spleen).

Many of the diseases depicted here are hereditary, but the blood may be affected by toxic, inflammatory, neoplastic, and other agents that are described in other chapters of this book.

Symptomatology can be divided into those symptoms due to anemia, those due to leukopenia, and those due to thrombocytopenia, or loss of one of the blood-clotting factors, and those due to hypertrophy of the blood-forming organs. Thus the anemia is manifested by pallor of the nails, skin, and conjunctiva, and by jaundice in some cases; the leukopenia, by ulcers of the tongue and mouth or frank signs of infection such as fever or chills; and, finally, the thrombocytopenia or the lack of a coagulation factor, by petechiae, ecchymoses, or frank bleeding from the nose, gastrointestinal tract, urinary tract, or into the joints.

The laboratory is essential for diagnosis, but a positive family history is also of immense help.

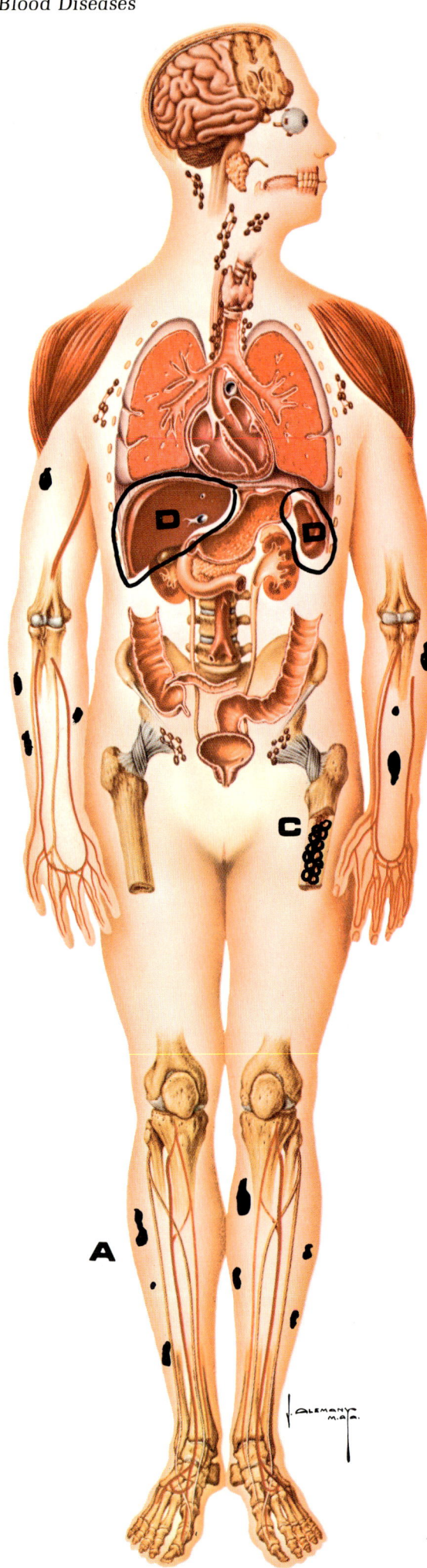

Aplastic Anemia

A 52-year-old white female complained of bruises of all 4 extremities, painful ulcers of the tongue, and intermittent fever of 1 week's duration. She had been treated with an antibiotic for a cold that had developed 3 weeks prior to admission.

Physical examination revealed pale skin and conjunctiva, numerous ecchymoses of all 4 extremities (A), necrotic ulcers of the tongue (B), but no lymphadenopathy or splenomegaly.

Laboratory examination revealed a RBC of 1,200,000 cells/cu. mm., a WBC of 2,000 cells/cu. mm., and a platelet count of 75,000 per cu. mm. The reticulocyte count was low, and the serum bilirubin was normal. Coombs' test was negative. Epinephrine failed to elevate the red cell count significantly. The spleen:liver ratio of chromium-tagged red cells was less than 2:1. Bone marrow examination revealed marked fatty infiltration (C) and occasional clusters of lymphocytes, but other elements were scarce.

Treatment with corticosteroids and testosterone was of no help.

Differential Diagnosis:
1. Myelophthisic anemia
2. Myelofibrosis
3. Primary hypersplenism
4. Aleukemic leukemia
5. Hodgkin's disease
6. Gaucher's disease
7. Lupus erythematosus
8. Cirrhosis of the liver

Clinical Note. The laboratory evaluation of these cases must be extensive to rule out other causes of anemia and to determine whether splenectomy is of any value. If the bone marrow is hypocellular, it is less likely that splenectomy will help. If the bone marrow is hypercellular, it is very likely that splenectomy will be beneficial. The determination of the spleen:liver ratio with chromium-tagged red cells will tell how damaging the spleen is to the patient's condition. There are an increasing number of drugs that can cause aplastic anemia; yet in a few cases the cause remains undetermined.

Pathology. The liver and spleen may be enlarged (D) by the extramedullary erythropoiesis in these organs. Mucosal ulcerations develop because of the lack of white cells to fight infection.

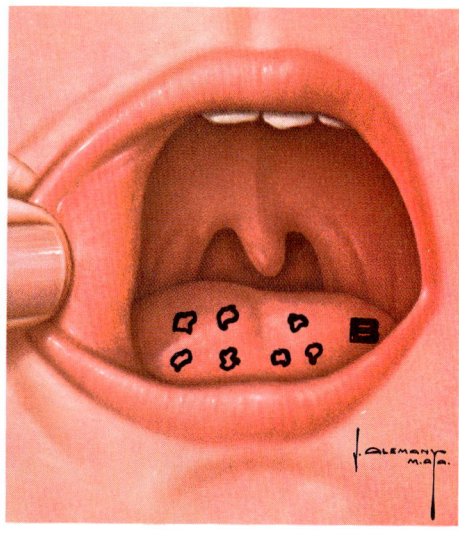

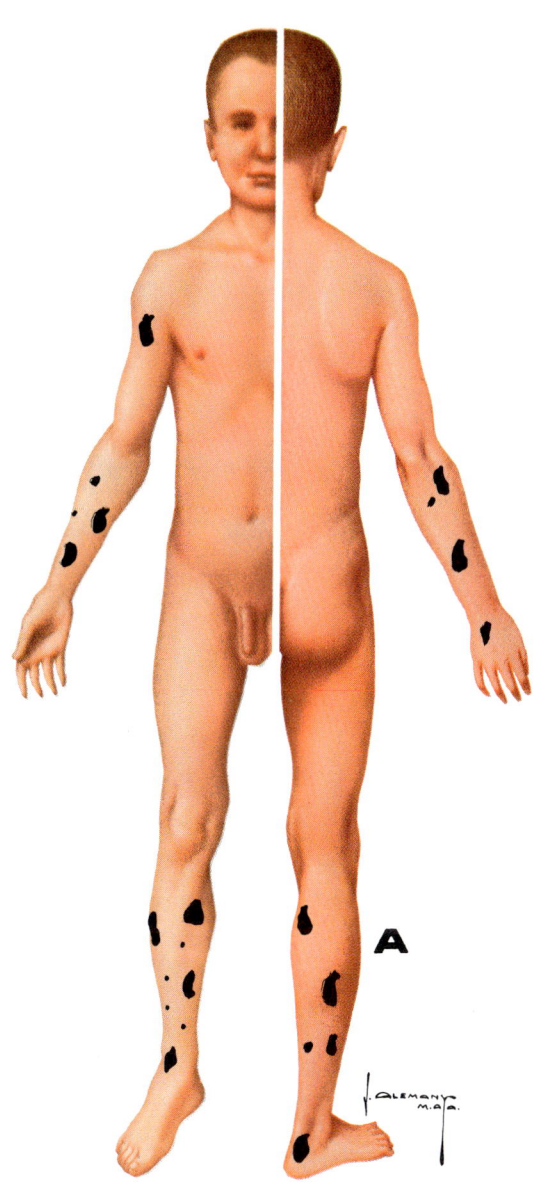

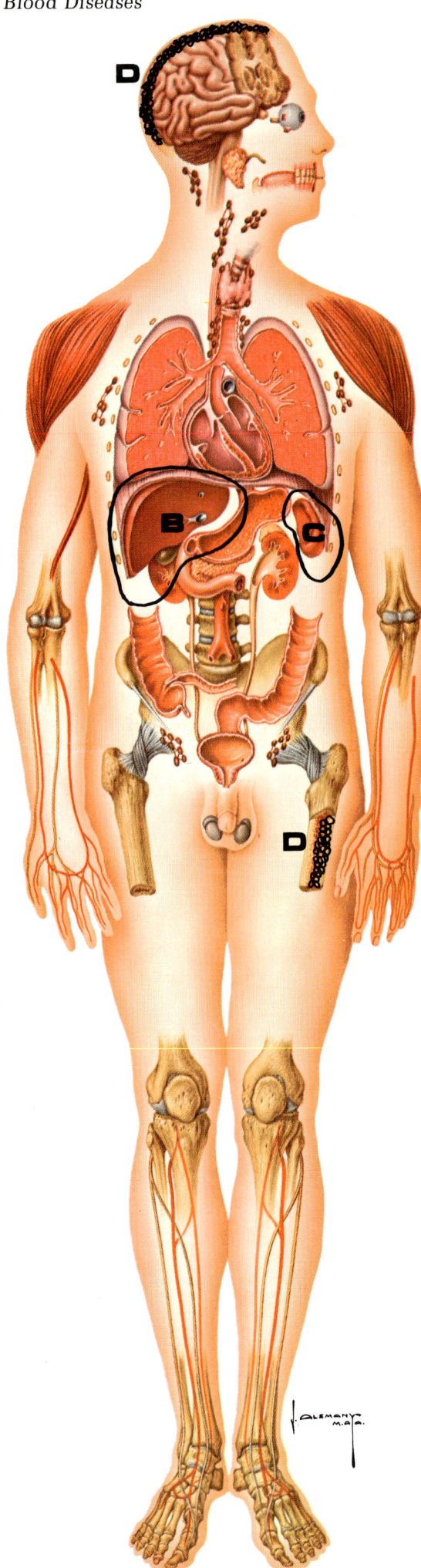

Mediterranean Anemia

A 13-month-old child presented at the emergency room with high fever and rigors, nausea and vomiting, and shortness of breath.

Physical examination revealed a listless, acutely ill, pale febrile infant with mongoloid face (A), icteric sclera, tonsillar exudates, enlarged liver (B) and spleen (C), and a grade II systolic murmur at the parasternal line in the 4th intercostal space.

Laboratory examination revealed a hemoglobin of 4.5 gm. per 100 ml.; microcytic red cells with anisopoikilocytosis and nucleated red cells; a reticulocyte count of 10 per cent; a WBC of 25,000 cells per cu. mm.; and a serum bilirubin of 7.5 mg./100 ml., most of which was of the indirect type. Hemoglobin electrophoresis revealed 60 per cent HbF.

Differential Diagnosis
1. Sickle cell anemia
2. Hemoglobin with anemia

3. Hereditary nonspherocytic hemolytic anemias
4. Hereditary spherocytosis
5. Acquired hemolytic anemia
6. Lupus erythematosus
7. Viral hepatitis
8. Infectious mononucleosis
9. Inclusion disease of the newborn
10. Common duct obstruction
11. Gargoylism

Clinical Note. As with most hemolytic anemias, acute exacerbations of the disease occur during infections—in this case, a streptococcal pharyngitis. It would have been easy to pass the infant off as a mongoloid with an upper respiratory infection if the icteric sclera had not been spotted. Hemoglobin electrophoresis is necessary for the diagnosis.

Pathology. The bone marrow is hyperplastic and occasionally megaloblastoid, and the enlargement of some bones, such as the skull, is due to intense erythropoiesis (D).

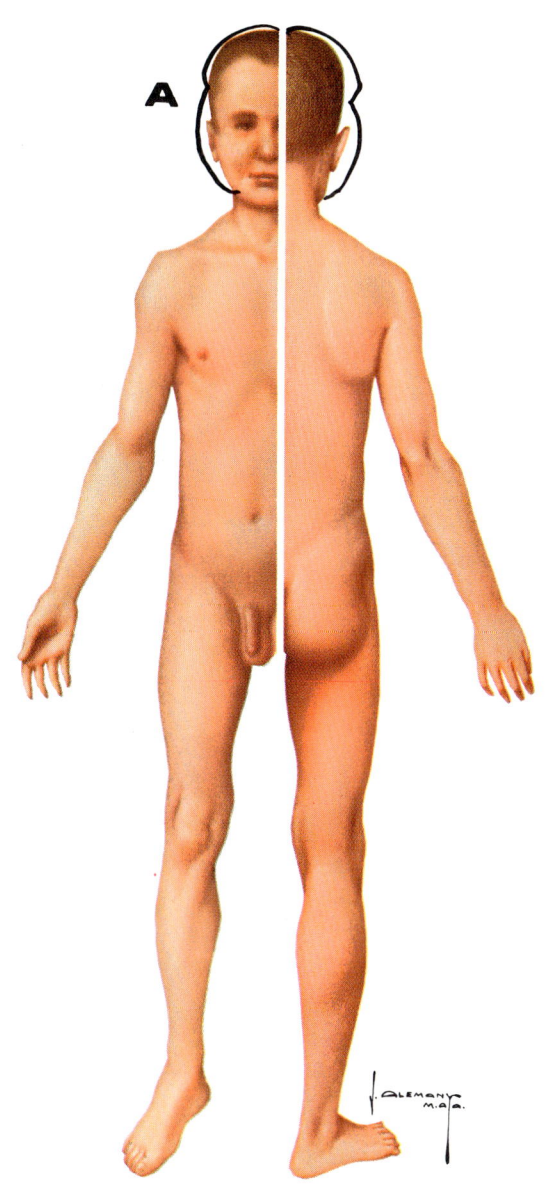

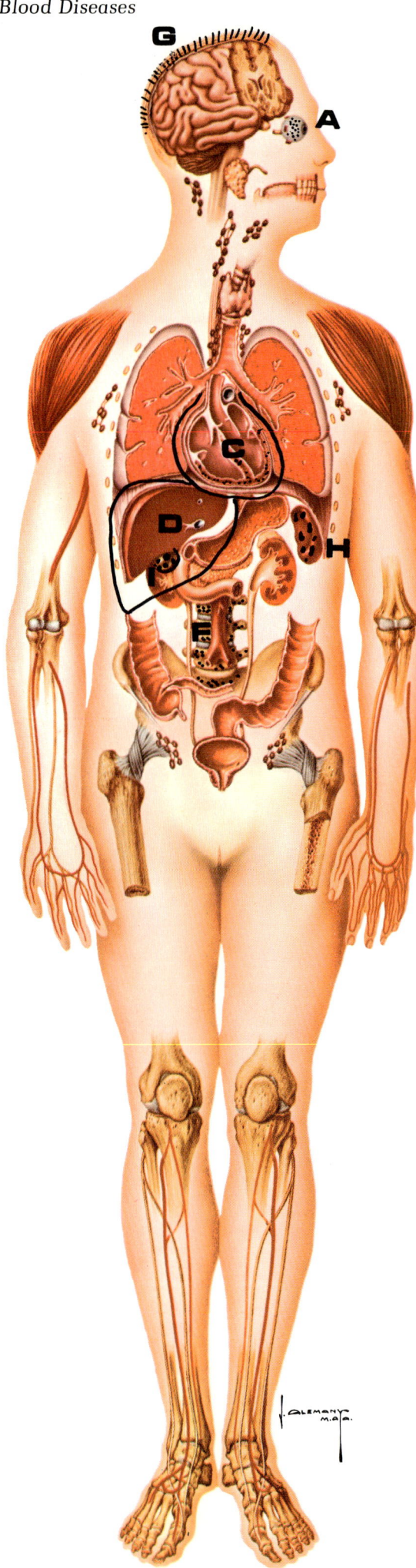

Sickle Cell Anemia

A 16-year-old Negro female was admitted to the hospital for treatment of a chronic leg ulcer. She had had at least 8 previous hospitalizations for fever, chills, abdominal and leg pains, during which a diagnosis of sickle cell crisis had been made. A younger sister was known to have sickle cell trait.

Physical examination revealed icteric sclera (A), retinal hemorrhages (B), and focal constriction of the retinal arteries, cardiomegaly (C), a grade II apical systolic murmur, hepatomegaly (D), and a large pretibial ulceration (E).

Laboratory examination revealed a normocytic, normochromic anemia, with a hemoglobin of 6.8 gm. per cent, an indirect bilirubin of 3.1 mg. per cent, 90 per cent sickling of blood cells on mixing with sodium metabisulfite, and an HbS on zone electrophoresis.

X-ray examination revealed osteoporosis of the spine with "fish-mouth" vertebrae (F) and a "hair-on-end" appearance of the skull (G).

Differential Diagnosis:
1. Rheumatic fever
2. Macroglobulinemia

3. Thalassemia
4. Hereditary spherocytosis
5. Malaria
6. Viral hepatitis
7. Collagen disease
8. Acute abdomen
9. Oroya fever
10. Acquired hemolytic anemia

Clinical Note. The crisis of sickle cell anemia is easily confused with rheumatic fever because of the cardiomegaly and auscultatory findings. The splenic and intestinal infarcts simulate the acute abdomen. After 10 years of age the spleen is not usually enlarged because of repeated infarcts (H).

Pathology. The reduced oxygen tension in the smaller vessels and capillaries that occurs in infections and other increased metabolic states leads to sickling of the red cells, increased viscosity of blood, and increased mechanical (but not osmotic) fragility of the red cells. This accounts for the multiple thromboses and infarcts in many organs, including the central nervous system, lungs, kidney, and long bones, and the hemolytic anemia associated with the disease. The large amount of pigment excreted in the bile may lead to bilirubin gallstones (I).

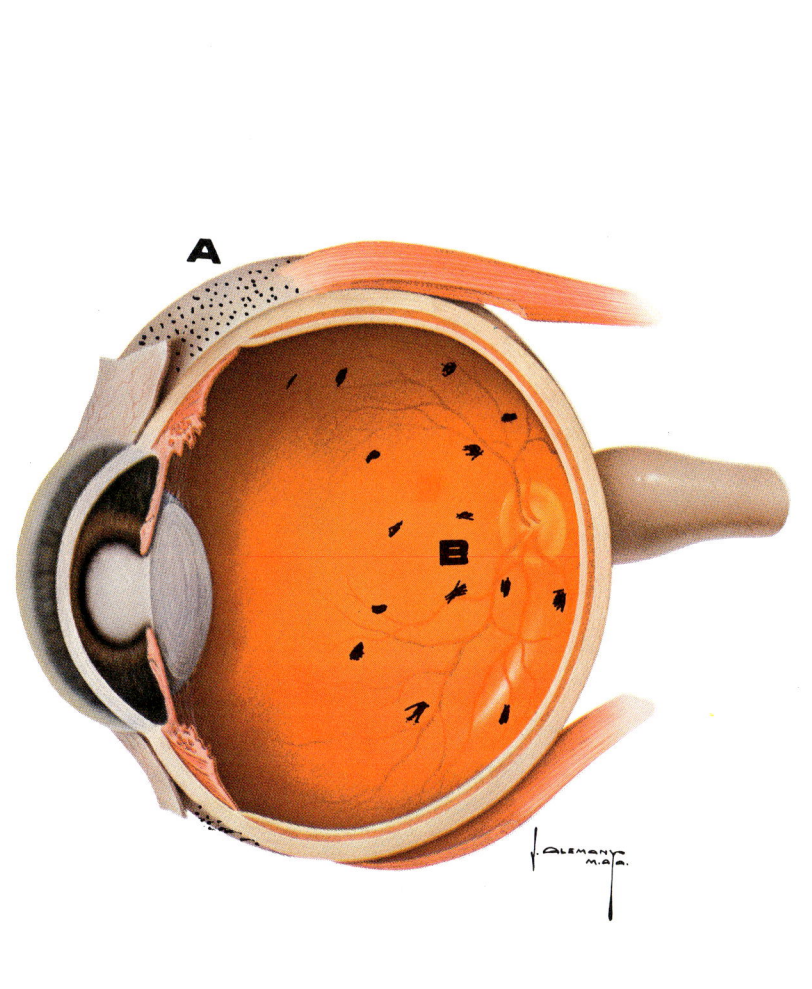

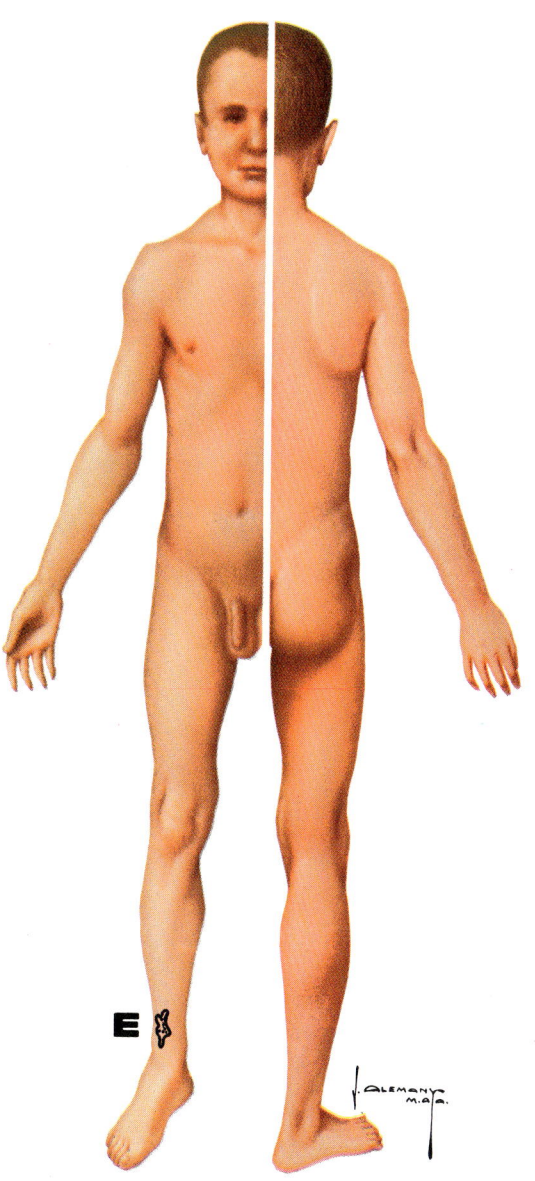

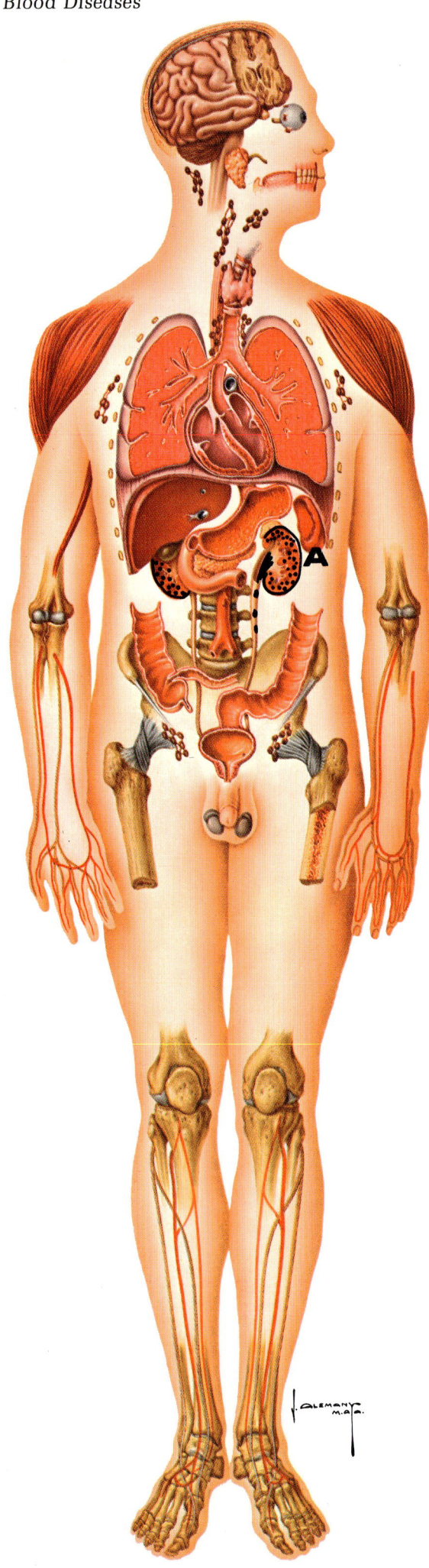

Henoch-Schönlein's Purpura

A 17-year-old white male was admitted to the hospital for gross hematuria (A). A careful history disclosed that 1 week prior to admission he had received an injection of penicillin for an acute streptococcal pharyngitis.

Physical examination revealed multiple petechiae on the distal portion of all 4 extremities (B). There was no lymphadenopathy or splenomegaly.

Laboratory examination revealed a positive tourniquet test, but there was a normal platelet count and CBC.

Treatment with corticosteroids led to an uneventful recovery.

Differential Diagnosis:
1. Acute leukemias
2. Acute glomerulonephritis
3. Collagen diseases
4. Subacute bacterial endocarditis
5. Aplastic anemia and agranulocytosis
6. Metastatic carcinoma or sarcoma
7. Meningococcemia
8. Vascular hemophilia
9. Renal stone or neoplasm
10. Scurvy
11. Hereditary hemorrhagic telangiectasia
12. Thrombocytopenic purpura

Clinical Note. There are numerous drugs that can cause this anaphylactoid purpura. Foods, various chemicals, and insect bites can also cause it.

Pathology. Aside from the multiple hemorrhages in the skin, kidneys, and other organs, there is no specific pathology.

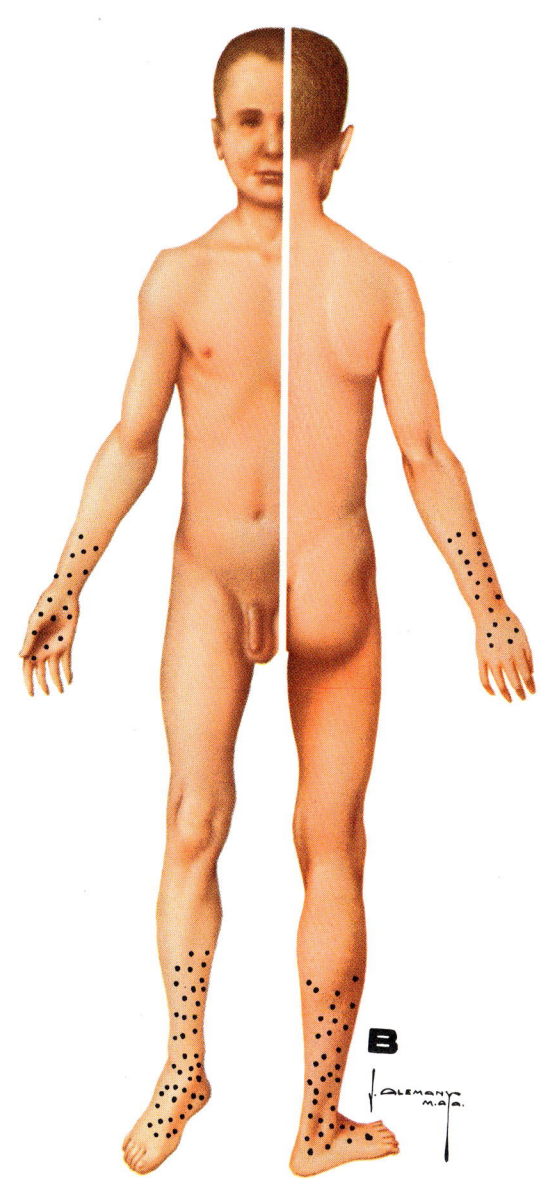

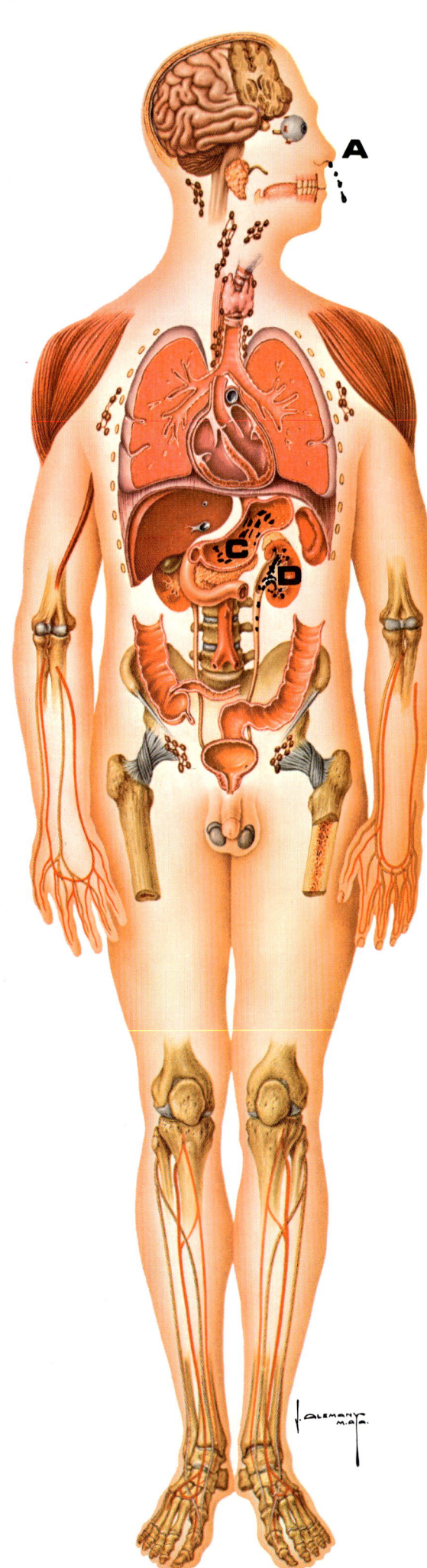

Idiopathic Thrombocytopenic Purpura

An 8-year-old boy was admitted to the hospital with severe uncontrollable epistaxis (A). He had had a severe cough and running nose 1 week prior to this. There was no history of drug ingestion.

Physical examination, aside from revealing the epistaxis, revealed multiple small petechiae on the lower extremities (B) from the knees down. Spleen or lymph nodes were not palpable.

Laboratory examination revealed a positive tourniquet test and prolonged bleeding time, but normal clotting time. The platelet count was 42,000/cu. mm.

Treatment with corticosteroids led to dramatic recovery. Splenectomy was not necessary.

Differential Diagnosis:
1. Acute leukemias
2. Lupus erythematosus
3. Aplastic anemia and agranulocytosis

4. Megaloblastic anemias
5. Gaucher's disease
6. Hypersplenism, of whatever cause
7. Metastatic carcinoma or sarcoma
8. Thrombotic thrombocytopenic purpura
9. Meningococcemia
10. Subacute bacterial endocarditis
11. Henoch-Schönlein's purpura
12. Infectious mononucleosis
13. Uremia

Clinical Note. While bleeding from the nose is often the first sign of this disease, gastrointestinal hemorrhage (C) and renal hemorrhages (D) may also occur. A history of drug ingestion should always be asked for. Splenomegaly and lymphadenopathy are rarely associated with this condition and, if present, should suggest leukemia or an infectious disease. This case is an example of the acute form. A chronic form is found in 10 per cent of the cases.

Pathology. The bone marrow reveals an increased number of megakaryocytes which are vacuolated and have fewer granules than normal. The spleen, which plays a role in the pathogenesis of this disease, shows very little change.

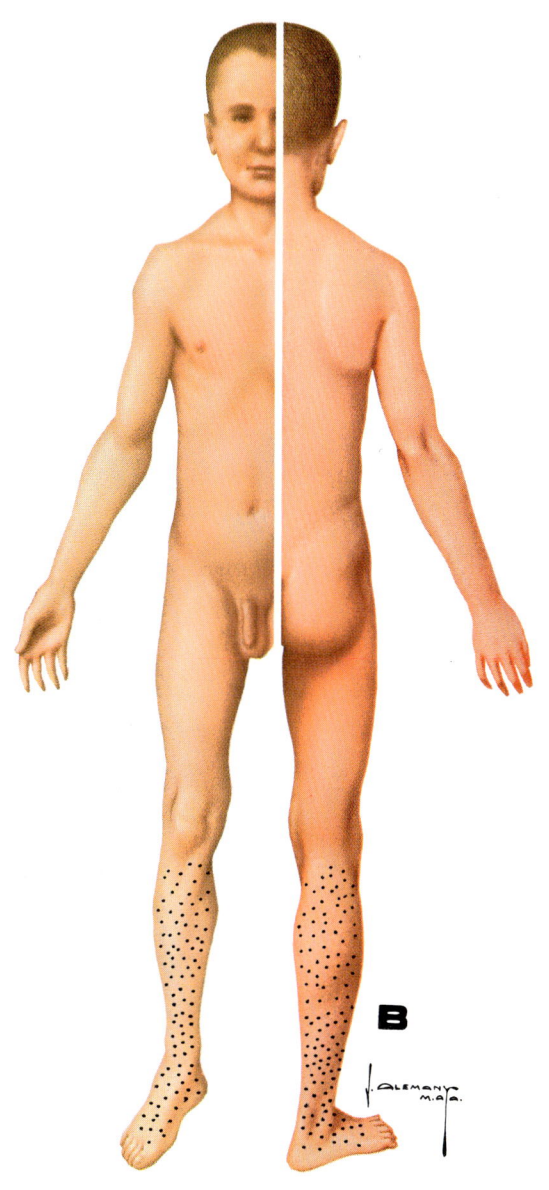

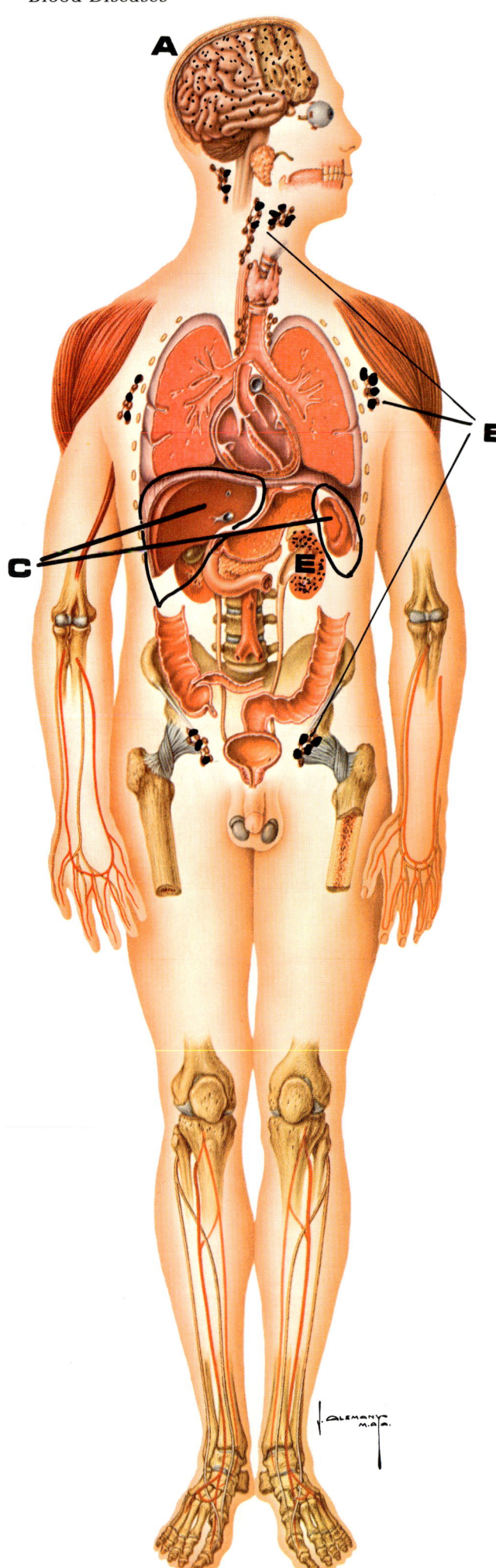

Thrombotic Thrombocytopenic Purpura

A 56-year-old white male was admitted to the neurology service because of recent hallucinations and hostile reactions (A). His temperature had been elevated for 3 days, and prior to the onset of psychotic behavior he had complained of pain in his muscles and joints.

Physical examination revealed a febrile, pale-looking white male who was irritable and uncooperative. There were icteric sclera, generalized lymphadenopathy (B), hepatosplenomegaly (C), and petechiae on the lower extremities bilaterally (D). Weakness and hyperactive reflexes were found in both the right upper and right lower extremities.

Laboratory examination revealed a hemoglobin of 9.2 gm./100 ml., a platelet count of 65,000/cu. mm., and an indirect bilirubin of 3.2 mg. There was poor clot retraction, together with a prolonged bleeding time and a positive Rumpel-Leede test. There was hematuria, indicating renal involvement (E).

Treatment with steroids was unsuccessful, and the patient went into a coma and died 3 weeks later.

Differential Diagnosis:
1. Idiopathic thrombocytopenic purpura
2. Hemolytic anemia, of whatever cause
3. Cirrhosis of the liver
4. Pernicious anemia
5. Wegener's granulomatosis
6. Lupus erythematosus
7. Periarteritis nodosa
8. Subacute bacterial endocarditis
9. Metastatic carcinoma
10. Leukemia

Clinical Note. Purpuric manifestations, neurologic signs and symptoms, and hemolytic anemia are the outstanding features of this disease. Although most cases are acute and fatal, a few become chronic for years. Steroids and splenectomy are usually worthless. The finding of hyaline thrombi in the capillaries from bone biopsies may establish the diagnosis.

Pathology. The hyaline thrombi are numerous throughout the brain, myocardium, renal cortex, adrenals, and pancreas. A proliferative glomerulonephritis may be present.

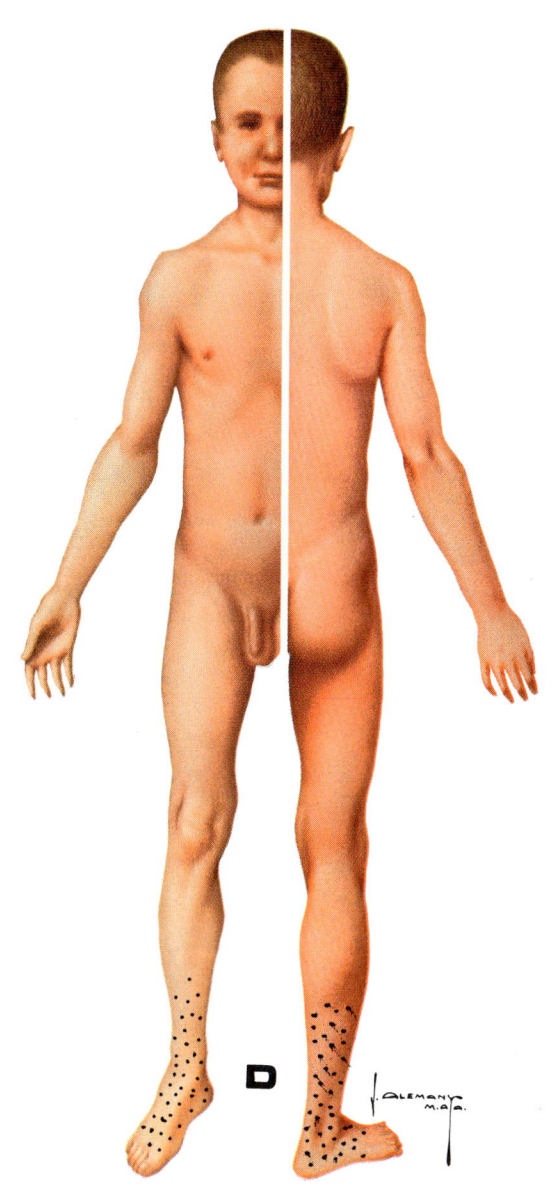

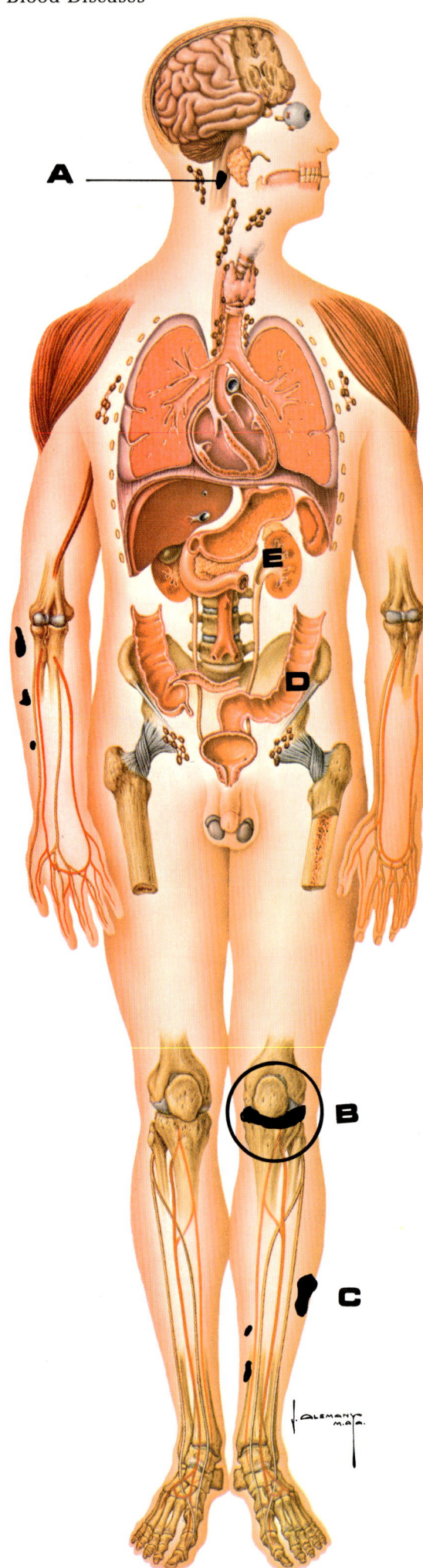

Hemophilia

A 7-year-old white male was admitted to the neurology service with sudden onset of paraplegia (A). Past history revealed he had had sudden swelling of the left knee joint (B) on one occasion and frequent bruises. He had always bled for a prolonged time from minor cuts. His uncle had a similar problem.

Physical examination revealed a few ecchymoses of right arm and left leg (C), weakness, and hyperactive reflexes of both lower extremities with bilateral Babinski signs and a sensory level at C-6 (A).

Laboratory examination was remarkably normal except for prolonged coagulation time and a short prothrombin consumption time. Thromboplastin generation test was also abnormal. A spinal tap was not done until after transfusion of fresh blood.

Differential Diagnosis:
1. Transverse myelitis
2. Acute disseminated encephalomyelitis
3. Epidural abscess
4. Occlusion of anterior spinal artery
5. Neurovascular syphilis
6. Guillain-Barré syndrome
7. Hodgkin's disease
8. Leukemia

Clinical Note. This is a case of factor VIII (AHG) deficiency, but factor IX (Christmas factor) and factor XI deficiency can present with the same picture. Gastrointestinal (D) and renal (E) bleeding are less common than in cases of thrombocytopenia.

Pathology. Other than in hematomas in various organs, these are normal findings.

Chapter 3

Collagen Diseases

Connective tissue is found in every organ of the body, and so here again one expects that collagen diseases would be classified as systemic diseases.

In the early stage of illness, however, only one organ may be affected clinically. Thus scleroderma may manifest only with skin involvement, dermatomyositis may present with muscle involvement alone, and Wegener's granulomatosis may present with only rhinitis. Hence these diseases do not "blitz" the body as frequently as the infectious systemic diseases do.

The etiology of these diseases is uncertain, but all are felt to have an autoimmune basis. Some, such as lupus erythematosus, have been observed as a reaction to a specific etiologic agent (hydralazine, etc.). There is so much overlap of the clinical manifestations of one collagen disease and another that some authorities have proposed they be considered one disease. All cases seem to have exacerbations and remissions. The diagnosis is usually dependent on a good biopsy of the affected organ except in lupus erythematosus, in which "L.E. preps" are important. Corticosteroids have been tried in all these disorders with varying degrees of success, but the prognosis in all remains generally guarded except in specific cases in which the disease actually seems to be burned out for good.

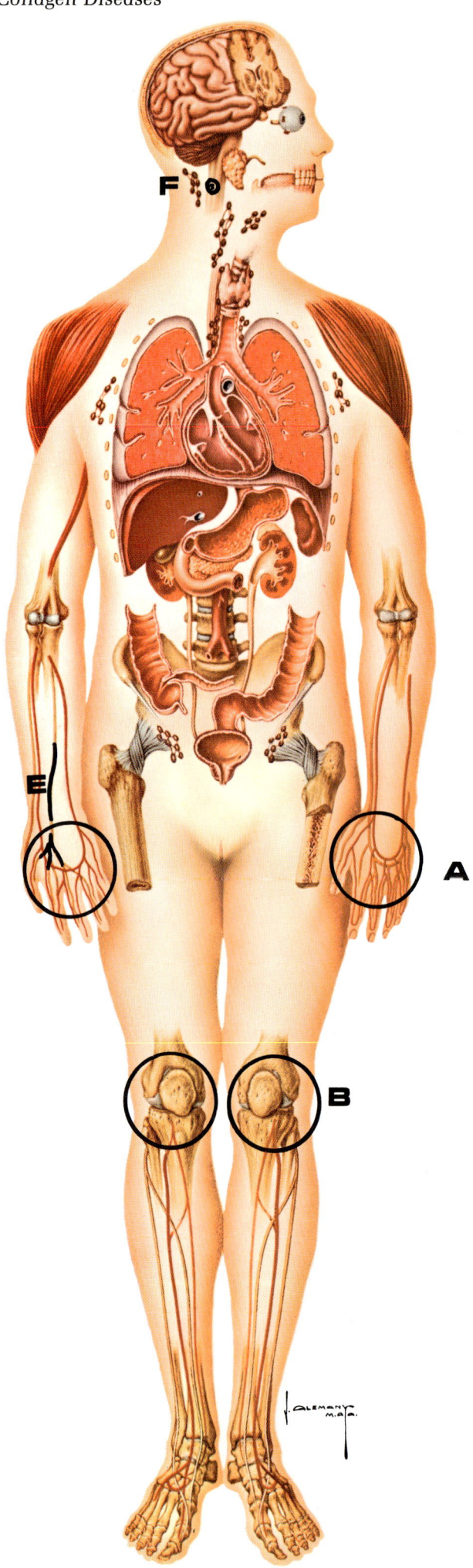

Rheumatoid Arthritis

A 44-year-old white female with a 5-year history of rheumatoid arthritis complained of a painful red left eye. She had had numbness and tingling of the first 3 digits of the right hand.

Physical examination revealed swollen and tender metacarpophalangeal and proximal interphalangeal joints of both hands (A), swollen knee joints (B), and rheumatoid nodules on the extensor surface of both forearms (C). The left eye showed an intense episcleritis (D). Neurologic examination revealed loss of sensation to touch and pain in the distribution of the right median nerve (E).

Laboratory examination revealed a positive latex fixation test, an elevated sedimentation rate, and, in an analysis of synovial fluid, an elevated protein and white count and poor quality of the mucin clot. X-ray examination of the hands and knees revealed osteoporosis of the metacarpal bones bilaterally and narrowing of the knee joints.

Treatment with corticosteroids cleared the episcleritis, and local injection of cortisone into the right carpal tunnel cleared the median nerve neuropathy.

Differential Diagnosis:
1. Gonococcal arthritis
2. Reiter's syndrome
3. Ulcerative colitis

4. Tuberculosis
5. Osteoarthritis
6. Rheumatic fever
7. Torn semilunar cartilages
8. Gout
9. Lupus erythematosus
10. Bacterial endocarditis
11. Serum sickness
12. Syphilis
13. Diabetes mellitus
14. Ochronosis
15. Rat-bite fever

Clinical Note. Ocular involvement occurs in 5 to 10 per cent of cases of rheumatoid arthritis. Neurologic involvement of the carpal tunnel is not uncommon. In addition, disease of the occipito-atlanto or atlanto-axial joint may cause spinal cord compression (F). Less commonly, involvement of other vertebral joints causes nerve root or cord compression. Polymyositis and a fibrinous pericarditis have been reported. The presence of vasculitis and positive L.E. preparations in this disorder indicates the overlapping with collagen diseases. Secondary amyloidosis may occur.

Pathology. The synovial membranes are infiltrated with a granulation tissue composed of hypertrophied stroma and lymphocytes. Later there is replacement with a fibrous scar. There is nothing pathognomonic about this picture.

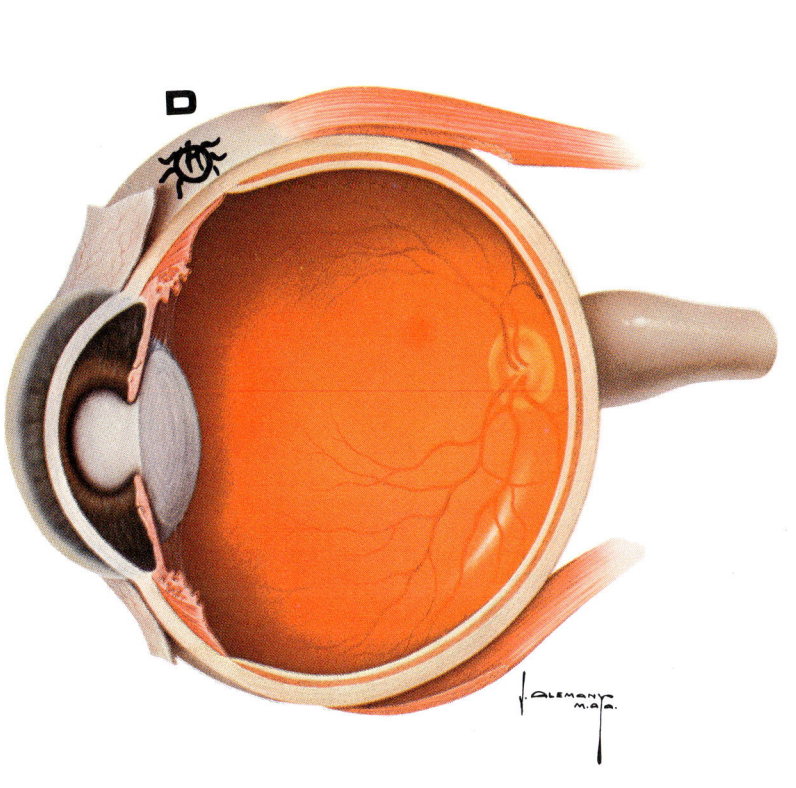

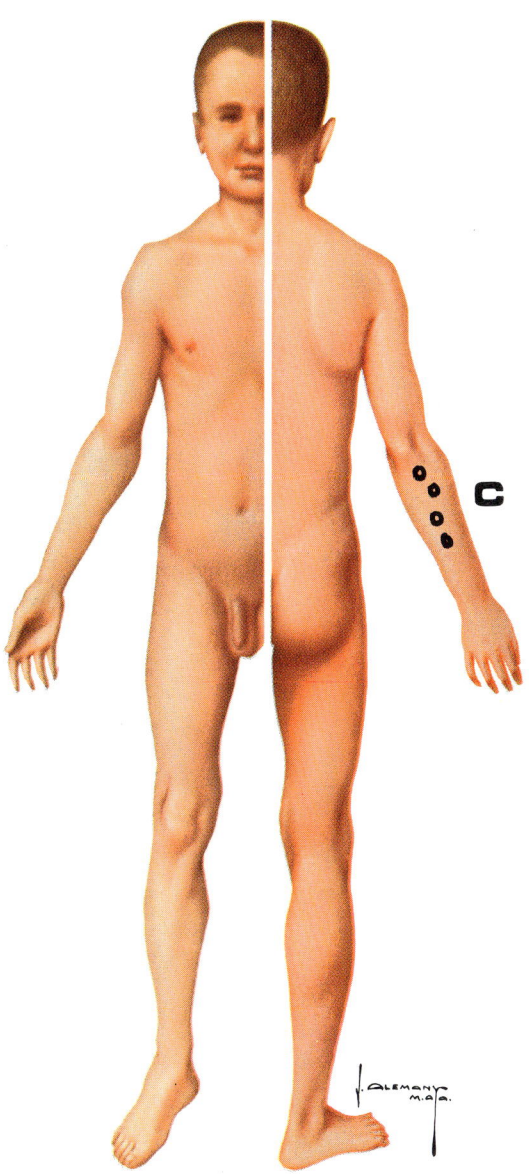

Collagen Diseases

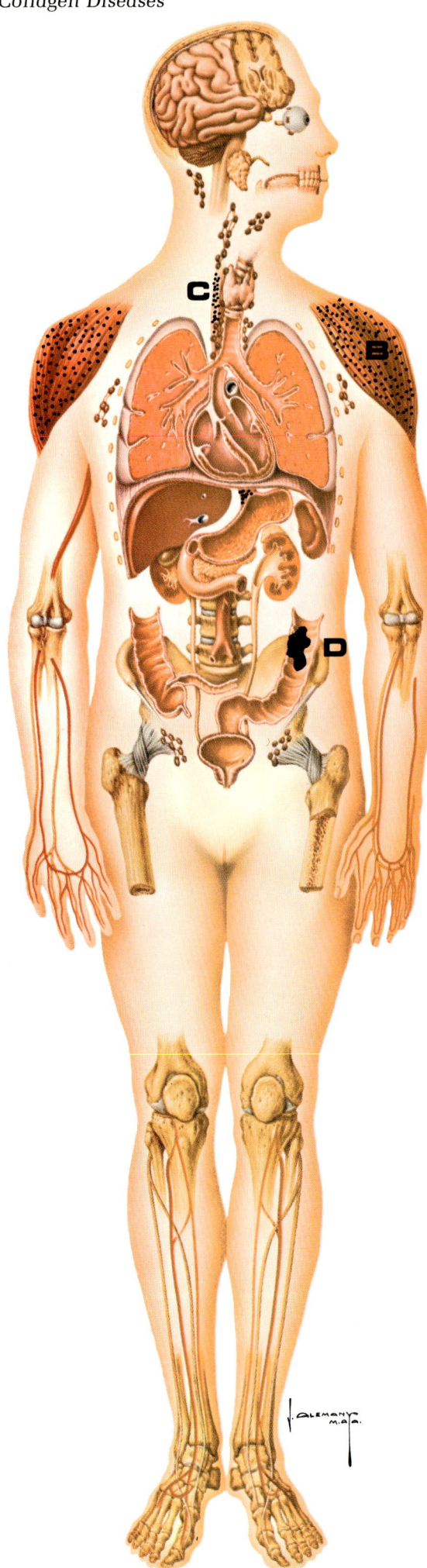

Dermatomyositis

A 42-year-old white female was referred for evaluation by her local physician because of persistent pain and weakness in her shoulder and pelvic muscles, associated with fever. She also had difficulty in swallowing.

Physical examination revealed a temperature of 102° F., periorbital edema with a heliotropic discoloration of the eyelids, face and neck (A) and firm, tender doughy muscles in the proximal portions of all 4 extremities (B).

Laboratory examination revealed a leukocytosis, elevated serum transaminase and aldolase. A muscle biopsy was compatible with the diagnosis.

X-ray examination of the esophagus revealed extremely poor peristalsis, indicating involvement of the esophageal muscle (C). A carcinoma of the colon (D) was found on barium enema.

Treatment with corticosteroids brought about remission.

Differential Diagnosis:
1. Trichinosis
2. Polyneuritis
3. Porphyria
4. Muscular dystrophy
5. Hyperthyroidism
6. Myasthenia gravis
7. Lupus erythematosus
8. Rheumatoid arthritis
9. Diphtheria

Clinical Note. This disease characteristically involves the muscles and skin, but there may be overlapping with the other collagen diseases so that the spleen, liver, heart, and joints may be affected. At least half the cases have a gradual onset. The muscle involvement may precede or follow the skin lesions. This case illustrates the frequent association of this disease with a malignancy.

Pathology. There is necrosis of muscle, and the sarcoplasm becomes highly refractile and eosinophilic, with loss of striations and shrinking of nuclei. There is interstitial edema with mononuclear infiltration and perivascular cuffing of white cells. Later fibrous tissue replaces muscle, and calcification occurs.

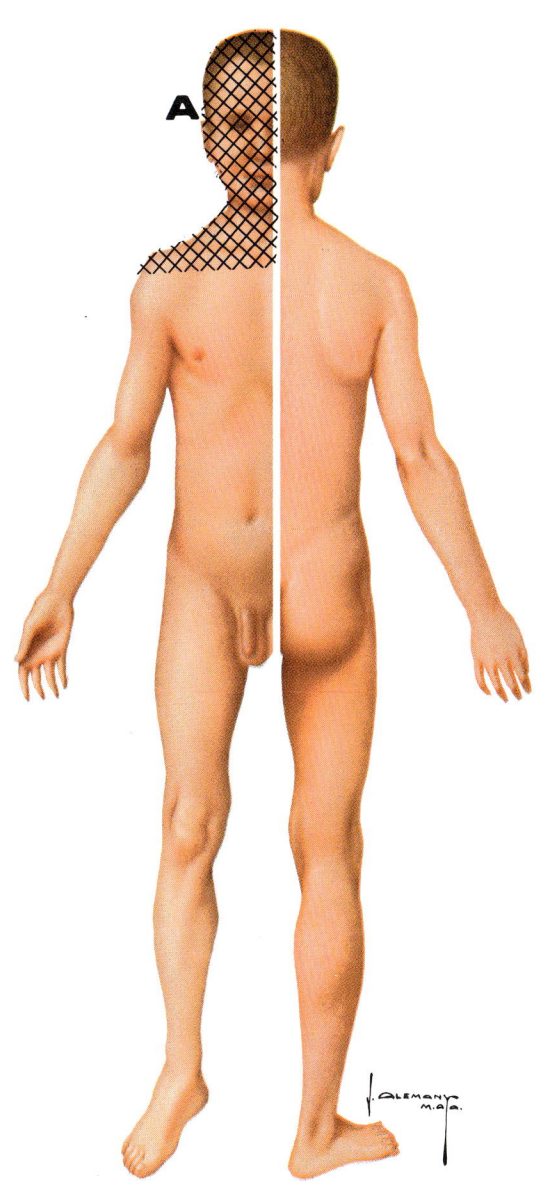

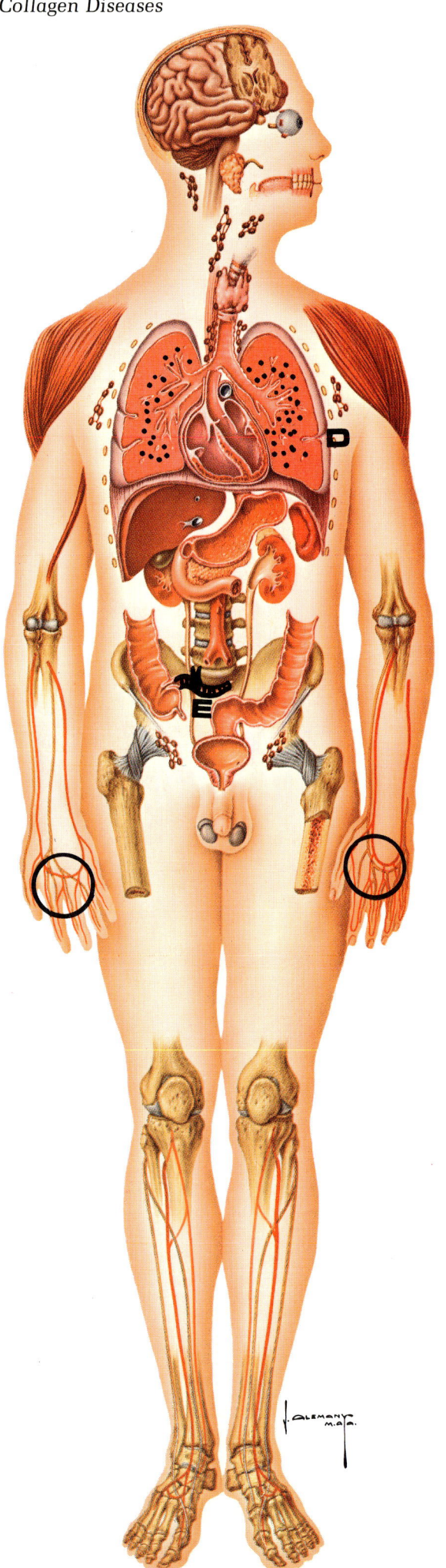

Periarteritis Nodosa

A 37-year-old known-hypertensive male developed sudden violent abdominal pain and nausea. He had had an episode of edema and hematuria 3 years previously diagnosed as glomerulonephritis.

Physical examination revealed swollen metacarpophalangeal joints bilaterally (A), grade II hypertensive retinopathy (B), subcutaneous nodules of the forearms and finger pads (C), and a distended tympanitic abdomen.

Laboratory examination revealed a white count of 22,500 cells/cu. mm. with 20 per cent eosinophils, a BUN of 36 mg. per cent, and numerous red cells, red cell and granular casts in the urine. A muscle biopsy was diagnostic.

X-ray examination of the chest revealed perivascular nodular densities throughout both lungs (D).

Laparotomy revealed a mesenteric artery thrombosis at the terminal ileum (E). Corticosteroids were helpful.

Differential Diagnosis:
1. Lupus erythematosus
2. Subacute bacterial endocarditis
3. Diabetes mellitus
4. Malignant hypertension
5. Rheumatoid arthritis

6. Porphyria
7. Wegener's granulomatosis
8. Macroglobulinemia
9. Intestinal obstruction
10. Lead intoxication
11. Rheumatic fever
12. Brucellosis
13. Sickle cell anemia

Clinical Note. Although this disease may involve any organ, it usually manifests as a mesenteric thrombosis, a glomerulonephritis, a peripheral neuropathy, a myocardial infarct, or bronchial asthma. Central nervous system involvement with convulsions and occasional hemiplegia may occur. The mesenteric artery thromboses may involve the appendix, pancreas, or liver. There may be typical signs of rheumatoid arthritis, as in this case. Hematuria is not always due to glomerulonephritis as there may be extensive vasculitis of the bladder. Skin lesions occur in 25 per cent of the cases and include urticaria and dermatitis gangrenosa. In this patient apparently the onset of periarteritis was accompanied by glomerulonephritis and secondary hypertension. This disease may also cause retinal perivasculitis with retinal detachment and episcleritis.

Pathology. Medium- and small-caliber arteries develop necrosis, fibrinoid degeneration, and leukocytic infiltration in all 3 layers of their walls. There may be thrombosis in the lumen or weakening of the wall, with aneurysm formation or perforation. No single set of vessels is typically involved.

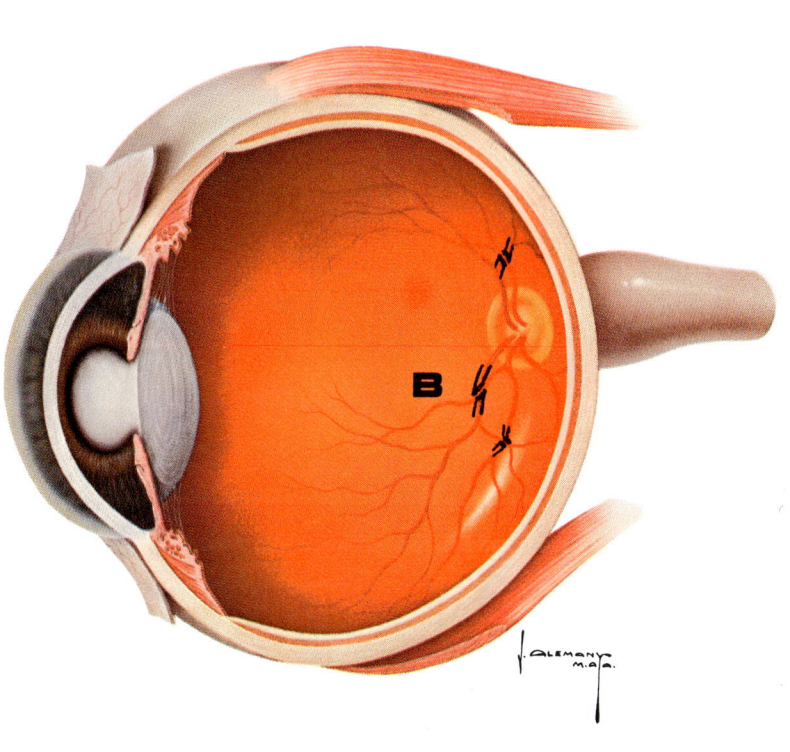

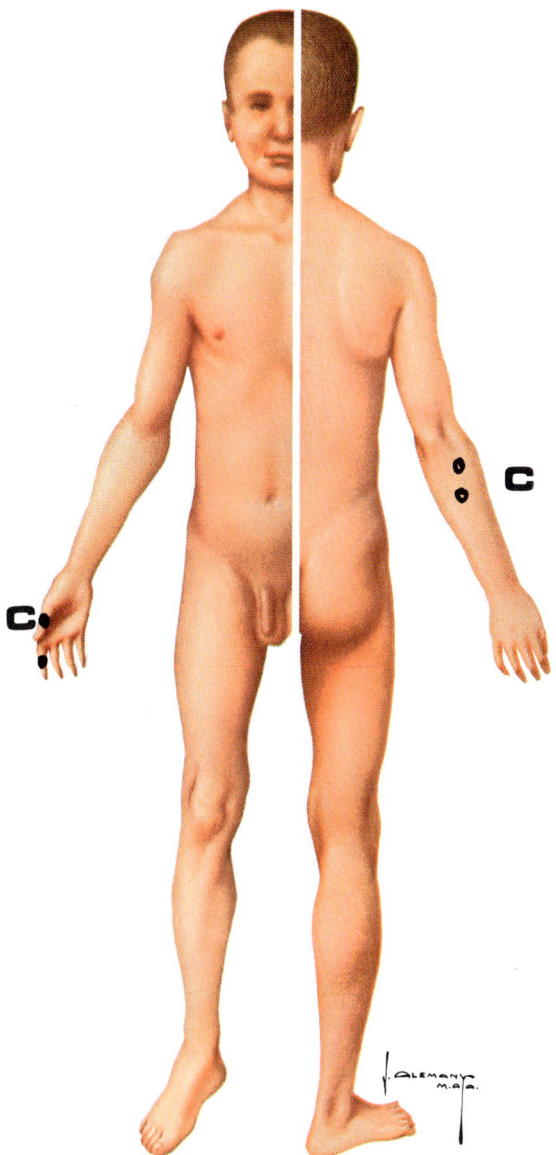

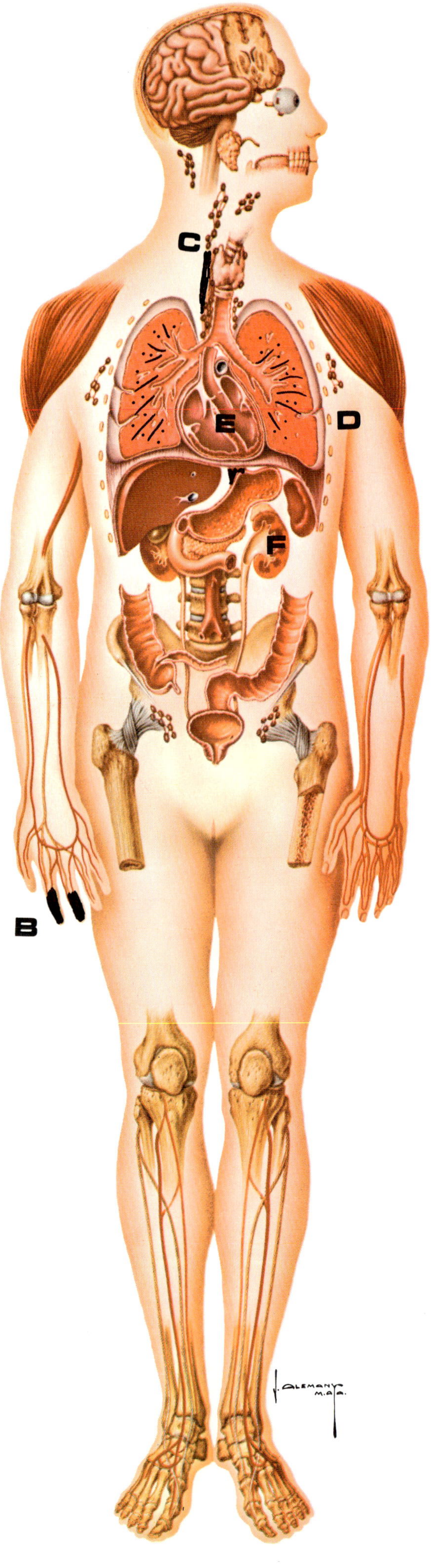

30 · *Collagen Diseases*

Scleroderma

A 43-year-old white female had complained for some time of episodes of cold painful fingers occasionally leading to gangrene. One month prior to admission she complained of dysphagia and increasing swelling of the hands and feet.

Physical examination revealed brawny, non-pitting edema of her hands and feet, which showed some hyperpigmentation (A). There was also gangrene of the 2nd and 3rd fingers of the right hand (B).

Laboratory examination revealed an increased serum gamma globulin, but it was otherwise unremarkable.

X-ray examination of the esophagus showed loss of motility and of normal peristalsis, indicating involvement (C).

Treatment with corticosteroids was unsuccessful, but para-aminobenzoic acid helped considerably.

Differential Diagnosis:
1. Scleredema
2. Dermatomyositis

3. Malabsorption syndrome
4. Pulmonary fibrosis
5. Addison's disease
6. Hypothyroidism
7. Werner's syndrome
8. Rothmund's syndrome

Clinical Note. This patient was in an early stage before frank atrophy of the skin and muscles and fixation of the joints occurred. The esophageal lesions also progress to chronic esophagitis and obstructive fibrosis. Although this patient manifested only skin and esophageal changes, there may be pulmonary fibrosis (D), a malabsorption syndrome, myocarditis (E), pericarditis, and occasionally polymyositis. Unlike other collagen diseases, there are no consistent laboratory findings, and the response to steroids is poor. In occasional cases renal involvement (F) with severe hypertension develops, and death follows in a matter of weeks.

Pathology. There is swelling of intercellular collagen tissue which later becomes dense and sclerotic. The blood vessels show intimal thickening and fibrinoid degeneration. Occasionally vessels are occluded by this process.

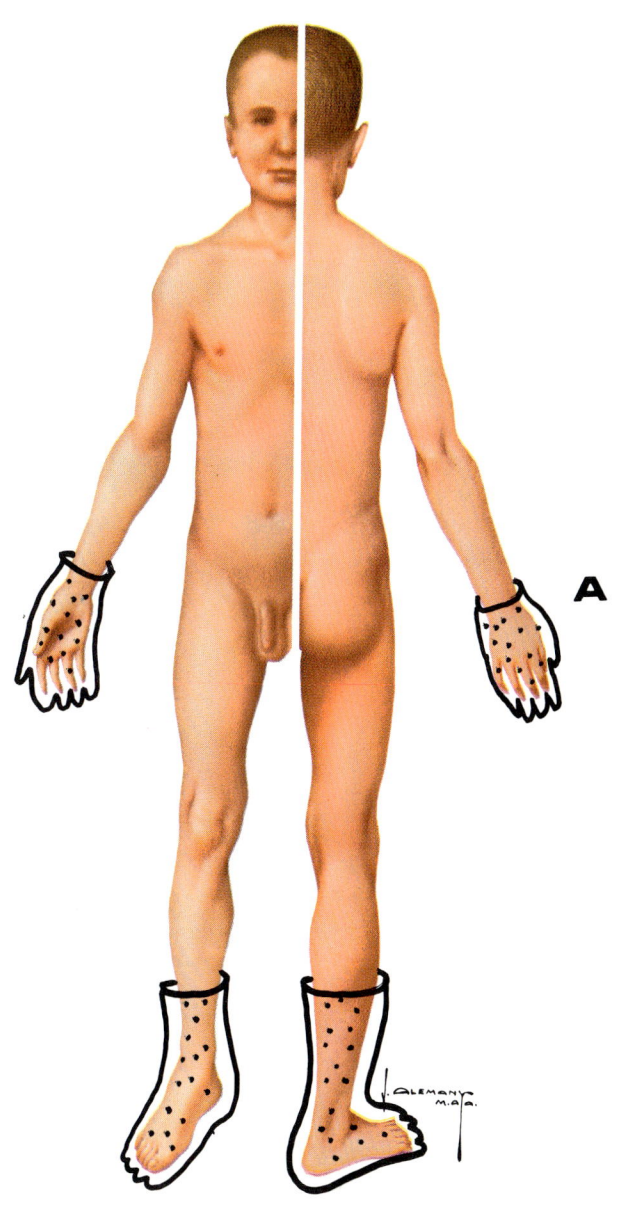

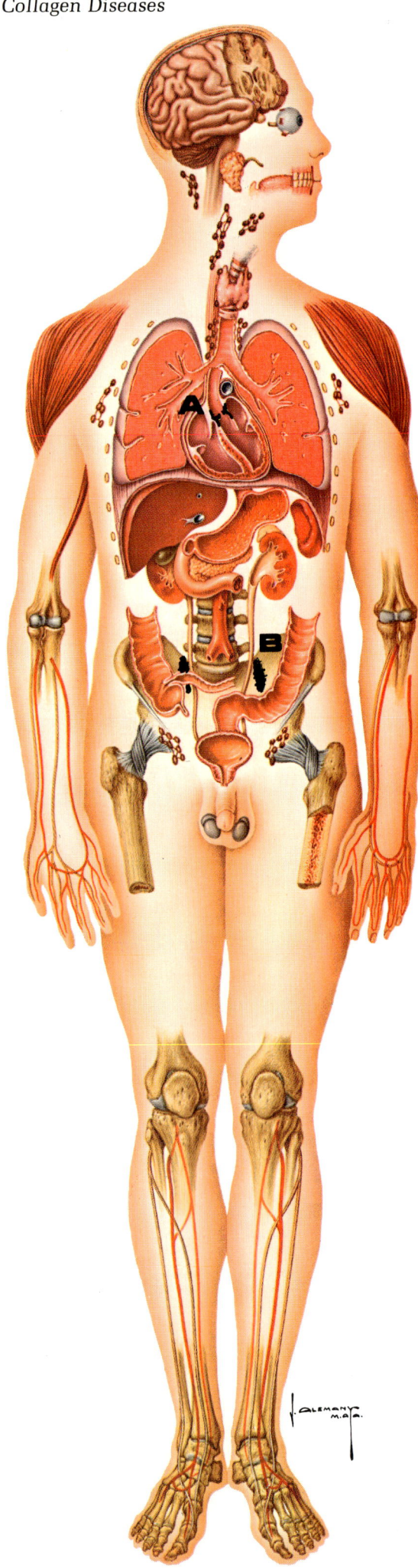

Ankylosing Spondylitis

A 27-year-old white male complained of persistent low-back pain and stiffness, particularly in the morning, for several months. A diagnosis of herniated disk had been made by another physician, but was not confirmed radiographically. His father had had rheumatoid spondylitis.

Physical examination revealed tenderness over the sacroiliac joints bilaterally and a grade II protodiastolic murmur at the aortic area, indicating aortic insufficiency due to aortic valvulitis (A). No subcutaneous nodules were found.

Laboratory examination revealed an elevated sedimentation rate but a negative latex flocculation test.

X-ray examination of the lumbosacral spine revealed sclerosis and blurring of the margins of the sacroiliac joints bilaterally (B).

Treatment with intermittent steroids brought about remission.

Differential Diagnosis:
1. Ochronosis
2. Ruptured intervertebral disk
3. Metastatic carcinoma

4. Cauda equina tumor
5. Multiple myeloma
6. Osteoporosis and osteoarthritis
7. Osteomalacia, of whatever cause
8. Gout
9. Paget's disease
10. Syphilis
11. Tuberculosis

Clinical Note. Although this condition is less frequently associated with systemic symptoms, aortic valvulitis does occur. In addition, uveitis and iritis (C) occur more frequently than in rheumatoid arthritis. Subcutaneous nodules do not occur. Frequently the laboratory is of no help in the diagnosis because the sedimentation rate may be normal, anemia is uncommon, and the latex flocculation test is positive in only 10 per cent of cases. Here was presented an early case of ankylosing spondylitis. As the disease progresses, there may be peripheral joint involvement, and the entire spine is involved, with, in some cases, complete limitation of motion in a "poker spine." This leads to pulmonary complications of emphysema. X-ray changes which appear later are sclerosis of the apophyseal joints and calcification of the intervertebral disks and longitudinal ligaments.

Pathology. The pathology is similar to that of rheumatoid arthritis, with a different location.

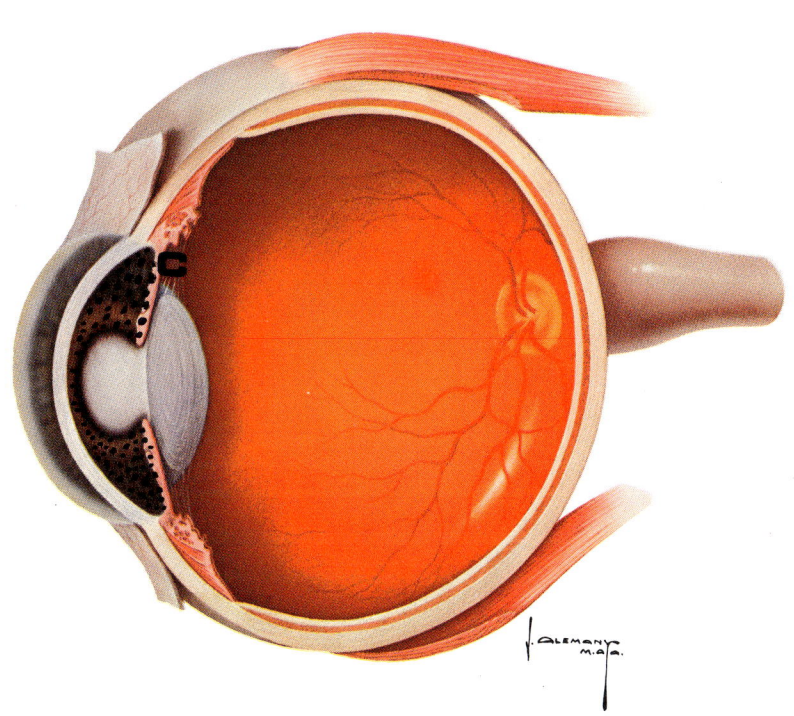

Collagen Diseases

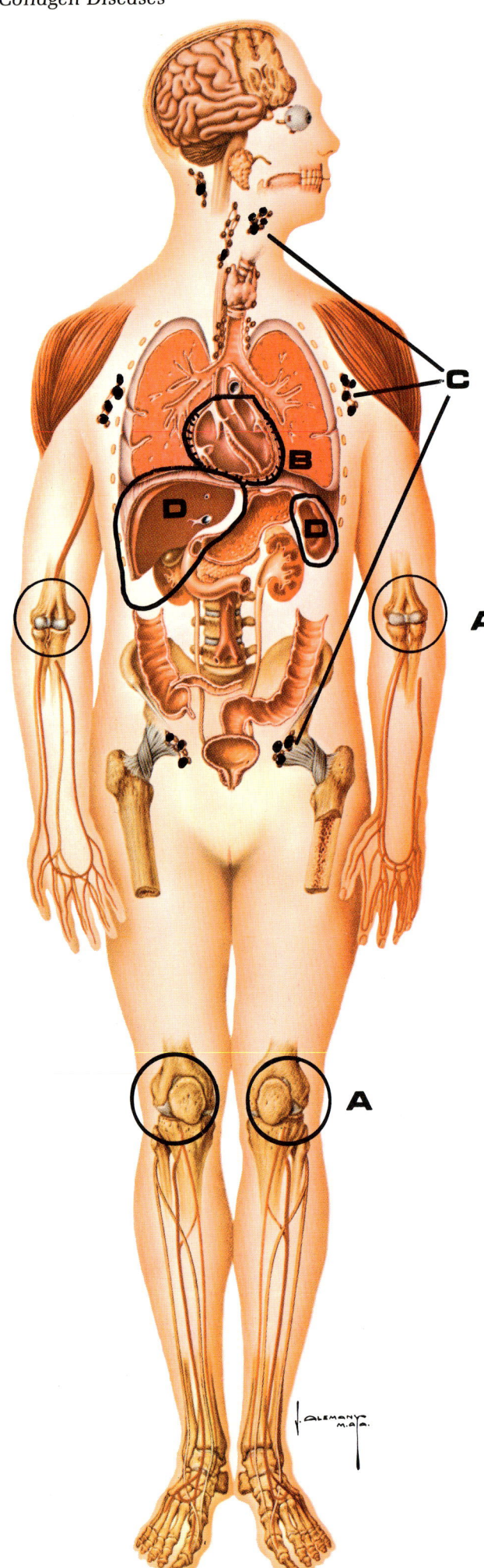

Still's Disease (Juvenile Rheumatoid Arthritis)

An 8-year-old white female developed a spiking temperature and swollen painful knee and elbow joints bilaterally.

Physical examination revealed swollen tender and red-hot elbow and knee joints bilaterally (A), a pericardial friction rub, suggesting pericarditis (B), generalized lymphadenopathy (C), and hepatosplenomegaly (D).

Laboratory examination revealed a positive latex fixation test, increased ESR, and a sample of synovial fluid revealed an elevated white count, protein, and poor mucin clot formation.

Treatment with corticosteroids was successful.

Differential Diagnosis:
1. Rheumatic fever
2. Subacute bacterial endocarditis
3. Infectious mononucleosis
4. Brucellosis
5. Tuberculosis
6. Lupus erythematosus
7. Gonorrhea
8. Leukemia

Clinical Note. Involvement of the cervical spine is common in this variety of rheumatoid arthritis, and lymphadenopathy and hepatosplenomegaly are frequent. Pericarditis and even valvular lesions are frequent. Rheumatoid nodules are rare, as in ankylosing spondylitis. When massive splenomegaly and an associated pancytopenia are present, the condition is referred to as Felty's syndrome.

Wegener's Granulomatosis

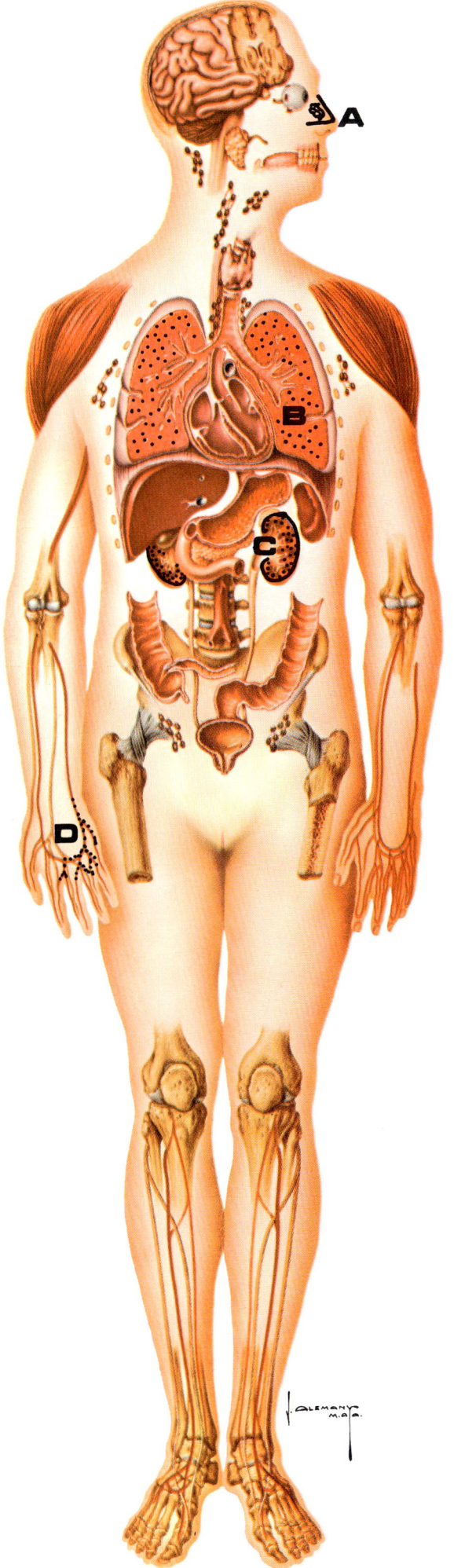

A 38-year-old white female complained of chronic stuffy nose and yellowish and occasionally bloody nasal discharge for 3 months prior to admission. Two weeks prior to admission she developed a cough, hemoptysis and night sweats.

Physical examination revealed ulceration and perforation of the nasal septum (A) and sibilant and sonorous rales throughout the lungs (B).

Laboratory examination revealed numerous red blood cells, red cell casts, and granular casts in the urine; a BUN of 42 mg. per cent, indicating renal involvement (C); eosinophilia and a high serum globulin.

X-ray examination revealed some opacification of both maxillary antra and scattered small densities throughout the lungs.

The course was progressively downhill despite steroid therapy, and the patient died in renal failure.

Differential Diagnosis:
1. Tuberculosis
2. Mucormycosis
3. Macroglobulinemia
4. Periarteritis nodosa
5. Asthma
6. Amyloidosis
7. Lupus erythematosus
8. Syphilis
9. Sarcoidosis
10. Histoplasmosis
11. Lethal midline granuloma

Clinical Note. Almost all cases eventually involve the upper respiratory tract and lungs, the peripheral arteries, and veins, and the kidneys. The small arteries and veins are involved with a necrotizing vasculitis (D), which was not present in this case. There may be a hemorrhagic skin eruption, musculoskeletal abnormalities, and peripheral neuropathy. In the separation of the respiratory phase from the systemic phase this disease is almost like rheumatic fever. This aids in diagnosis.

Pathology. Wherever the lesions occur there is an inflammatory necrosis of the small blood vessels with giant cell formation and destruction of neutrophils. Glomerular epithelial crescents develop.

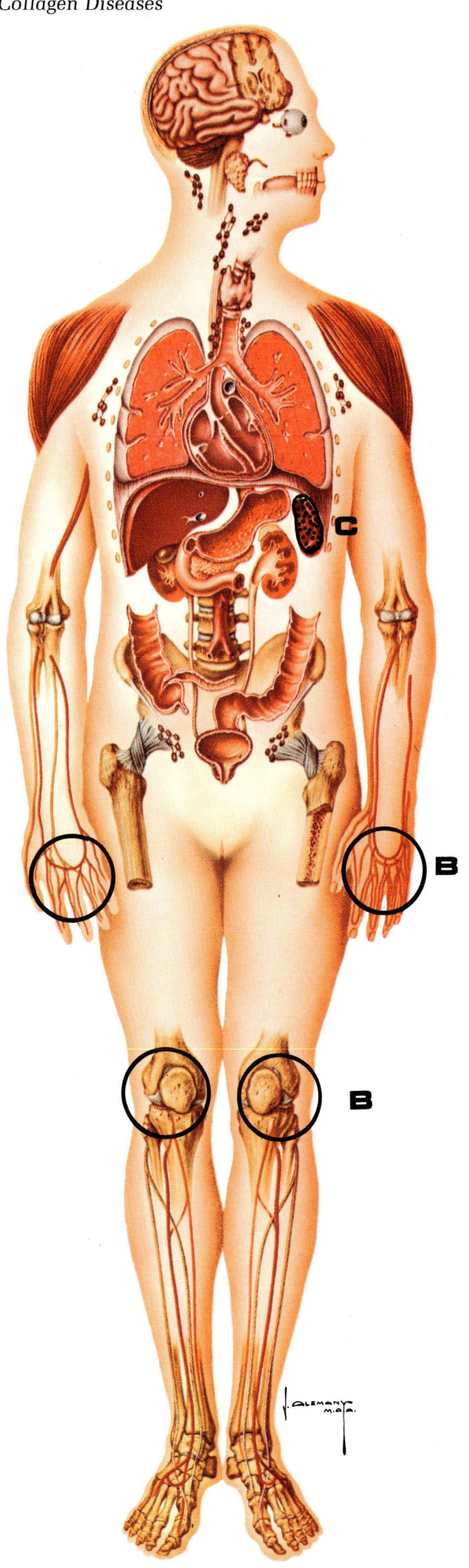

Lupus Erythematosus, Case 1

A 19-year-old white female was admitted to the hospital with a 12-day history of a rash beginning on the lower portion of the legs and spreading to involve thighs, hips, and the distal portion of the upper extremities. For some months prior to admission she had experienced pain and stiffness of her fingers and knees.

Physical examination revealed multiple petechiae of legs and arms (A), and swollen tender knee, interphalangeal and metacarpophalangeal joints bilaterally (B).

Laboratory examination revealed anemia, leukopenia and thrombocytopenia, numerous red blood cells and granular and hyaline casts in the urine, and a positive L.E. preparation. A renal biopsy was also helpful in the diagnosis.

Differential Diagnosis:
1. Rheumatic fever
2. Acute glomerulonephritis
3. Rheumatoid arthritis
4. Gonococcal arthritis

5. Multiple myeloma
6. Gout
7. Hemophilia
8. Thrombocytopenia purpura
9. Sickle cell anemia
10. Periarteritis nodosa

Clinical Note. A polyarthritis is the most common initial sign of lupus erythematosus, followed by significant skin manifestations. Ninety per cent of cases occur in women. This case demonstrates signs of hypersplenism (C) (pancytopenia), but there was no enlargement on physical examination. The pancytopenia and presence of formed elements in the urine frequently help to differentiate this from other disorders.

Pathology. There are fibrinoid degeneration, occasional necrosis, hematoxylin bodies, and collagenous sclerosis in the heart, lymph nodes, kidneys, lungs, and, most frequently, the spleen. In the kidney there is fibrinoid thickening of the basement membrane in the glomeruli, giving a wire-loop appearance. In the spleen there is sclerosis of the collagen, leading to an onion-skin appearance around the small arteries.

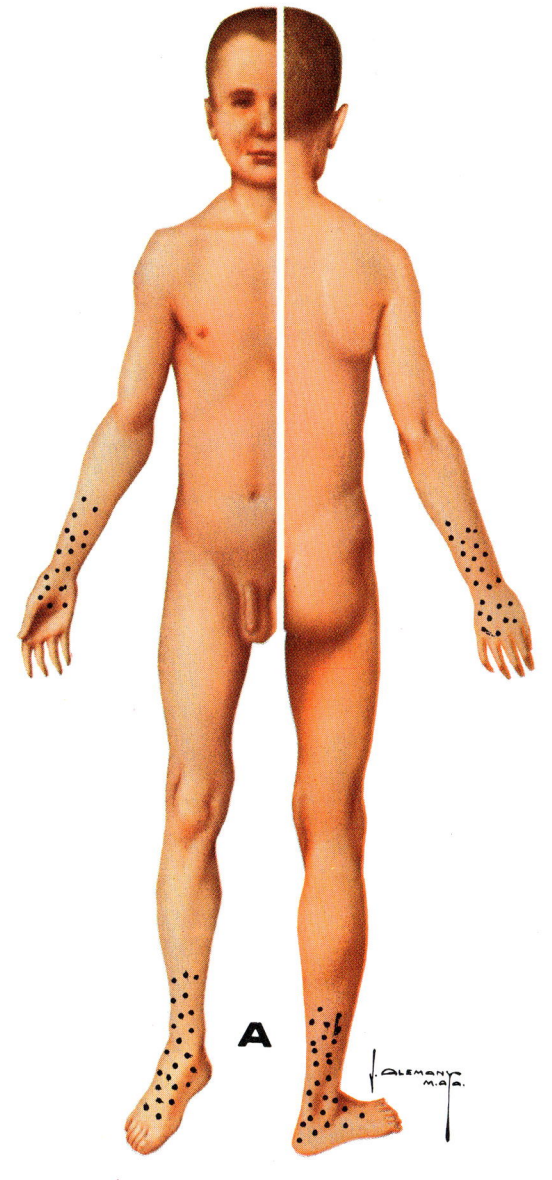

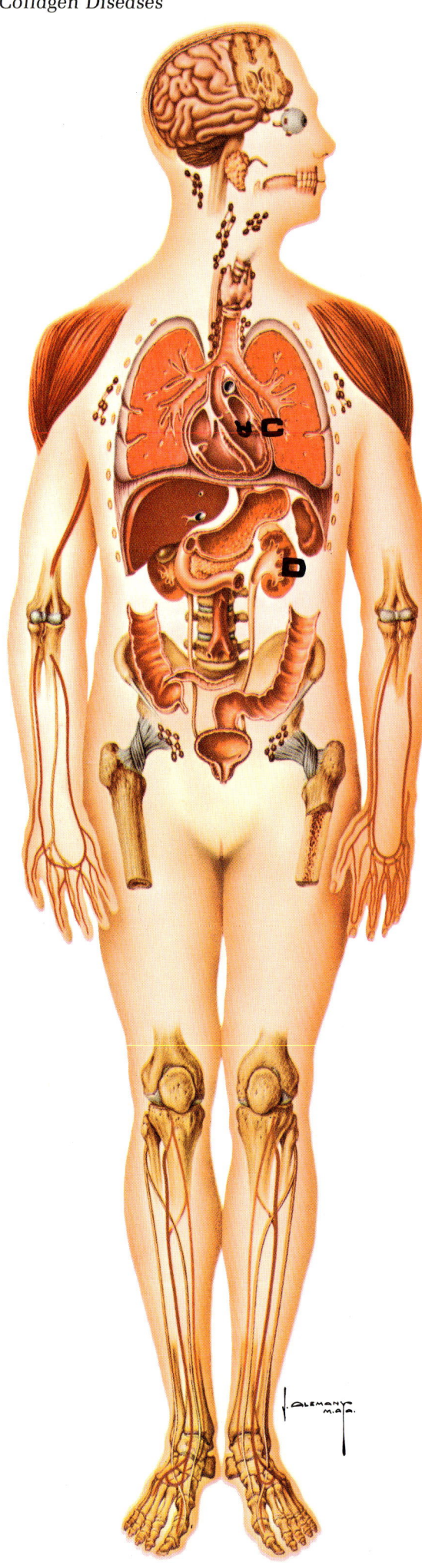

Lupus Erythematosus, Case 2

A 28-year-old white female who was 5 months pregnant developed swelling of the eyelids and all 4 extremities 2 weeks prior to admission. She had suffered from a recurring rash of the face, ears, and thorax for the past 2 years. There was also a history of migratory arthralgias.

Physical examination revealed a butterfly erythematous scaling rash of the face (A), periorbital and pretibial edema (B), and a grade III apical systolic murmur suggesting mitral valve involvement (C). The blood pressure was normal.

Laboratory examination revealed 4+ albuminuria; numerous red cells, red cell casts, and granular casts in the urine; hypoproteinemia and hypercholesterolemia. Repeated L.E. preparations were negative, but a renal biopsy revealed the characteristic wire-loop appearance of the glomeruli (D).

Clinical Note. Here is the nephrotic syndrome with skin involvement and only a suggestion of joint involvement. The sudden onset of edema in a pregnant woman suggests toxemia, but the rash and the normal blood pressure rule against it. The kidneys are involved in 75 per cent of the cases of lupus erythematosus. This case illustrates the difficulty in finding L.E. cells in every case, but by using the best methods it is possible to find them in 98 per cent of the cases. The presence of systolic murmurs does not always mean verrucous endocarditis of Libman-Sacks as the anemia is frequently the cause of these murmurs.

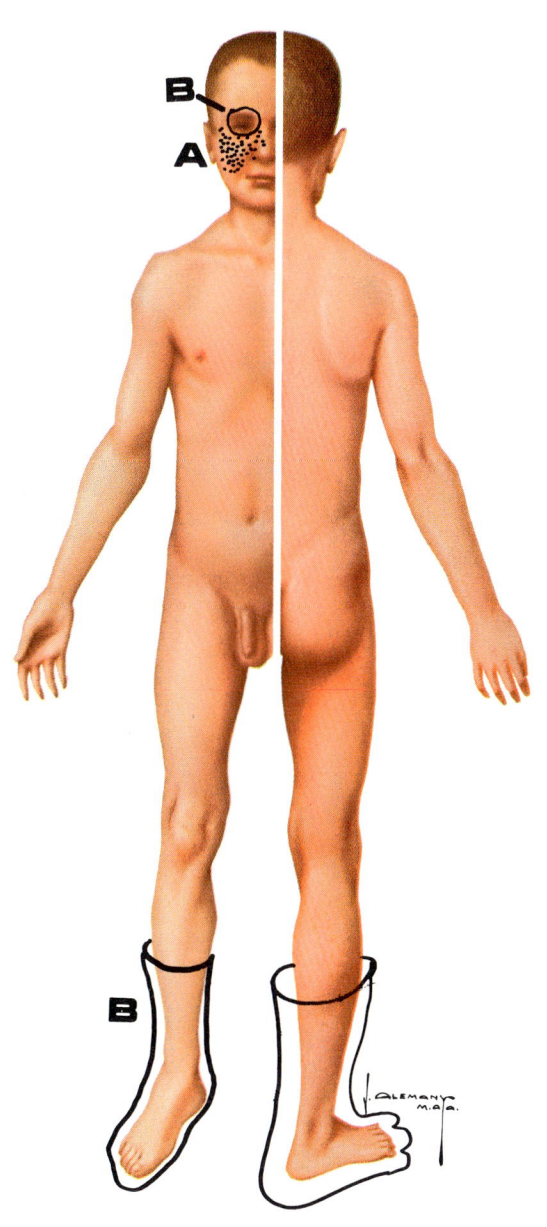

Lupus Erythematosus, Case 3

A 64-year-old white male had experienced an irregularity of the heart beat for 9 months prior to admission. Two weeks prior to admission he became severely ill with fever, swelling of the finger and ankle joints bilaterally, and shortness of breath.

Physical examination revealed a pericardial friction rub, cardiomegaly, bilateral pleural effusion (A), swollen, tender metacarpophalangeal joints, and tender ankle joints (B). A pericardial tap produced 300 ml. of serosanguinous fluid (C), explaining the cardiomegaly.

Laboratory examination revealed a weakly positive Wassermann, anemia, leukopenia and thrombocytopenia, and, on the peripheral smear, L.E. cells.

Treatment with corticosteroids produced a dramatic remission.

Clinical Note. There is a pancarditis like that of rheumatic fever, joint involvement, and pleural involvement in this case. Polyserositis is commonly encountered in this disorder. The myocarditis produces arrhythmias and conduction disturbances.

Summary. The presentation of only 3 types of lupus erythematosus are given here. It would take a whole volume to illustrate all the many ways in which it may present. Mental and neurologic disturbances occur in one fourth of these patients. It may present with jaundice, as in lupoid hepatitis. We could go on.

Chapter 4

Congenital Diseases

Although most of these diseases are hereditary in etiology, by using the classification *congenital,* mongolism and Sturge-Weber syndrome can be included. There is much less overlap from one disease to another than in the collagen disorders. Clinical diagnosis is more important here than in any other group of disorders. A careful examination of the eye, skin, and nervous system will make a specific diagnosis in most cases. The laboratory is helpful in a few, such as fibrocystic disease and porphyria.

There is no useful treatment for the vast majority of these disorders, and genetic counseling seems to be the only way of reducing the incidence of these diseases.

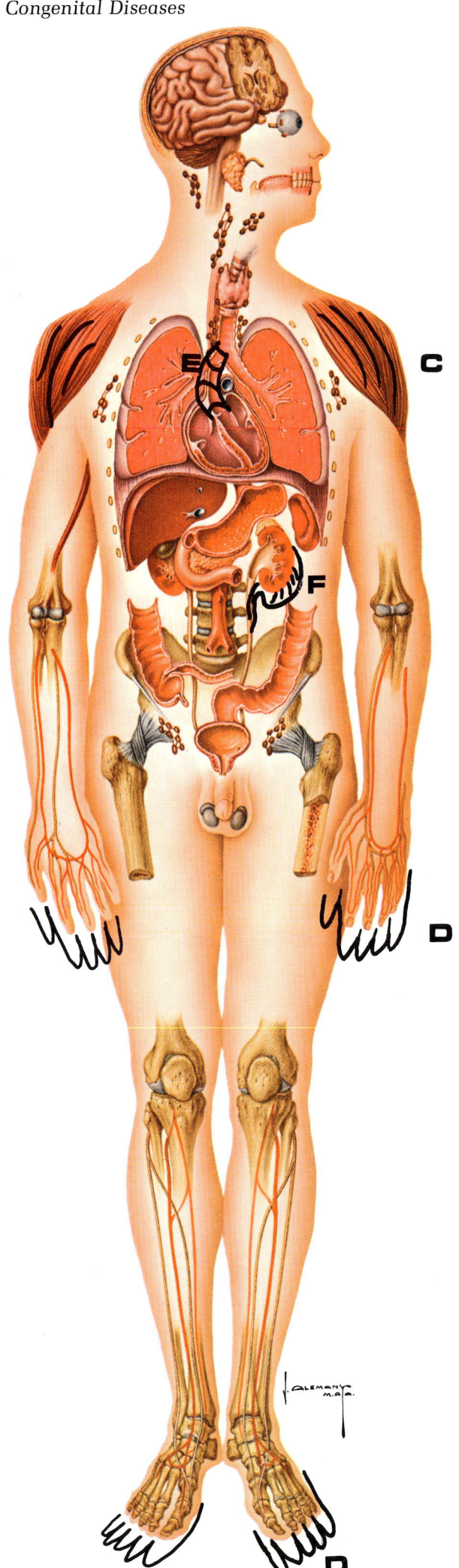

Arachnodactyly

A 14-year-old white male was brought for ophthalmologic examination because of blurred vision. Other members of the family manifested long arms, and one sibling had died of a ruptured aorta.

Physical examination revealed ectopia lentis (A), severe myopia, a high-arched palate (B), generalized hypotonia (C), long arms and legs (D), and a grade III aortic systolic murmur.

Laboratory examination revealed pyuria and an increased urinary hydroxyproline.

X-ray examination of the chest revealed marked dilatation of the ascending aorta (E), fusion of the 1st and 2nd lumbar vertebra of the spine, and a double left kidney (F) on intravenous pyelogram.

Differential Diagnosis:
1. Congenital heart disease
2. Syphilis

3. Hypertensive cardiovascular disease
4. Aortic aneurysm, atherosclerotic

Clinical Note. Very few illnesses can give this combination of eye, cardiovascular, and skeletal changes on a hereditary basis. Gargoylism is one. Rheumatic fever causes no ocular involvement. This diagnosis should be made easily on physical examination; but *formes frustes* of the disease occur with perhaps only aortic or ocular involvement, and the diagnosis becomes difficult.

Pathology. There is diffuse connective tissue disease with cystic medionecrosis of the aorta, which may lead to dissection, rupture, aneurysm, or aortic insufficiency. The pulmonary artery is less commonly involved by the same process. Pyelonephritis is frequent. The elongation of the bone does not usually give rise to any gross pathologic change. There may be associated congenital heart lesions such as patent foramen ovale or patent ductus arteriosus.

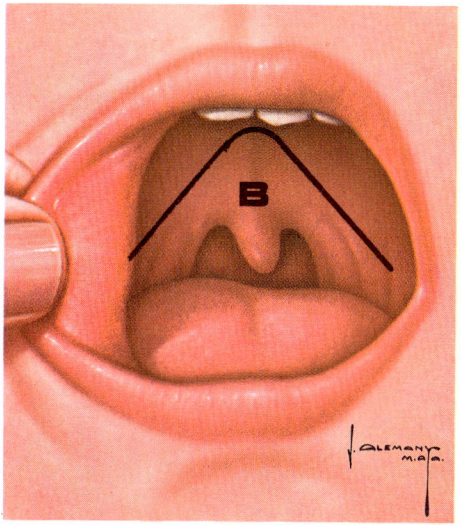

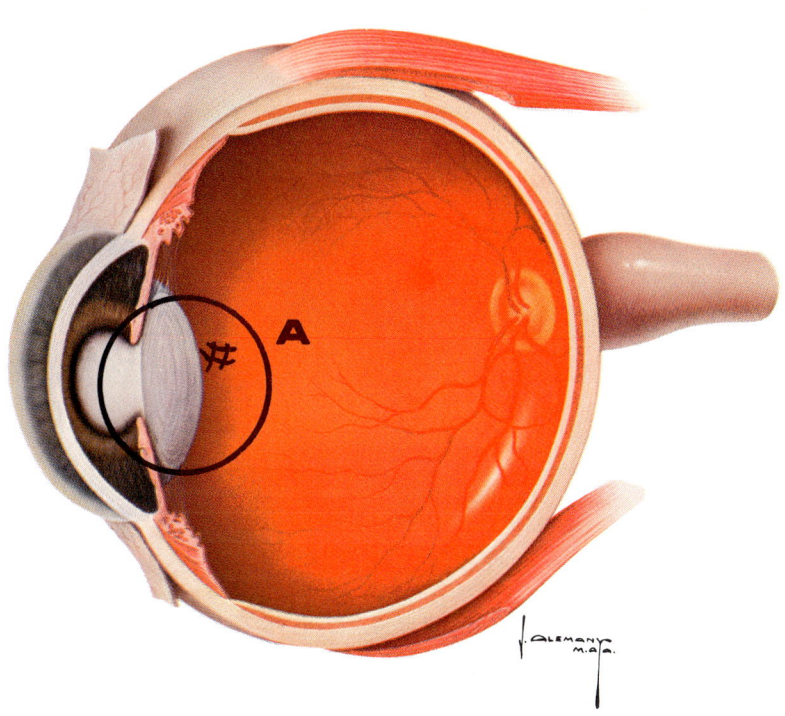

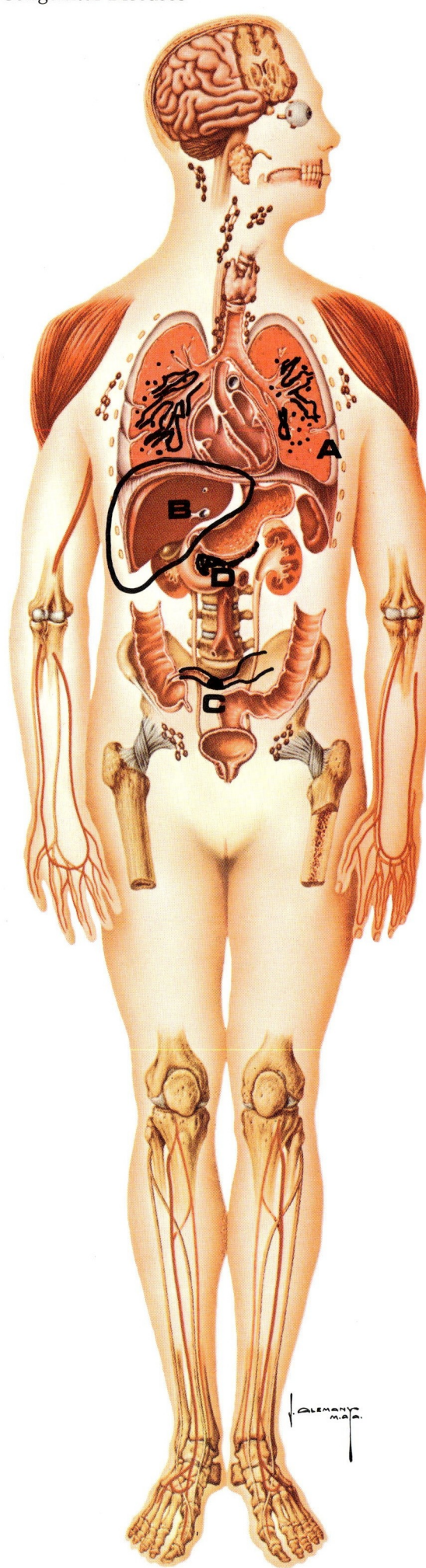

Fibrocystic Disease

An 11-year-old white female complained of shortness of breath and increasing cough productive of yellowish sputum for 1 week prior to admission. Past history revealed she had had repeated respiratory infections for a number of years. Her brother had died of cystic fibrosis in early childhood.

Physical examination revealed rapid pulse, tachypnea, barrel chest, sibilant and sonorous rales throughout both lung fields (A), and hepatomegaly (B).

Laboratory examination revealed high sodium and chloride concentrations in the sweat test, diminished trypsin in the duodenal drainage and stools, and low serum carotene.

X-ray of the chest showed scattered areas of consolidation in both lungs (A) and changes suggesting bronchiectasis.

Treatment with antibiotics, multivitamins, diet, and pancreatin was helpful.

Differential Diagnosis:
1. Celiac disease
2. Bronchial asthma
3. Tuberculosis
4. Bronchiectasis
5. Foreign body in the lung
6. Histoplasmosis
7. Coccidioidomycosis

Clinical Note. Many cases die in infancy of meconium ileus (C). The pancreatic insufficiency (D) may manifest itself in older children with large bulky stools, abdominal distention, and cramps. Cirrhosis of the liver accounts for the hepatomegaly. The combination of chronic lung, liver, and pancreatic disease in children with a family history of the disorder rarely occurs in any other disease. Adult cases are being recognized more frequently.

Pathology. This is a disease of all the exocrine glands but particularly of the lungs and pancreas. Obstruction of the pancreatic ducts by amorphous eosinophilic concretions leads to dilatation of the acini, degeneration of the parenchyma, and fibrosis. Generalized bronchial obstruction in the lungs leads to pulmonary emphysema.

Gargoylism

A 5-year-old white male was brought to the neurology clinic for evaluation of mental retardation. One brother had been institutionalized for several years.

Physical examination revealed bilateral corneal opacities (A), minimal early papilledema (B), mental retardation, an aortic systolic murmur, cardiomegaly (C), hepatosplenomegaly (D), and kyphoscoliosis with a short stature.

Laboratory examination revealed acid mucopolysaccharide in the urine, which proved to be both chondroitin sulfate B and heparitin sulfate.

X-ray examination of the skull revealed marked enlargement, dolichocephaly, and elongation of the sella turcica (E). X-rays of the spine revealed hypoplasia and distortion of vertebrae (F). There were tubular enlargements of the long bones of the upper extremities.

Differential Diagnosis:
1. Arachnodactyly
2. Mongolism
3. Cretinism
4. Niemann-Pick disease
5. Gaucher's disease

Clinical Note. Certainly Niemann-Pick disease can give this combination of mental retardation, hepatosplenomegaly, eye and bone involvement; but instead of corneal opacities, there is a cherry red spot on the macula. In addition, there is no cardiovascular anomaly. Arachnodactyly does not cause mental retardation or hepatosplenomegaly, and the eye involvement is different. The laboratory is of great assistance in differentiating among these three disorders. There may be umbilical and inguinal hernias in gargoylism. Heredity is often sex-linked, but may not be.

Pathology. The major changes in all the organs are due to infiltration with the mucopolysaccharides and reactive fibrosis. The nerve cells of the brain are infiltrated by an unidentified lipid (G).

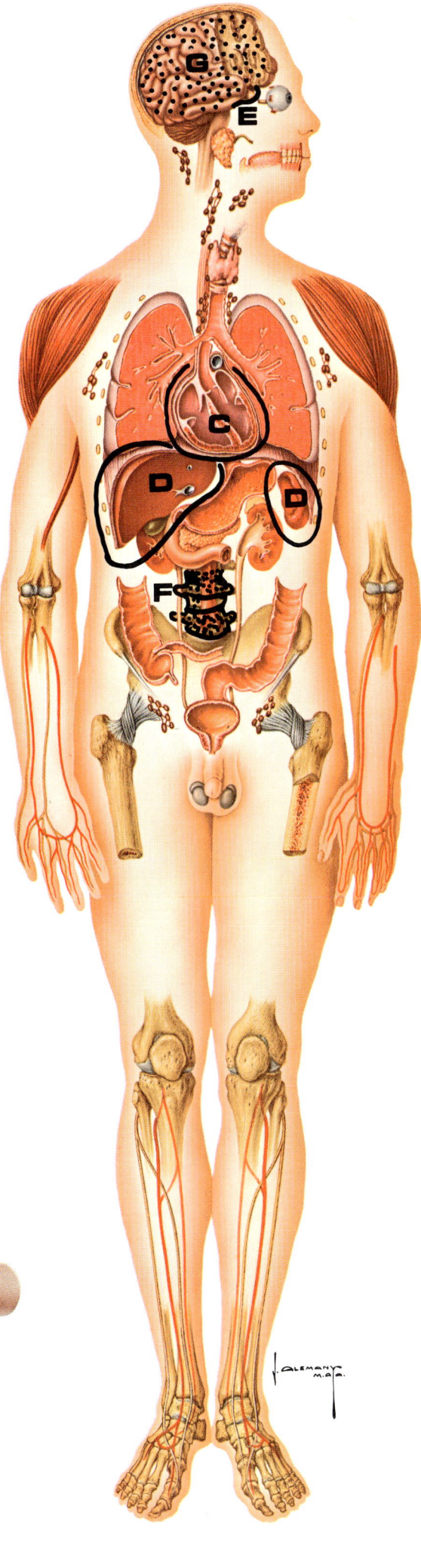

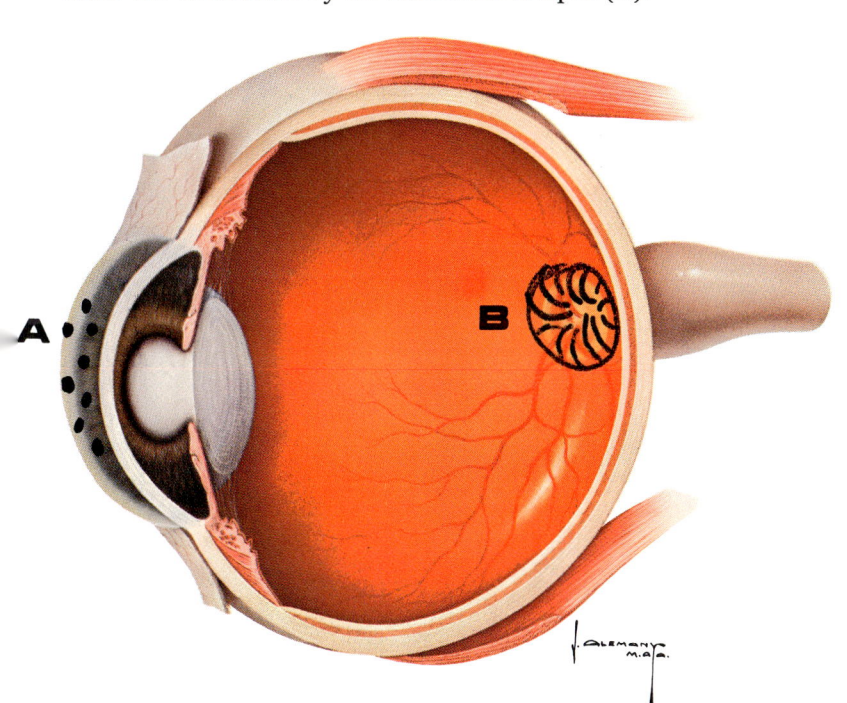

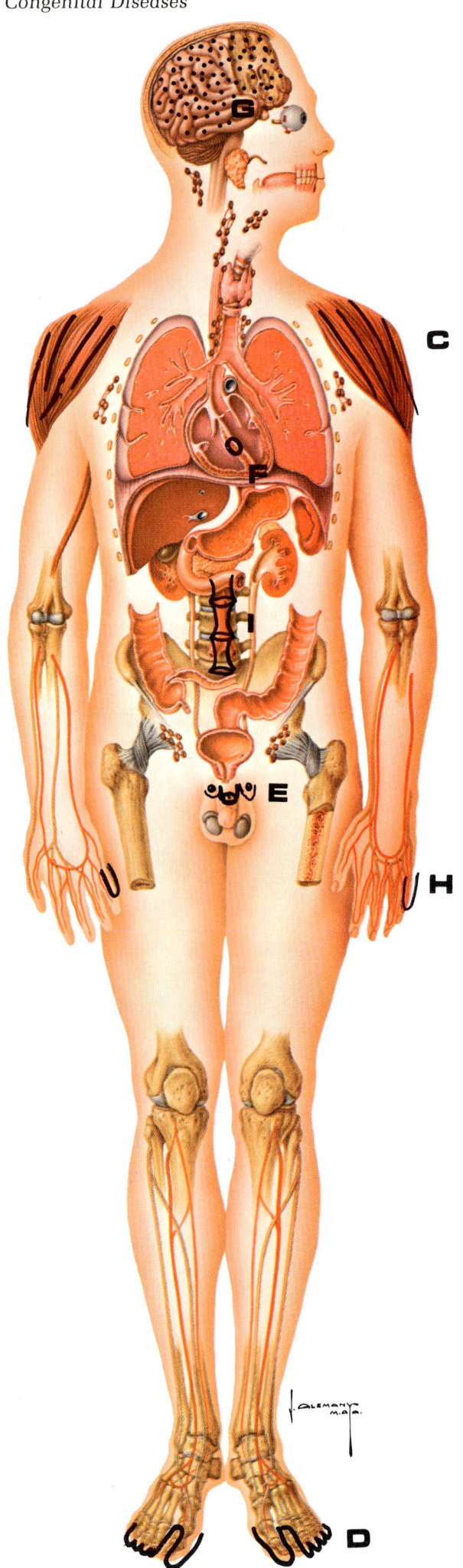

Mongolism

A 7-year-old white male was presented to the neurology clinic for evaluation of an I.Q. of 45.

Physical examination revealed narrow palpebral fissures and epicanthal folds (A), transverse straight palmar creases (B), generalized hypotonia (C), a large cleft between the 1st and 2nd toe (D), small genitalia (E), a grade III systolic murmur of the pulmonic area, indicating an interventricular septal defect (F), and mental retardation, indicating cerebral involvement (G).

Laboratory examination was unremarkable.

X-ray examination revealed hypoplastic middle and terminal phalanges of the 5th digit bilaterally (H) and elongation of the vertebral bodies (I). The angle formed by the slope of the lateral pelvis was very acute as was the acetabular slope.

Differential Diagnosis:
1. Cretinism
2. Gargoylism
3. Niemann-Pick disease
4. Cerebral palsy
5. Idiopathic mental retardation

Clinical Note. Here there is cerebral involvement with numerous skin changes but no rash, as is found in tuberosclerosis, and no actual ocular changes, as is found in gargoylism. In contrast to the others, this is not hereditary but is produced by a mutant gene. *Formes frustes* of this condition also occur.

Pathology. The brain is small, and there are shallow sulci. The microscopic pathology here is scanty and of doubtful significance.

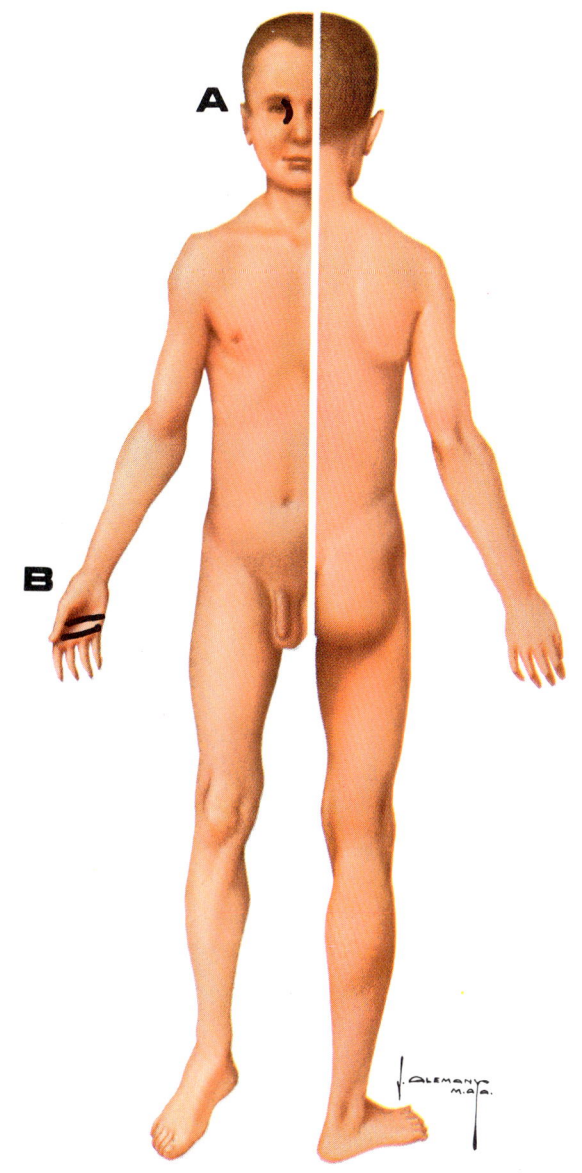

48 · Congenital Diseases

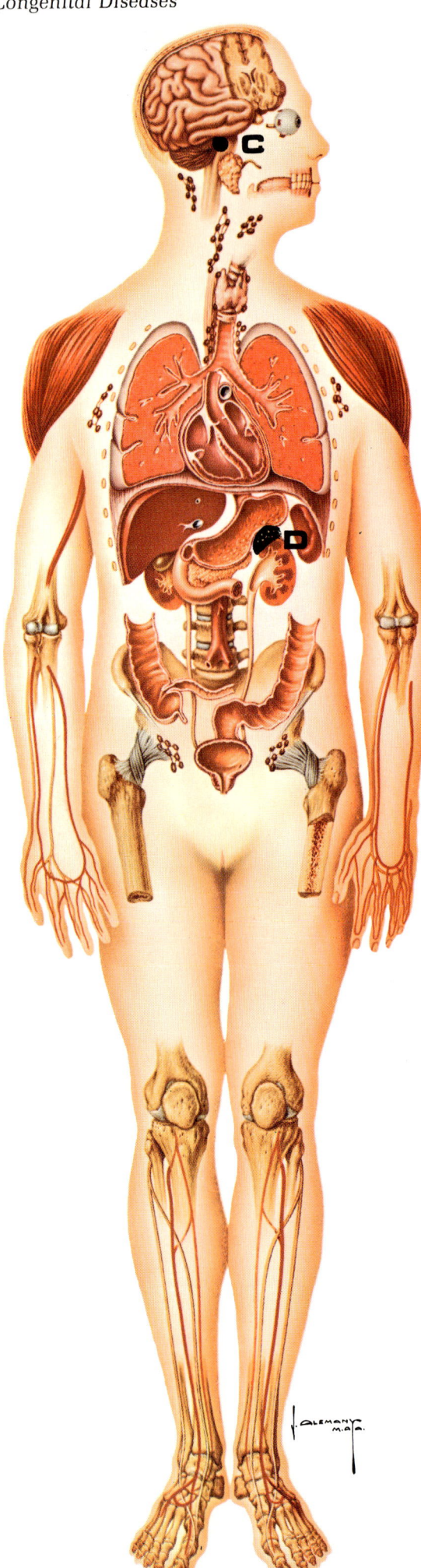

Neurofibromatosis

A 36-year-old white female complained of increasing tinnitis and deafness of the right ear for the past year. There was a family history of neurofibromatosis.

Physical examination revealed a blood pressure of 210/120, numerous brownish pigmented oval spots over the body (*café au lait* spots) (A) and fibromas of the skin (B), perceptive deafness in the right ear, and loss of the right corneal reflex.

Laboratory examination revealed a high spinal fluid protein, right canal paresis on caloric testing of the right ear, and an increased 24-hour urine VMA.

X-ray examination of the skull revealed erosion of the right petrous bone, suggesting an acoustic neuroma (C), and x-ray of the lumbar spine revealed erosion of the vertebrae.

The patient died during surgery for the acoustic neuroma, and an autopsy revealed a pheochromocytoma of the left adrenal gland as well (D).

Differential Diagnosis:
1. Petrositis
2. Tuberculosis with meningitis
3. Syphilis
4. Tuberosclerosis
5. Carcinomatosis
6. Lymphoma
7. Multiple myeloma

Clinical Note. Here there is involvement of skin, nervous system, and bone. Tuberculosis, lymphomas, and carcinomatosis may present this combination, but the hereditary history and the *café au lait* spots are a complete giveaway. Neuromas and gliomas may develop in other parts of the nervous system, in peripheral nerves, and in other internal organs. The fibromas may also undergo sarcomatous degeneration.

Pathology. The pathology is that of the neurofibroma. The tumors are firm and nodular on gross examination. Microscopically, they are made up of interlacing strands of elongated cells with very little collagen tissue in the stroma. There is prominent palisading of the nuclei. The neurofibromas found in this disorder are prone to become malignant.

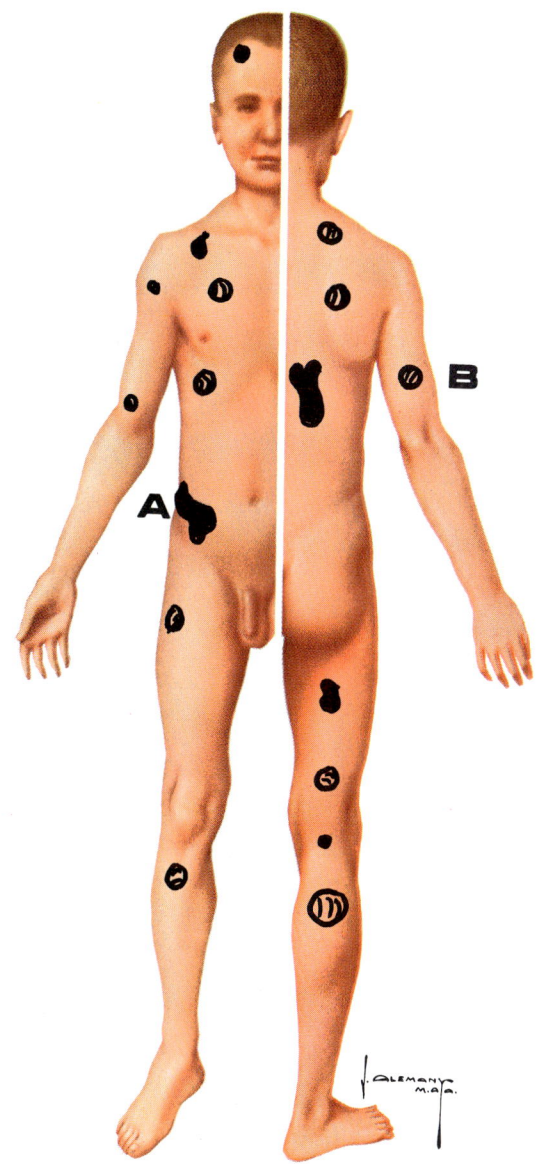

50 · *Congenital Diseases*

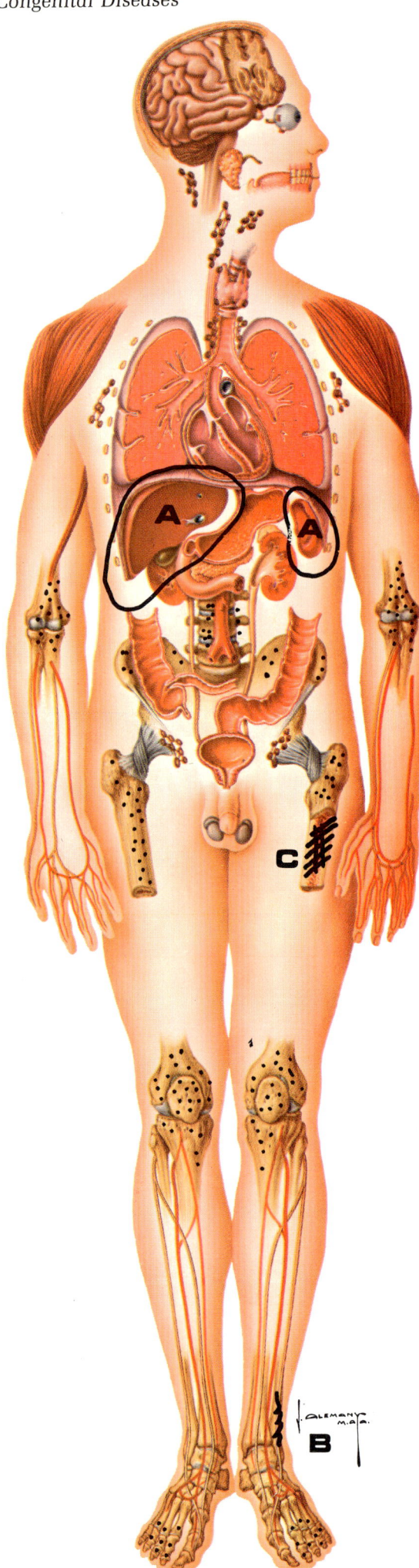

Osteopetrosis

A 4-year-old white male was brought to the emergency room after a minor fall.

Physical examination revealed pale conjunctiva and skin, hepatosplenomegaly (A), and suggested a fracture of the left fibula (B).

Laboratory examination revealed a hypochromic microcytic anemia with a few normoblasts in the peripheral blood.

X-ray examination revealed a generalized increase in density of the bones, with obliteration of the medullary cavity in many places (C), and confirmed the fracture of the left fibula. The orbital and facial bones were intensely sclerotic.

Differential Diagnosis:
1. Multiple myeloma
2. Osteogenesis imperfecta
3. Osteomalacia, of whatever cause
4. Renal rickets
5. Osteoporosis
6. Paget's disease

Clinical Note. The combination of blood and bone involvement is seen in numerous disorders, but particularly in osteogenesis imperfecta. The latter, however, is associated with blue sclerae and relaxation of the ligaments, with hypermotility of the joints, and x-rays show translucent bone with more numerous pathologic fractures. Both may be associated with deafness; but in osteopetrosis this is due to encroachment on the 8th nerve, whereas in osteogenesis imperfecta it is due to otosclerosis (conductive loss). Blindness may also occur in osteopetrosis due to encroachment on the optic foramina.

Pathology. The hepatosplenomegaly is due to extramedullary erythropoiesis since the anemia is myelophthisic.

Polycystic Disease

A 54-year-old white male was admitted to the hospital because of sudden onset of severe headache and stiff neck. One uncle had died of kidney disease.

Physical examination revealed a blood pressure of 220/110, a right subchoroidal hemorrhage of the retina (A), nuchal rigidity, and masses in both flanks (the enlarged polycystic kidneys) (B).

Laboratory examination revealed bloody spinal fluid, albuminuria, hematuria, and a BUN of 49 mg. per cent.

X-ray Examinations. A right carotid angiogram revealed an internal carotid aneurysm (C). An intravenous pyelogram revealed bilateral polycystic kidneys.

Surgery was unsuccessful, and the patient died a few days later.

Differential Diagnosis:
1. Hypernephroma with metastasis
2. Obstructive uropathy
3. Cerebral hemorrhage
4. Subacute bacterial endocarditis
5. Cerebral embolism or thrombosis

Clinical Note. One fifth of the cases of polycystic kidneys have associated cerebral aneurysms and may present with a subarachnoid hemorrhage. There are also, in some cases, cysts of the pancreas, liver (D), lungs, and spleen. A family history is obtained in the majority of cases. The disease may present in infancy as bilateral renal masses and uremia.

Pathology. The kidneys are enlarged and nodular, and on cross section the entire parenchyma is honeycombed by cysts of various sizes filled with serous, hemorrhagic, or pustular fluid.

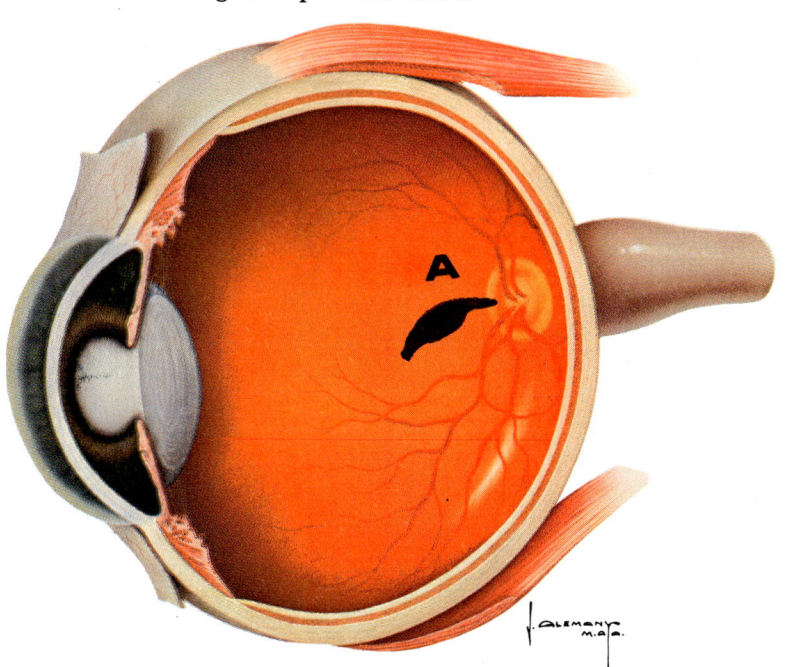

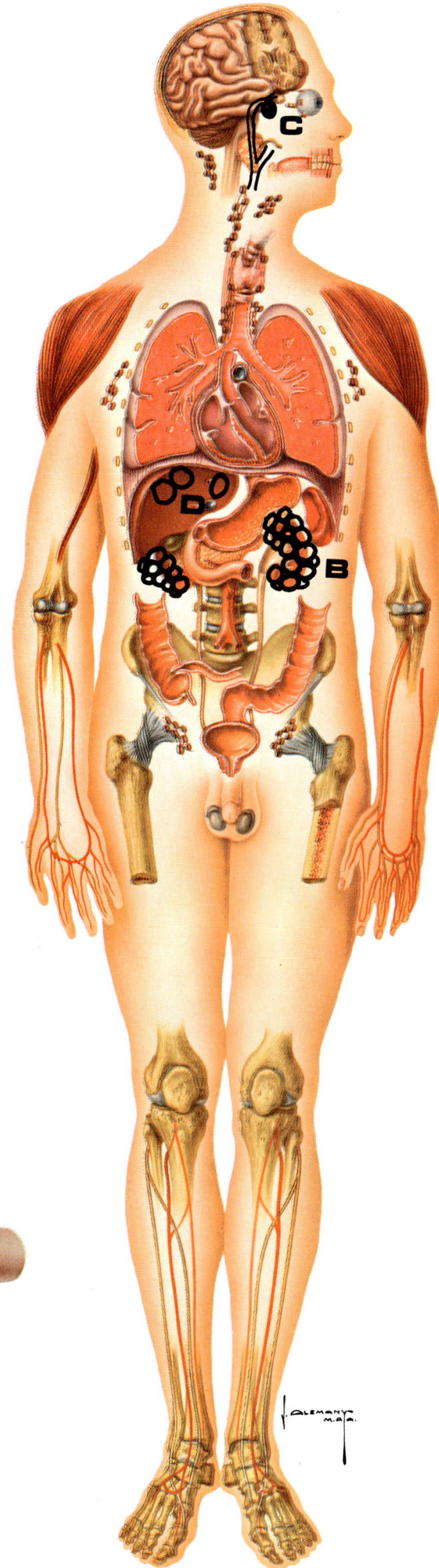

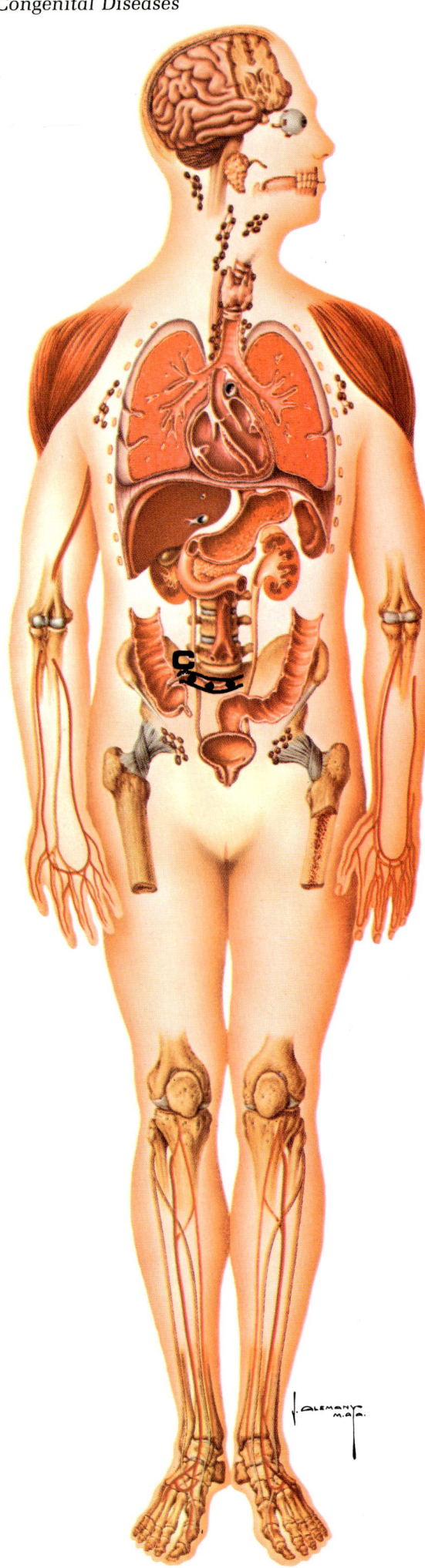

Peutz-Jegher's Syndrome

A 16-year-old white female complained of recurrent bouts of colicky abnormal pain following meals and loud, noisy embarrassing sounds coming from her bowels. She had been considered neurotic by her local physician. One brother had been found to have intestinal polyposis.

Physical examination revealed pigmented spots of the lips and buccal mucosa (A), the palms, fingers, and toes (B), and audible borborygmi of the intestines.

Laboratory examination revealed a microcytic hypochromic anemia.

X-ray examination of the small bowel revealed multiple polyps of the jejunum and ileum (C).

Treatment in the form of a stool softener was administered.

Differential Diagnosis:
1. Addison's disease
2. Regional ileitis
3. Renal calculus
4. G.I. malignancy
5. Intestinal obstruction
6. Porphyria
7. Lead intoxication
8. Ulcerative colitis

Clinical Note. Here we have bowel and skin manifestations together, which may be found in ulcerative colitis and regional enteritis. The combination of skin lesions and bowel tumors is also seen in acanthosis nigricans and in dermatomyositis. The embarrassing noisy bowel sounds may not be a laughing matter if intussusception develops. However, since these polyps do not become malignant, there is no reason to do elective bowel resection. The anemia is due to moderate gastrointestinal bleeding.

Pathology. The polyps may occur in the bladder, pharynx, colon, and stomach.

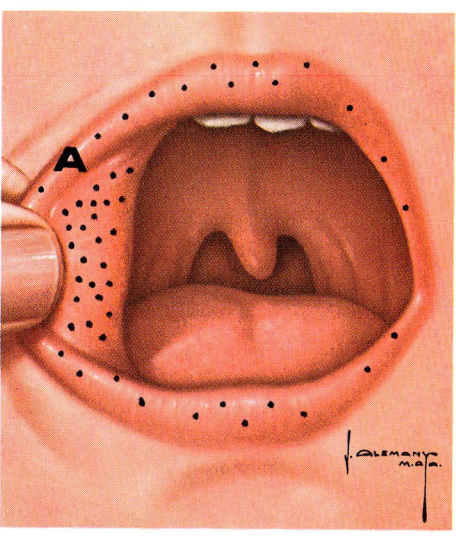

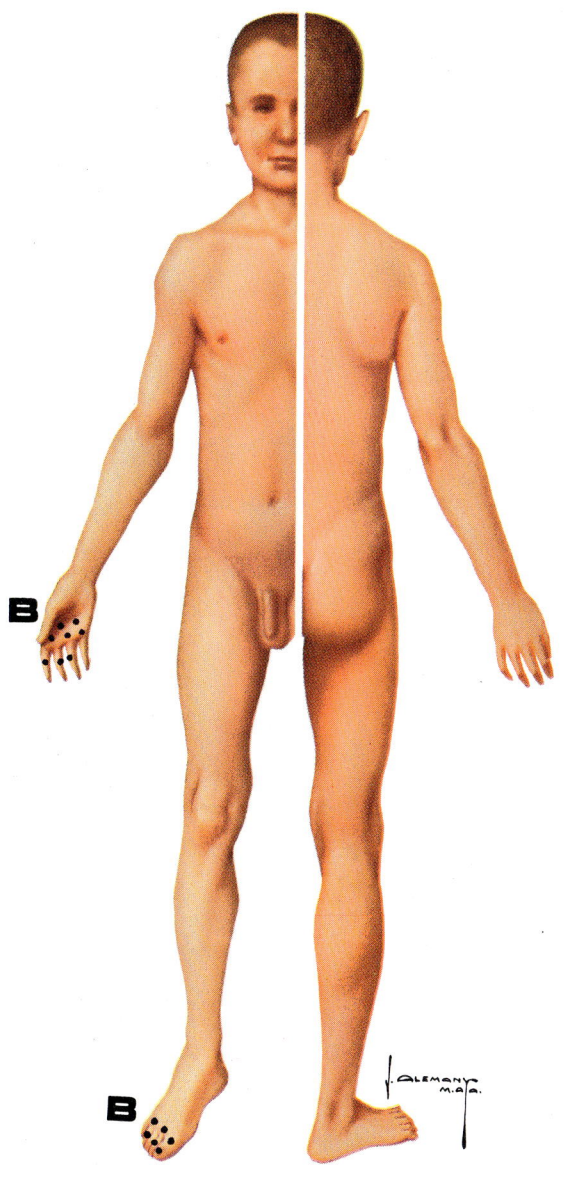

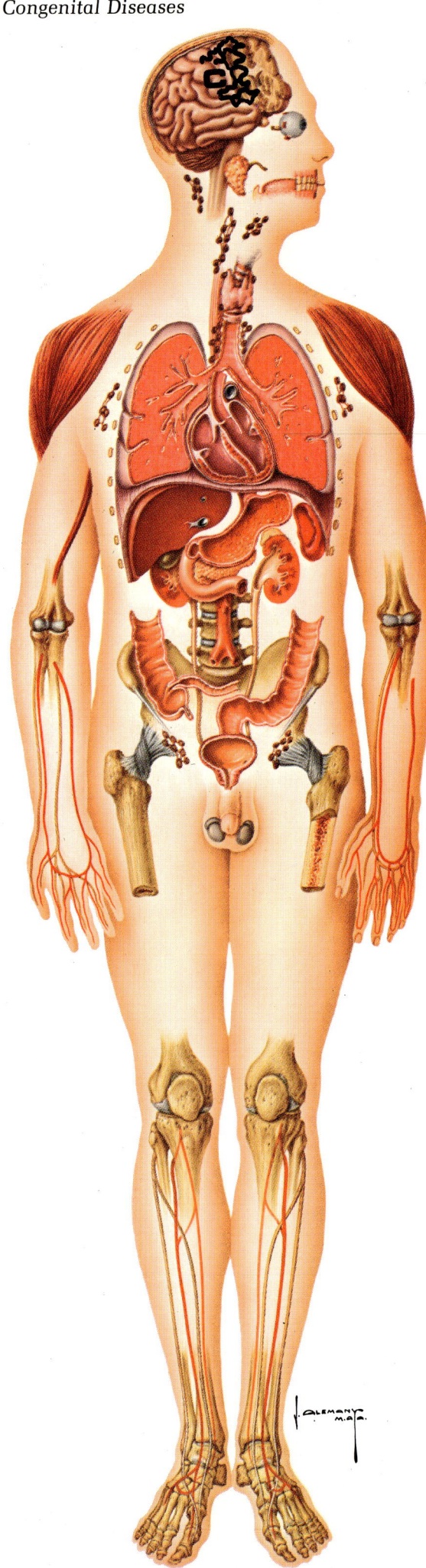

Sturge-Weber Syndrome

(Congenital but not Hereditary)

A 5-year-old white male began having left-sided jacksonian seizures in late infancy although there was no family history of these.

Physical examination revealed a macular port-wine stained lesion over the right side of the face (A), which proved to be a cavernous hemangioma, retinal angiomas (B), and contralateral hemiplegia with slight mental retardation (C).

Laboratory examination was unremarkable except the EEG revealed a persistent spike focus in the right occipital area.

X-ray examination of the skull revealed extensive convolutional calcification of the occipital and parietal cortex on the right. Both pneumoencephalography and arteriography demonstrated right cortical atrophy (C).

Differential Diagnosis:
1. Cerebral palsy
2. Tuberous sclerosis
3. Toxoplasmosis
4. Space-occupying lesion of cerebral cortex
5. Lead intoxication

Pathology. The angioma of the cortex is predominantly venous; and beneath the lesion the cortex becomes calcified, hard, and atrophic. Angiomas may involve many other organs and may account for hematemesis or hematuria.

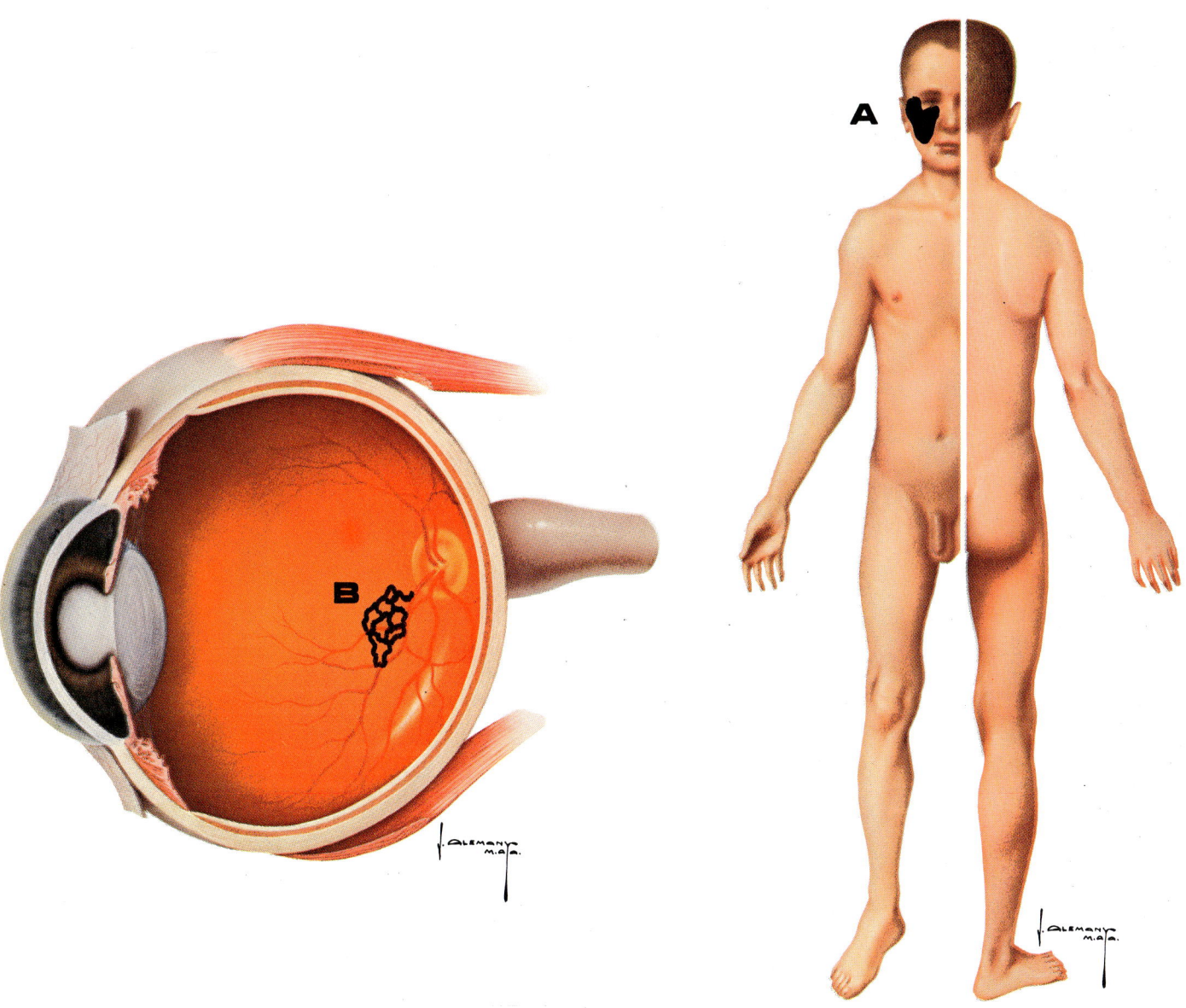

Tuberosclerosis

A 7-year-old white male was brought to the neurology clinic for evaluation of documented grand mal seizures. One sister with mental retardation had died in convulsions.

Physical examination revealed a butterfly-shaped, papular rash of the nose and cheeks and, to a lesser extent, the low back (adenoma sebaceum) (A) and obvious mental retardation.

Laboratory examination was unremarkable except for diffuse paroxysmal slowing on the electroencephalogram.

X-ray examination of the skull revealed numerous round calcifications in the region of the lateral ventricles (B). X-rays of the spine revealed osteosclerotic areas in the vertebral bodies (C).

Differential Diagnosis:
1. Acne dur to prolonged use of Dilantin
2. Space-occupying lesion of the brain
3. Sturge-Weber syndrome
4. Tuberculous meningitis
5. Toxoplasmosis
6. Niemann-Pick disease

Clinical Note. Here is a hereditary or congenital disease that presents with skin and nervous system involvement. Niemann-Pick disease may do this, but it develops earlier in life, and the course is more rapid; in addition, a cherry-red spot is present in the macula. The rash in tuberosclerosis is quite typical.

Pathology. There are whitish areas of glial sclerosis throughout the cortex. These become calcified in the walls of the lateral ventricles. They may undergo malignant transformation. Neurolemmoblastomas may develop in the kidneys and other organs. Rhabdomyomas may develop in the heart.

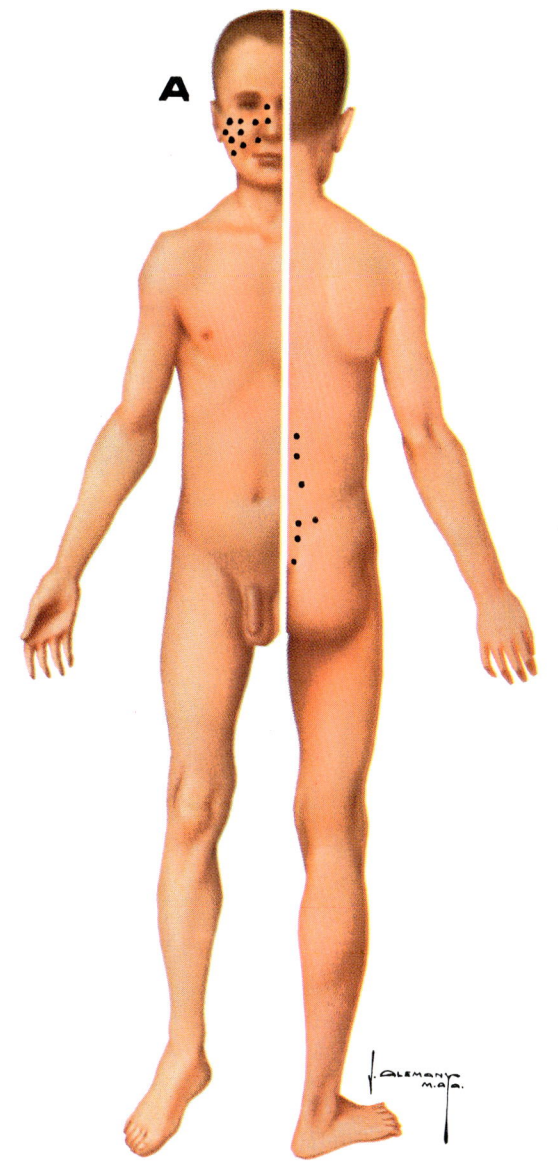

58 · Congenital Diseases

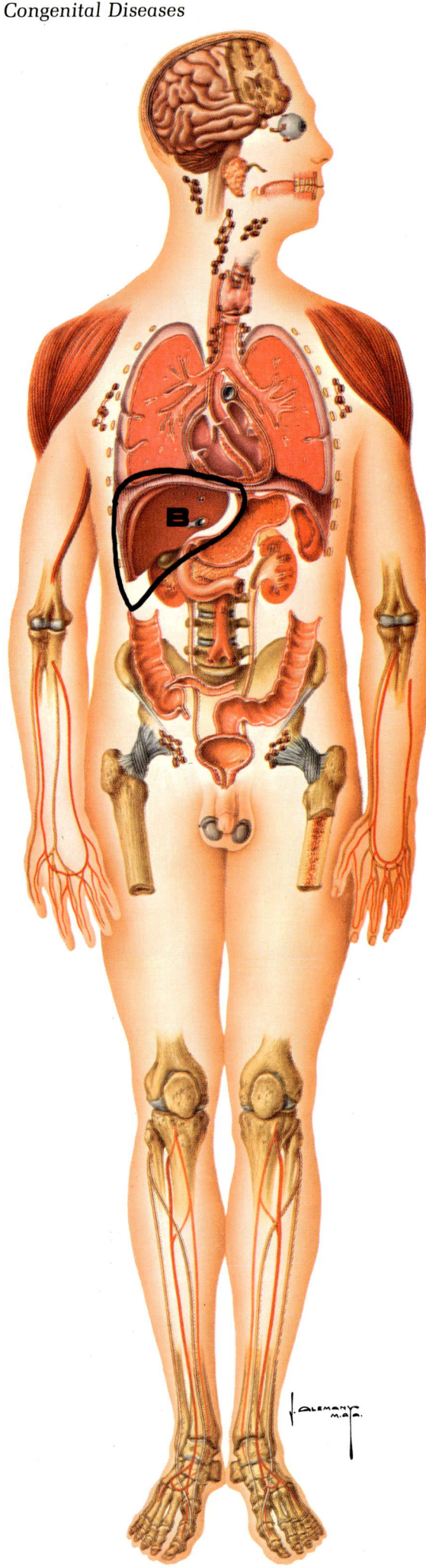

Porphyria Cutanea Tarda

A 32-year-old male, South African, complained of recurrent blisters on his skin on exposure to sunlight.

Physical examination revealed bullae and vesicles of the face and back of the hands (A) and hepatomegaly (B).

Laboratory examination revealed dark urine with abundant porphyrins but no porphobilinogen. He had a high thymol turbidity, alkaline phosphatase, and transaminase as an indication of liver damage.

Differential Diagnosis:
1. Pemphigus
2. Epidermolysis bullosa
3. Infectious mononucleosis
4. Other forms of porphyria
5. Hydroa aestivale

Clinical Note. This form may be acquired or hereditary. It is the most common form of cutaneous porphyria among Americans and Europeans and among non-Europeans of Southern Africa, who use to excess a home-brewed alcohol.

Pathology. There is fatty infiltration of the liver, together with bullous and vesicular lesions of the affected areas of the skin.

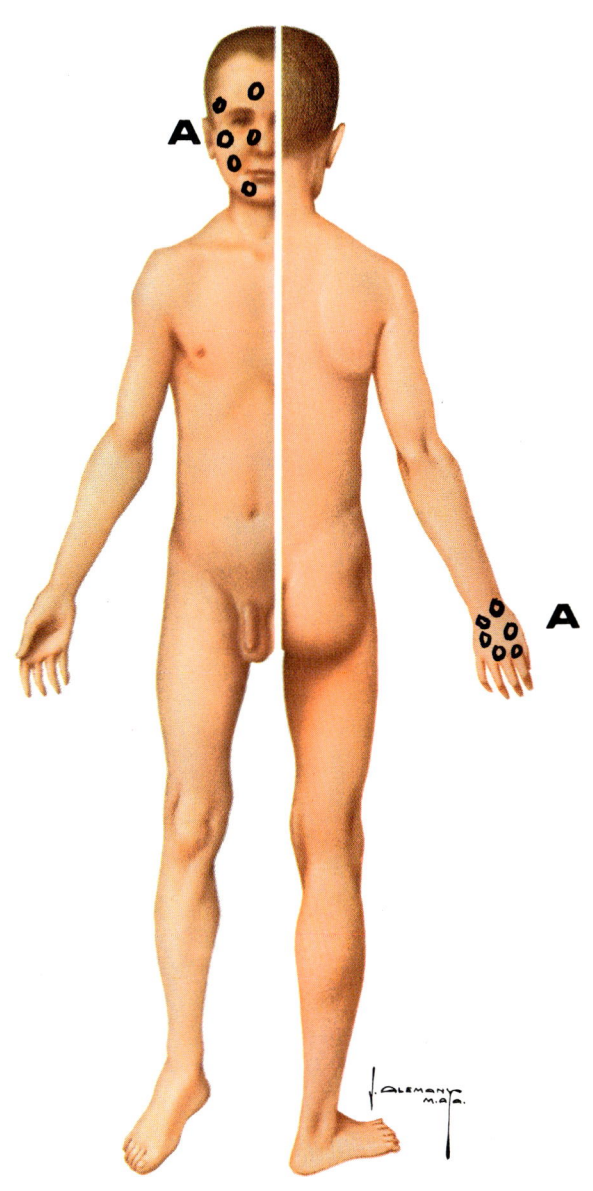

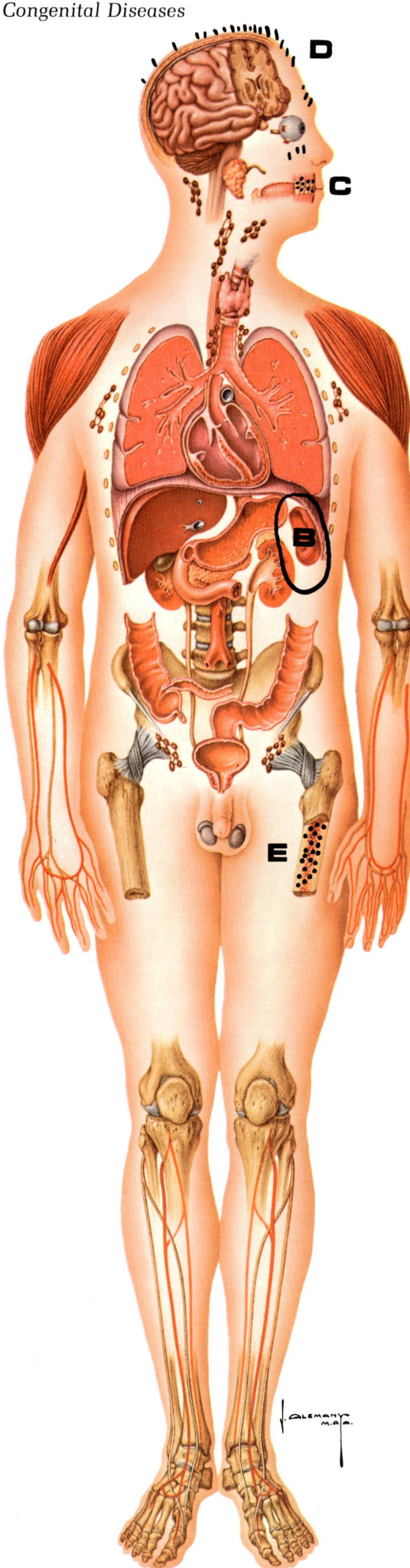

Porphyria Erythropoietica

A 14-year-old white male was admitted for consideration for splenectomy. He had a bullous dermatitis, hemolytic anemia, and port-wine color to his urine since infancy.

Physical examination revealed bullous and vesicular eruption of hands, face, and neck (A), brownish pigmentation of the skin in these areas, splenomegaly (B), pinkish-staining of the teeth (C), and hirsuitism (D).

Laboratory examination revealed large amounts of uroporphyrins in the bone marrow, blood, and urine with no significant porphobilinogen. There was a hemolytic anemia.

Treatment by splenectomy was helpful.

Differential Diagnosis:
1. Pemphigus vulgaris
2. Hemolytic anemia, of whatever cause
3. Hydroa aestivale
4. Typhoid fever
5. Meningococcemia
6. Bullous staphylococcus infection

Clinical Note. This type is now known to be very rare. Most of the cases of porphyria with cutaneous involvement are the hepatic cutaneous type (page 58). The urine in porphyria erythropoietica is colored red at the time of excretion; but since porphobilinogen is colorless, the urine is colorless in the intermittent abdominal type until exposure to sunlight.

Pathology. The porphyrin also accumulates in the red cells, bones (E), and spleen as well as the bone marrow.

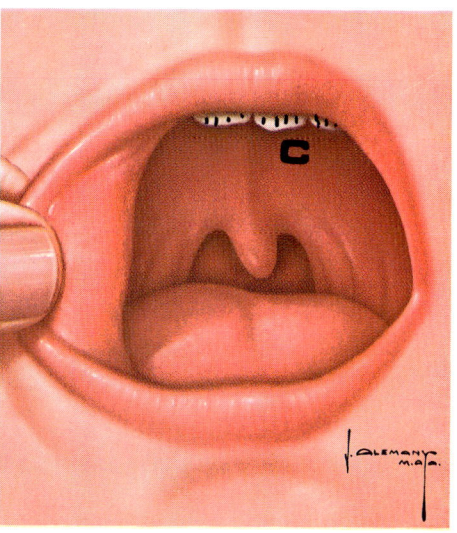

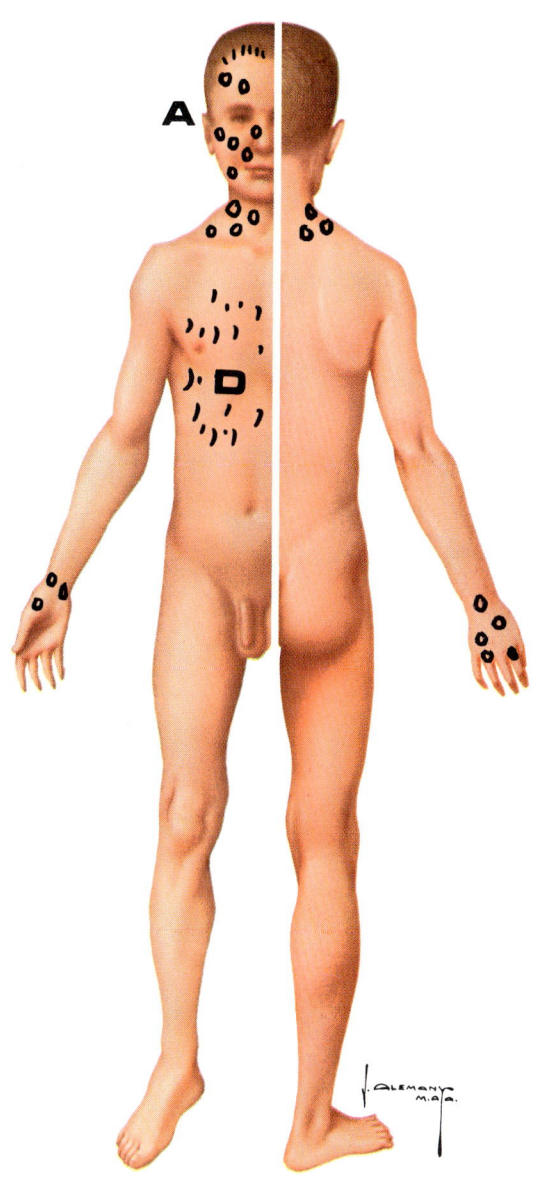

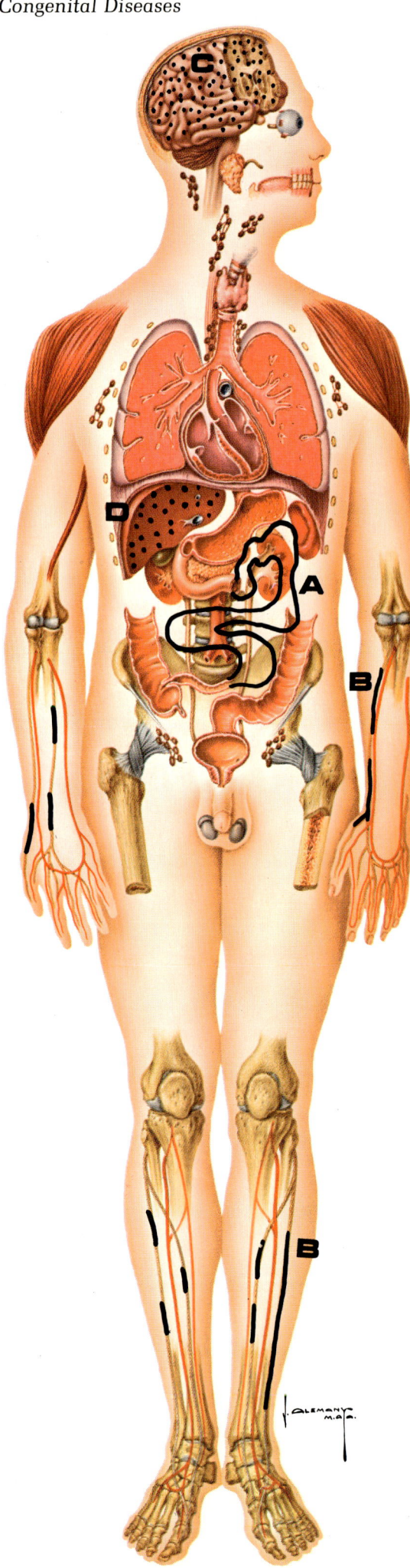

Porphyria, Intermittent Abdominal Type

A 29-year-old white male complained of severe colicky, midepigastric pain, and distention of the abdomen. Physical examination on that occasion was normal except for the distention. Two weeks later the patient developed increasing weakness, pain, and paresthesias in all 4 extremities. His family noted that at times he was delirious and manifested poor judgment. He had had an attack of abdominal pain 3 years previously, diagnosed as "acute hepatitis." His father and one brother had suffered similar symptoms.

Physical examination revealed a distended tympanitic abdomen (A), weakness and hypoactive deep-tendon reflexes in all 4 extremities with painful muscles and nerve trunks (B), and glove and stocking hypalgesia and hypesthesia bilaterally. The patient was disoriented in time and space and had a poor attention span (C).

Laboratory examination revealed a urine "urobilinogen" of 1:1000, which was not extracted with chloroform, an indication that it was indeed porphobilinogen.

Differential Diagnosis:
1. Acute pancreatitis
2. Perforated peptic ulcer
3. Cholecystitis
4. Intestinal obstruction
5. Nutritional neuropathy
6. Diabetic neuropathy and acidosis
7. Lead intoxication
8. Periarteritis nodosa
9. Renal calculus
10. Guillain-Barré syndrome
11. Pellagra

Clinical Note. Do not operate on atypical cases of abdominal pain unless the urine has been checked for porphobilinogen! This case emphasizes the abdominal and neurologic manifestations of this unique disorder. The skin may be involved in the combined type. Also note the familial occurrence of this disorder.

Pathology. The peripheral nerves undergo degeneration of the myelin sheaths and occasionally of the axis cylinders, with a moderate interstitial reaction. There are diffuse tiny ischemic lesions of the brain. The liver is loaded with porphobilinogen, and there is fatty metamorphosis with early cirrhosis (D).

Chapter 5

Deficiency Diseases

Today most of these diseases are rarely seen clinically except in alcoholics. However, pernicious anemia is now seen more frequently because of the increase in the aged population. Pernicious anemia is not usually due to a deficiency of vitamin B_{12} in the diet but rather to absence of the intrinsic factor of Castle.

Deficiency diseases affect principally one or two types of tissue in the body. Thus vitamin A deficiency affects the skin and eye. Vitamin D deficiency affects the bone. Thiamine deficiency affects the heart and nerves.

Mild subclinical deficiencies of various vitamins are probably present in a large segment of the population, particularly people who consistently eat in restaurants, where the vitamins may be steamed out of food sitting on hot plates for several hours.

To add daily multivitamin supplement to the diet is dictated by good common sense. Probably most avitaminoses seen today are mixed, and the clinical manifestations may not be clear-cut. Therefore in treatment multiple vitamins should be given, not just one vitamin.

With the advances of medical science has come iatrogenic vitamin deficiencies; thus tuberculosis patients given isoniazid may develop pyridoxine deficiency. A gastrectomy may produce pernicious anemia if too much stomach has been removed. Reducing diets often pay little attention to adequate vitamins.

Most community hospitals are limited in laboratory facilities for the diagnosis of avitaminosis. A serum iron, serum calcium (for rickets), and long bone x-rays are usually all that can be obtained.

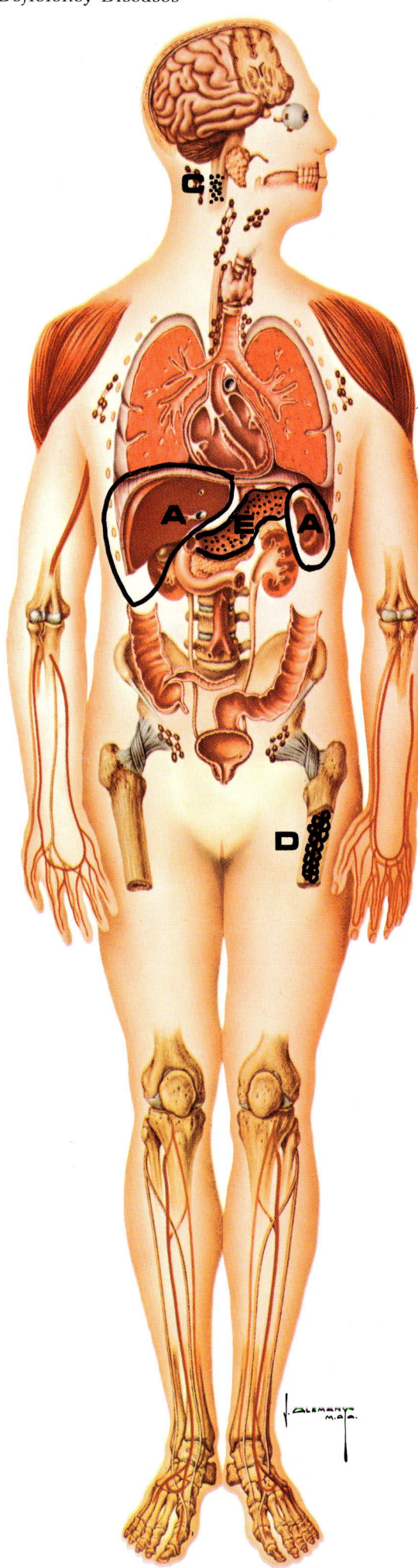

Pernicious Anemia

A 68-year-old white female complained of anorexia, nausea, and occasional vomiting over a 3-month period. An elaborate diagnostic workup at another hospital had been negative. A review of systems disclosed that she also experienced shortness of breath, numbness, and tingling of the extremities.

Physical examination revealed a pale, slightly icteric, blue-eyed, white-haired lady with mild hepatosplenomegaly (A), a smooth tongue (B), and loss of vibratory and position sense in both lower extremities, indicating spinal cord involvement (C).

Laboratory examination revealed a macrocytic, hyperchromic anemia, leukopenia with hypersegmented neutrophils, and thrombocytopenia. The serum bilirubin was 2.5 mg. per cent, and a gastric analysis with histamine revealed achlorhydria. The bone marrow was megaloblastic and hypercellular (D). A Schilling test confirmed the diagnosis.

Treatment. She experienced a rapid reticulocytosis and eventual recovery on 200 mcg. of B_{12} every other day.

Differential Diagnosis:
1. Multiple myeloma
2. *Diphyllobothrium latum*
3. Celiac disease
4. Tabes dorsalis
5. Hemolytic anemias
6. Lupus erythematosus
7. Gastric malignancy
8. Spinal cord tumor

Clinical Note. The classical picture with multisystem involvement and severe anemia is only occasionally found today. The low incidence is the result of diets rich in meat and vitamins that frequently contain folic acid supplement, which improves the anemia but may make the cord involvement worse. The peripheral blood may show a microcytic, hypochromic picture or no anemia at all. The disease is rare before 40 years of age although a juvenile form may occur and is usually hereditary. All patients with a so-called negative gastrointestinal work-up should be studied for this disease.

Pathology. In addition to the bone marrow changes, there are atrophy of the gastric mucosa (E) and degeneration of the posterior and lateral columns of the spinal cord. Carcinoma of the stomach may develop.

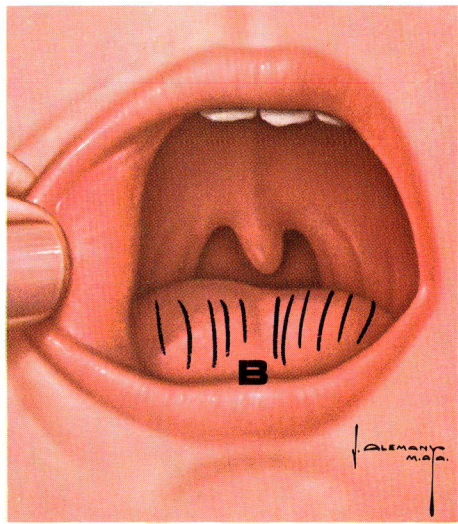

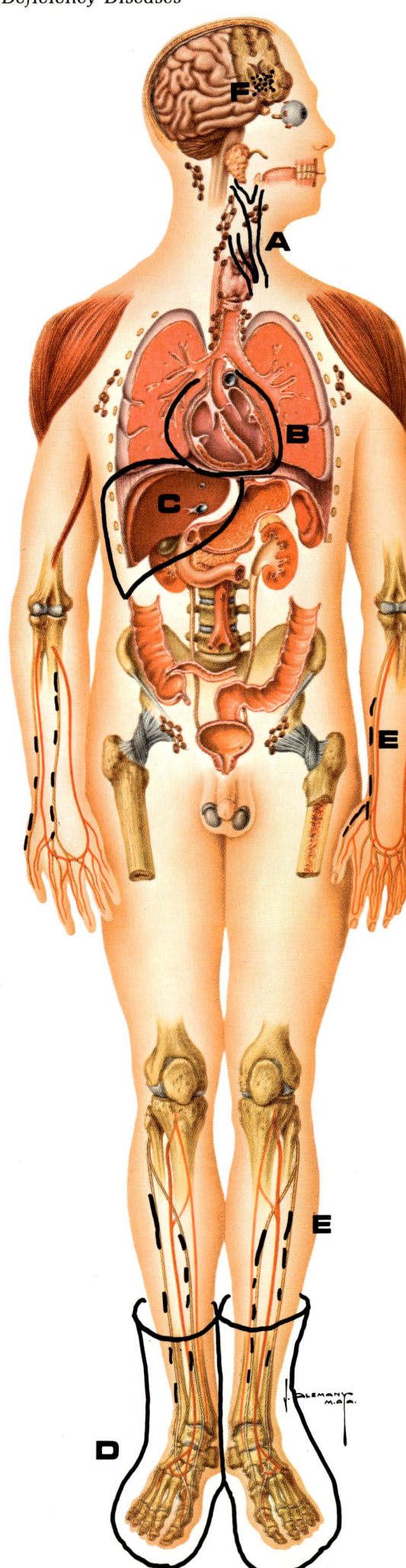

Beriberi

A 38-year-old Negro male alcoholic was admitted to the medical service because of severe shortness of breath and swelling of his legs.

Physical examination revealed 2+ neck vein distention (A), cardiomegaly (B), hepatomegaly (C), and pitting edema of both lower extremities (D). There were glove and stocking hypesthesia and hypalgesia and decreased deep-tendon reflexes of the extremities, indicating peripheral nerve involvement (E).

Laboratory examination revealed a high blood pyruvic acid but a low blood and urine thiamine even after a loading dose of the vitamin.

Treatment with thiamine brought about complete remission.

Differential Diagnosis:
1. Hypothyroidism
2. Alcoholic neuropathy and myocardiopathy
3. Rheumatic or congenital heart disease
4. Atherosclerotic heart disease
5. Constrictive pericarditis
6. Diabetic neuropathy

Clinical Note. With the exception of alcoholics, this disease is rare. Yet it must be considered in all patients with so-called "atherosclerotic heart disease." Although this case presents signs of both wet (cardiac) and dry (neuropathic) beriberi, the clinical picture is usually not mixed to this extent.

Pathology. Microscopic examination of the peripheral nerves reveals that the axons and myelin sheaths are in various stages of degeneration, extending to complete fragmentation. There is very little interstitial reaction. The thalamic and hypothalamic nuclei and mammillary bodies may be involved with congestion and hemorrhages (F) (Wernicke's encephalopathy). There may be similar lesions throughout the brain, with demyelinization in Korsakoff's psychosis.

Plummer-Vinson Syndrome

A 33-year-old white female complained of weight loss, fatigue, and increasing difficulty in swallowing without heartburn for the past 3 to 4 months.

Physical examination revealed spoon nails (A), smooth tongue (B), and pale conjunctivae, skin, and nailbeds. *Esophagoscopy* revealed webbing of the upper esophagus (C).

Laboratory examination revealed a hypochromic, microcytic anemia and a serum iron of 22 mcg. per cent.

Treatment with vitamins and iron was instituted.

Differential Diagnosis:
1. Foreign body of esophagus
2. Cardiospasm of esophagus
3. Reflux esophagitis and hiatal hernia
4. Neoplasm of the esophagus
5. Esophageal diverticulum
6. Scleroderma

Clinical Note. It must not be forgotten that iron deficiency is a systemic disease. These patients should be watched later for carcinomas of the oral cavity and larynx. Most cases of dysphagia today are related to hiatal hernias and esophagitis, but this condition must not be forgotten.

Pathology. The web is composed of esophageal mucosa. The mucosa of the mouth and pharynx, however, is atrophied.

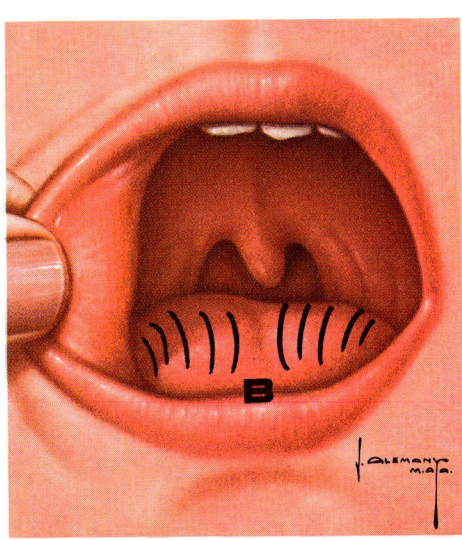

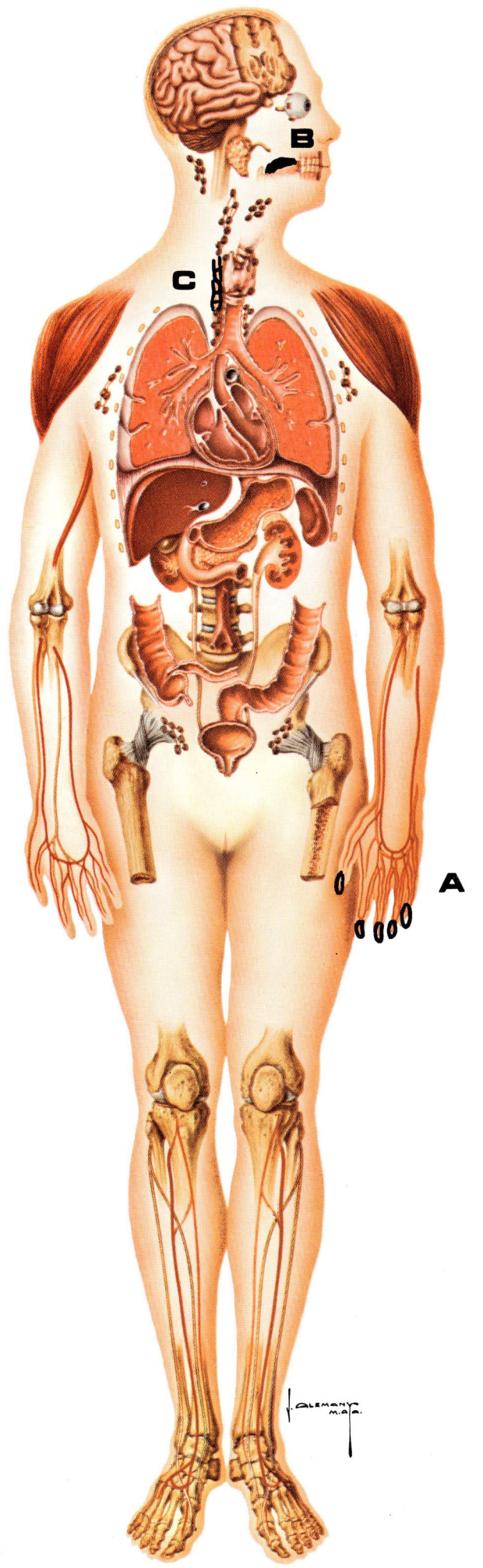

68 · *Deficiency Diseases*

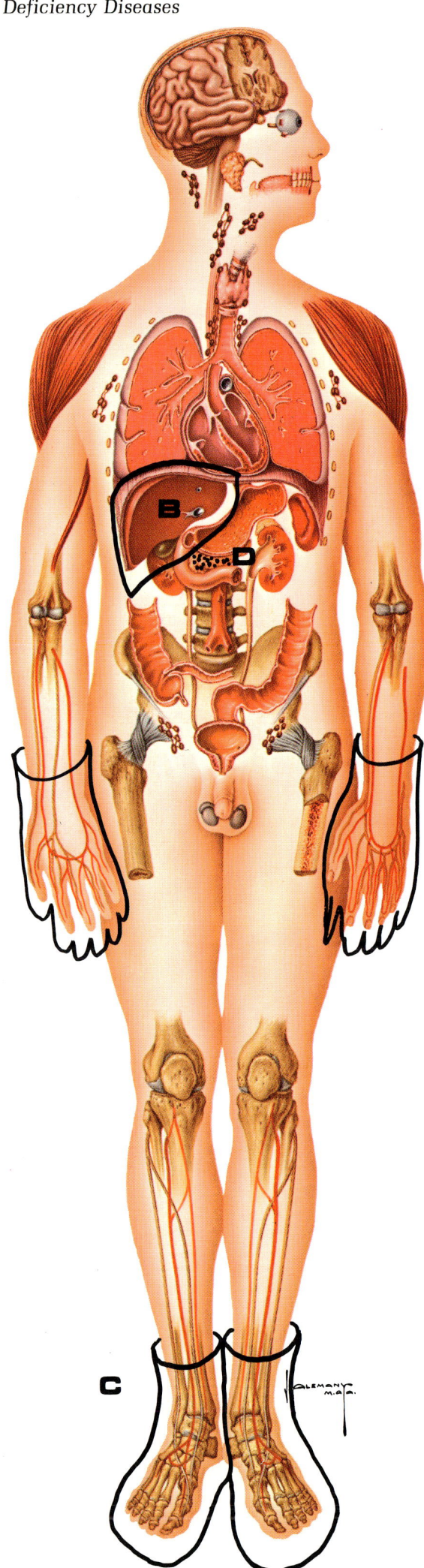

Kwashiorkor

An 18-month-old Negro South African child was brought to the pediatric clinic with a known history of poor nourishment.

Physical examination revealed hyperpigmentation and hyperkeratosis on the chest, axillae and groins (A), thinning of the hair, which was crinkly and reddish in places, hepatomegaly without jaundice (B), and pitting edema of the extremities (C). The child was apathetic and irritable.

Laboratory examination revealed a low serum albumin and macrocytic anemia. Liver biopsy revealed a fatty metamorphosis but only a slight increase in fibrous tissue.

Treatment with a well-balanced diet and milk brought about remission.

Differential Diagnosis:
1. Marasmus
2. Glycogen storage disease
3. Galactosemia
4. Pellagra
5. Celiac disease
6. Fibrocystic disease of the pancreas

Clinical Note. The skin changes resemble those of pellagra but do not respond to vitamins. This disease is probably due to deficient quality and quantity of protein in the food. Thus, instead of the extreme emaciation of severe undernutrition, there is often pancreatic insufficiency due to atrophy of the acinar cells of the pancreas (D). The fatty liver in this condition resembles that of alcoholism, and is reversible.

Pathology. Microscopic examination of the liver reveals extensive fatty infiltration, and this may progress to fibrosis. Both the acinar and islet cells of the pancreas may be atrophied, and the islet cells may undergo cyst formation.

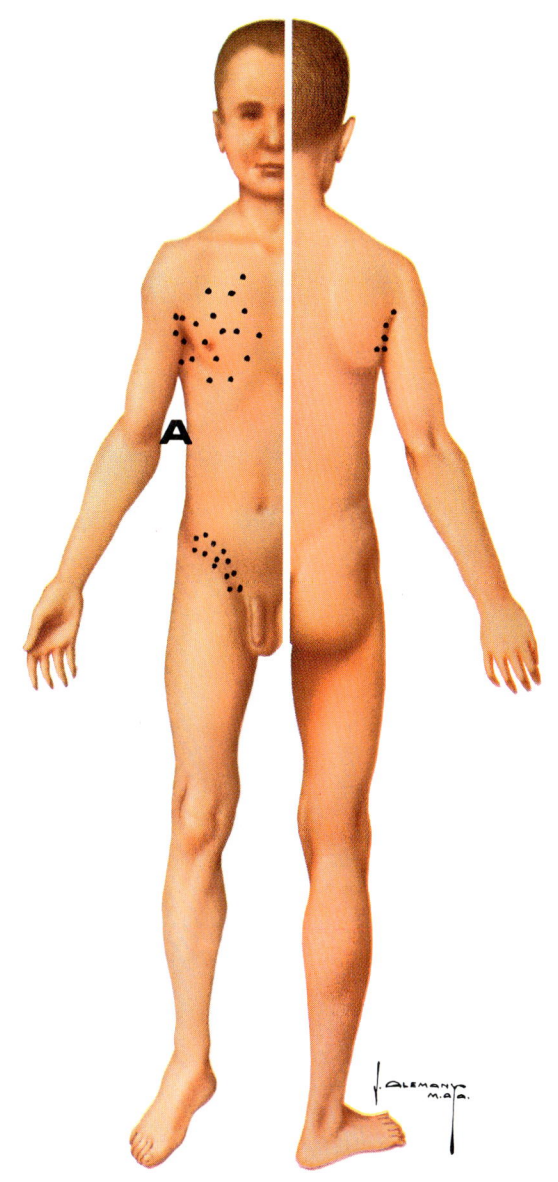

70 · *Deficiency Diseases*

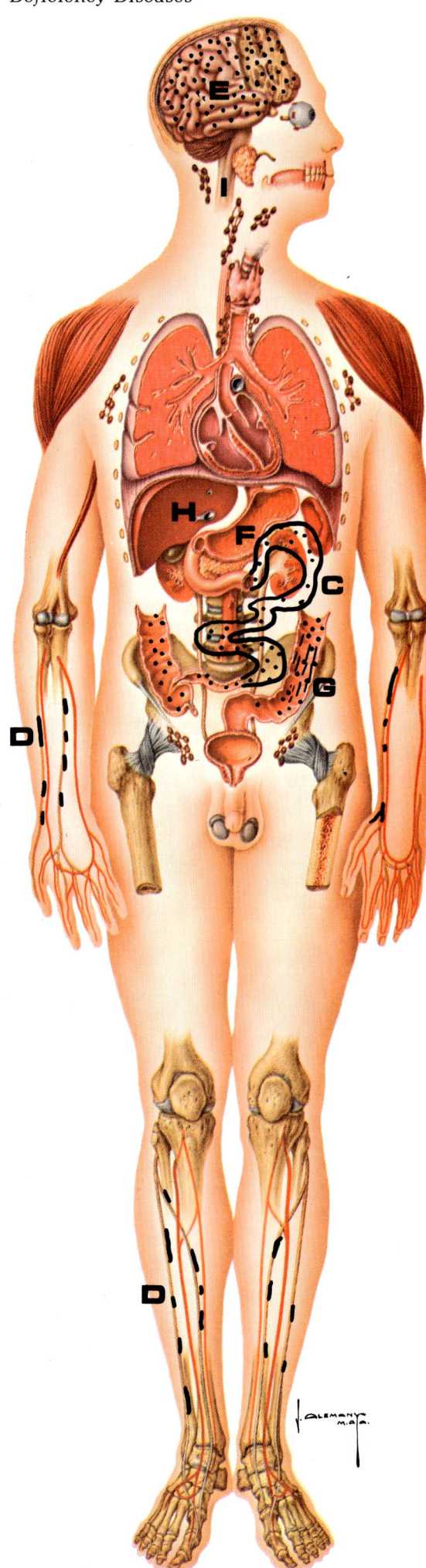

Pellagra

A 65-year-old Puerto Rican male with a history of alcoholism underwent a prostatectomy for benign prostatic hypertrophy. Postoperatively he failed to eat and had paralytic ileus intermittently for 23 days. His weight declined. On the 28th hospital day he developed a rash on the face, neck, and dorsum of the distal portions of all 4 extremities. A few days later he began having severe diarrhea and confusion.

Physical examination revealed erythematous, vesicular eruption of the face, neck, and distal extremities (A) with desquamation. The lips were swollen, red, and cracked at the angles (angular stomatitis) (B). Slight distention of the abdomen and hyperactive bowel sounds indicated gastrointestinal involvement (C). Diminished sensation to touch and pain on the distal portions of all 4 extremities indicated peripheral neuropathy (D). He was disoriented in time and space and could not interpret proverbial phrases, giving evidence of central nervous system involvement (E).

Laboratory examination revealed an increase in urinary N^1-methylnicotinamide.

Treatment with a high-protein diet, niacin, thiamine, and pyridoxine led to dramatic improvement.

Differential Diagnosis:
1. Porphyria
2. Lupus erythematosus
3. Lead intoxication
4. Diabetic neuropathy

Clinical Note. This condition is most commonly seen in alcoholics, but must be considered in elderly and debilitated people with dementia as well as people with chronic gastrointestinal disease (sprue) and those whose nutrition is poor postoperatively. It may also be seen in affluent people who deliberately restrict their diet. There is usually deficiency of the other B-vitamins as well as niacin.

Pathology. There are vesicular and inflammatory changes of the skin, mouth, tongue, rectum, and vagina. The gastric mucosa is often atrophied (F), and the large intestinal musculature may be fibrosed (G). There may be necrosis and fatty infiltration of the liver (H). There is degeneration of the posterior and posteromedian columns of the spinal cord (I). The bone marrow may be megaloblastic.

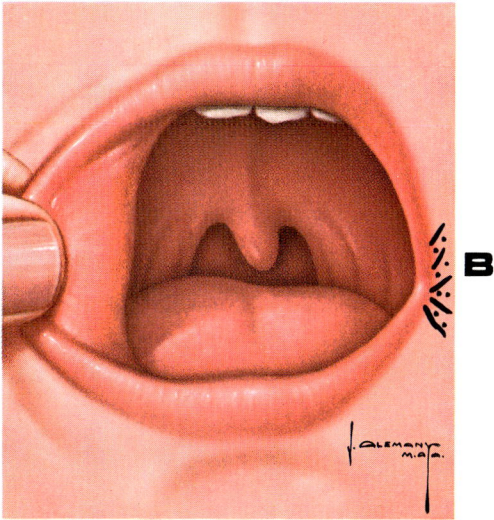

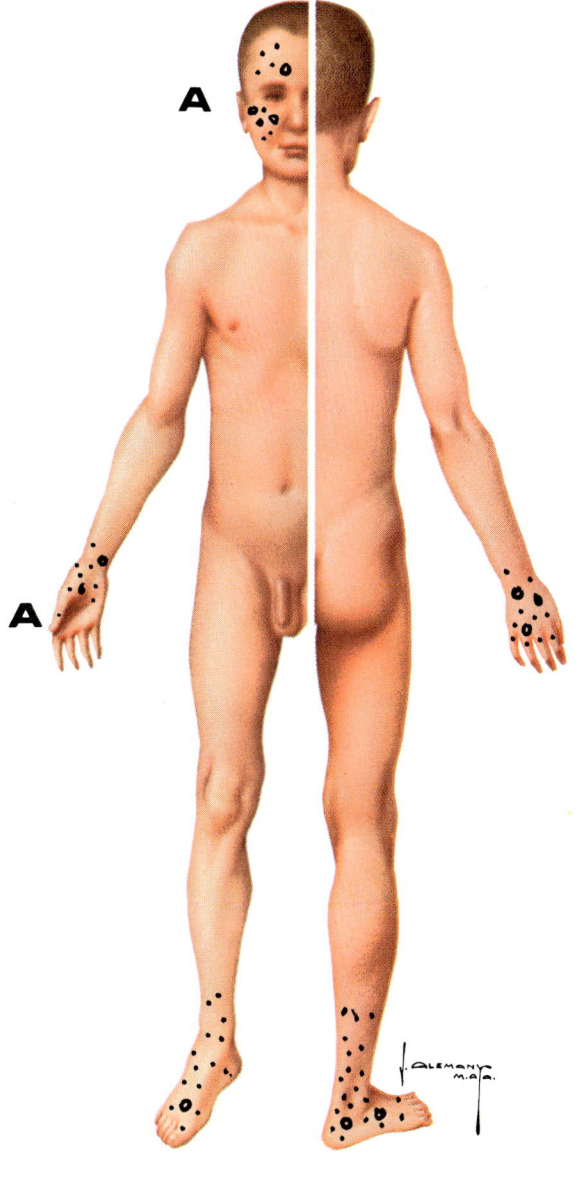

Scurvy

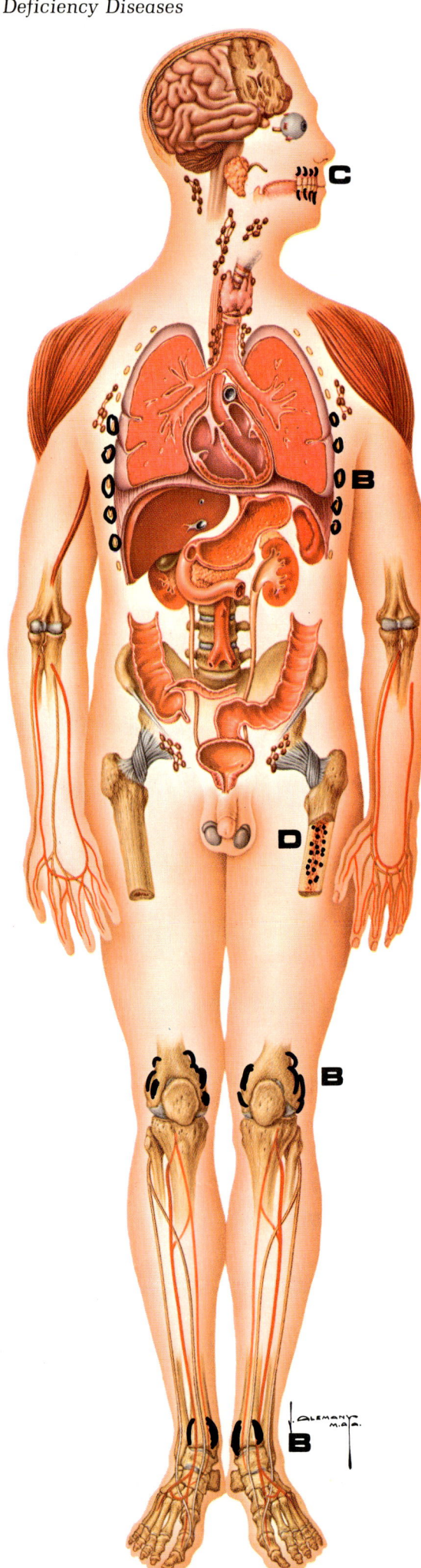

A 17-month-old white infant was brought for examination because of loss of appetite and listlessness.

Physical examination revealed hyperkeratosis and perifollicular hemorrhages of the skin of the thighs, forearms, and abdomen (A). There were tender swellings of the distal femur, tibia, and costochondral junctions (scorbutic rosary) as evidence of subperiosteal hemorrhages (B). The gums were swollen and inflamed, and bled easily (C).

Laboratory examination revealed anemia and leukopenia as evidence of hemorrhages and bone marrow involvement (D). Plasma and leukocyte concentrations of ascorbic acid were low. There was a positive Rumpel-Leede Test.

Treatment with ascorbic acid produced dramatic improvement.

Differential Diagnosis:
1. Thrombocytopenic purpura
2. Henoch-Schönlein's purpura
3. Acute leukemia
4. Aplastic anemia
5. Meningococcemia
6. Hemophilia

Clinical Note. Subperiosteal hemorrhages are less frequent in the adult form of scurvy. The bone marrow involvement is the result of a decrease in the conversion of folic acid to folinic acid, producing an occasional case of macrocytic anemia. This is one of the few deficiency states which may occur without associated deficiency of other vitamins.

Pathology. Deficient or defective ground substance in the collagen tissues, bones, teeth, and blood vessels leads to capillary fragility and hemorrhages throughout the body as well as a suppression of the orderly growth of bone and conversion of cartilage to bone.

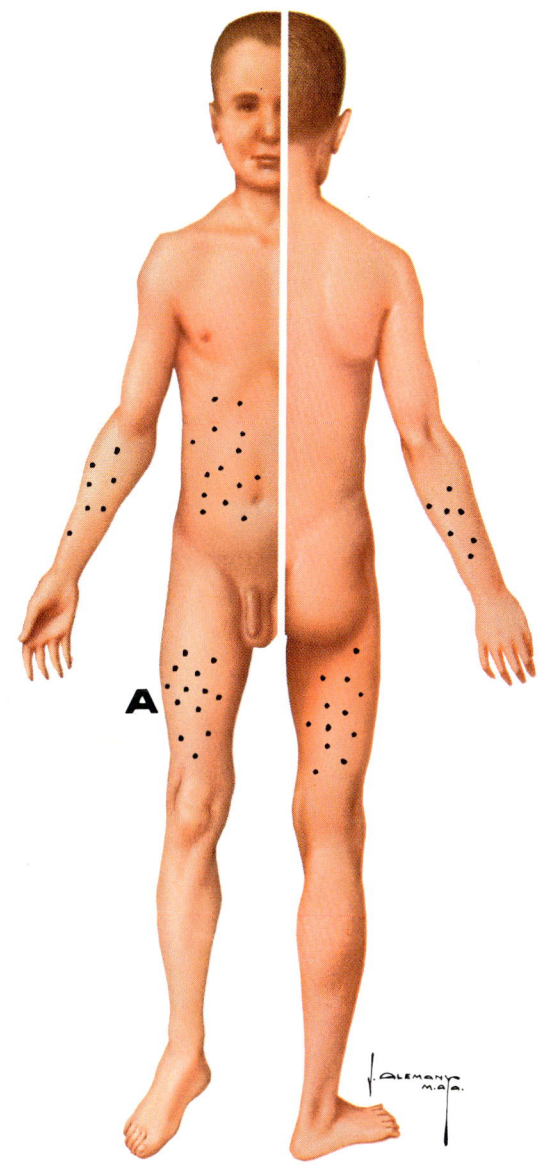

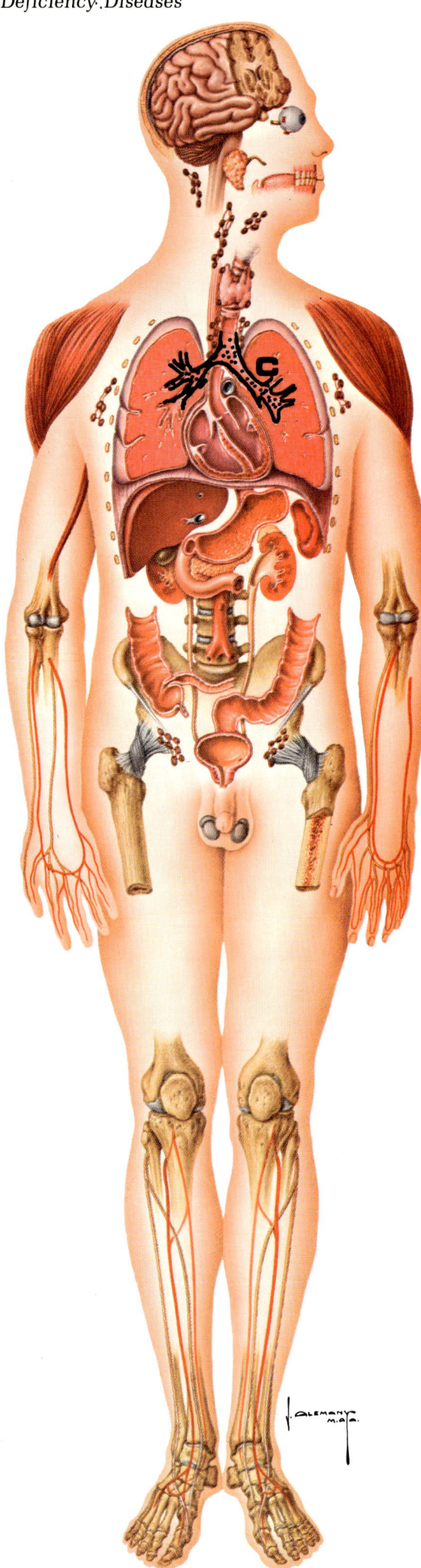

Vitamin A Deficiency

An 11-year-old East African boy complained of pain in his eyes, blurring of vision, and frequent colds. He had a history of nutritional deficiency.

Physical examination revealed drying of the conjunctiva (xerosis conjunctivae) and cornea (xerophthalmia) (A) with Bitot's spots and ulcerations. In addition, there was follicular hyperkeratosis of the skin throughout the body (B). There were sibilant and sonorous rales over the lungs, indicating the involvement of the bronchi (C).

Laboratory examination revealed a low serum vitamin A and carotene, and biopsy confirmed the hyperkeratosis of the follicles and squamous metaplasia of epithelial cells.

Differential Diagnosis:
1. Scurvy
2. Trachoma
3. Uveitis secondary to sarcoidosis and systemic disease
4. Fibrocystic disease of the pancreas
5. Gargoylism
6. Hyperparathyroidism
7. Gonorrhea
8. Syphilis
9. Sjögren's syndrome

Clinical Note. This condition is now rare in this part of the world; but, like the other avitaminoses, it can be found in the aged and debilitated in nursing homes and state hospitals. Cystic fibrosis is associated with vitamin A deficiency because vitamin A is not absorbed.

Pathology. The squamous metaplasia and hyperkeratosis of the epithelial cells in the conjunctiva, cornea, skin, and bronchial mucosa are the basis of the clinical picture in this disease. The Bitot's spots are due to collections of keratin debris and bacteria in the limbus of the cornea.

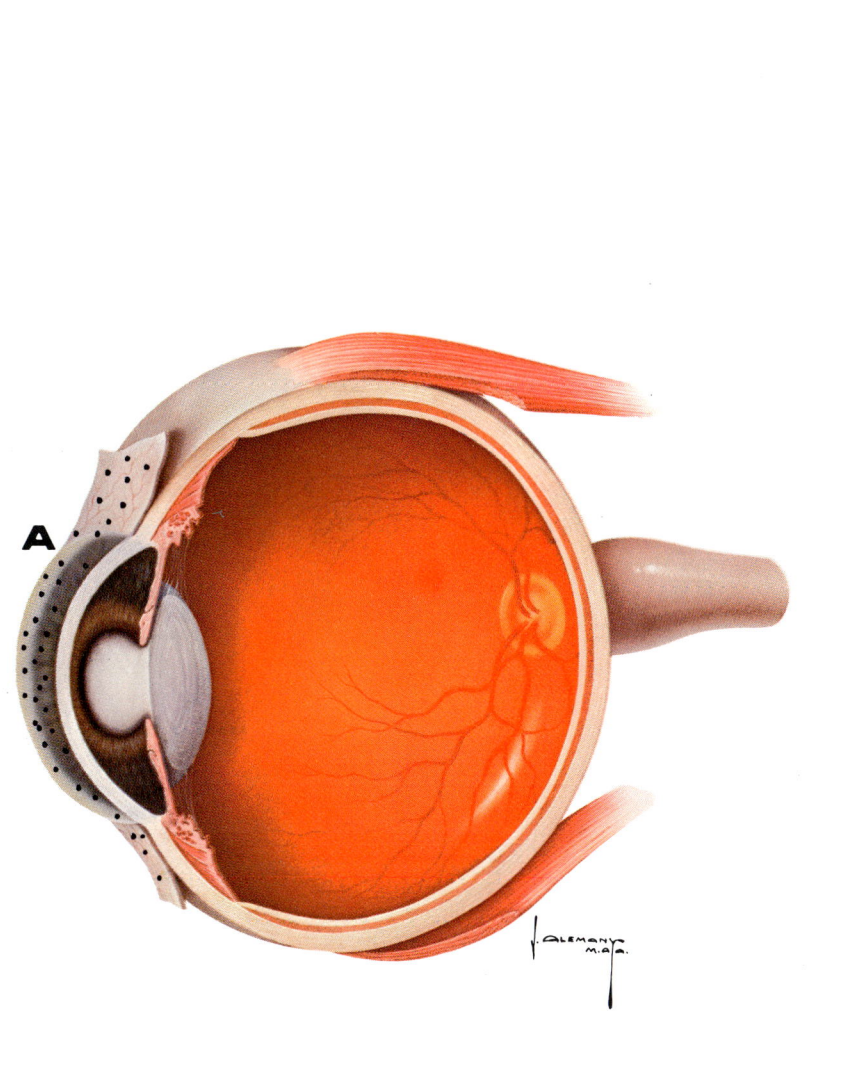
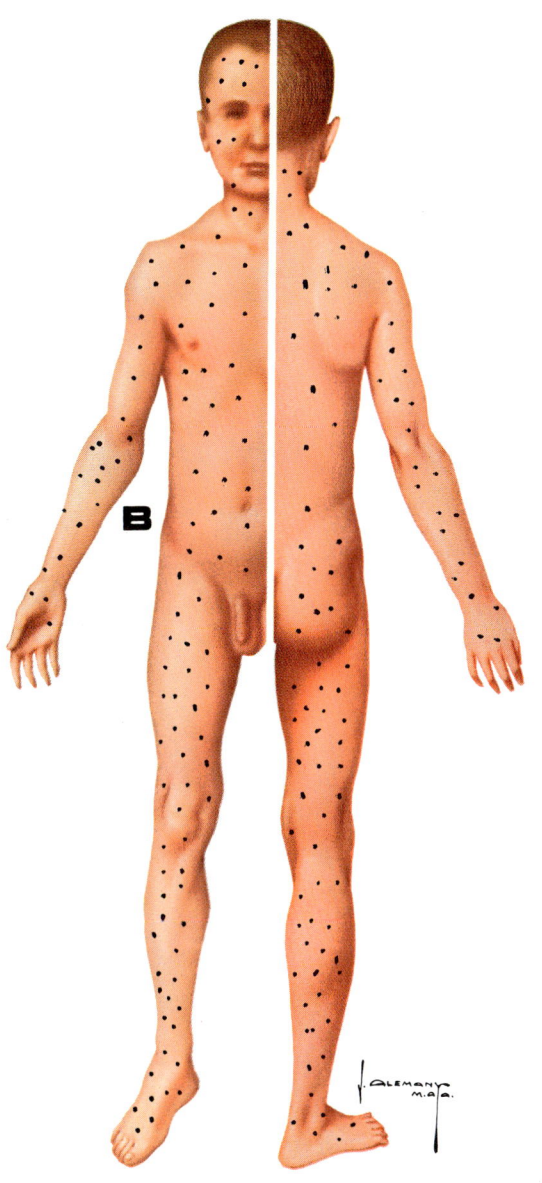

Deficiency Diseases

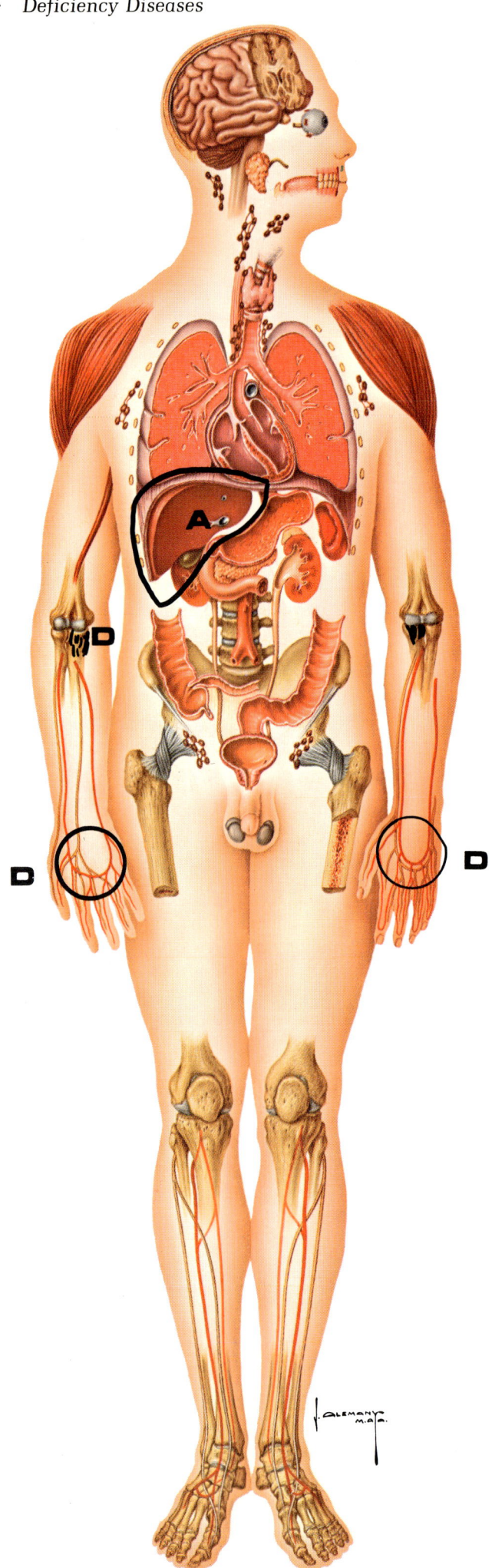

Hypervitaminosis A

A 23-month-old infant was brought in for evaluation because of irritability, pain in the arms and legs, and failure to thrive.

Physical examination revealed an irritable child with hepatomegaly (A), brawny swelling of the extremities and occiput (B), coarse hair and dry skin (C).

Laboratory examination revealed a high serum vitamin A level.

X-ray examination revealed periosteal elevation and new bone formation, particularly in the ulna and metatarsal bones (D).

Differential Diagnosis:
1. Infantile cortical hyperostosis
2. Hypoparathyroidism
3. Hypothyroidism
4. Kwashiorkor
5. Lead intoxication

Clinical Note. The skin, bone, and liver involvement is typical. This syndrome is rare today.

Pathology. Maturation and degeneration of the epiphyseal cartilage is accelerated, and multiple fractures may occur.

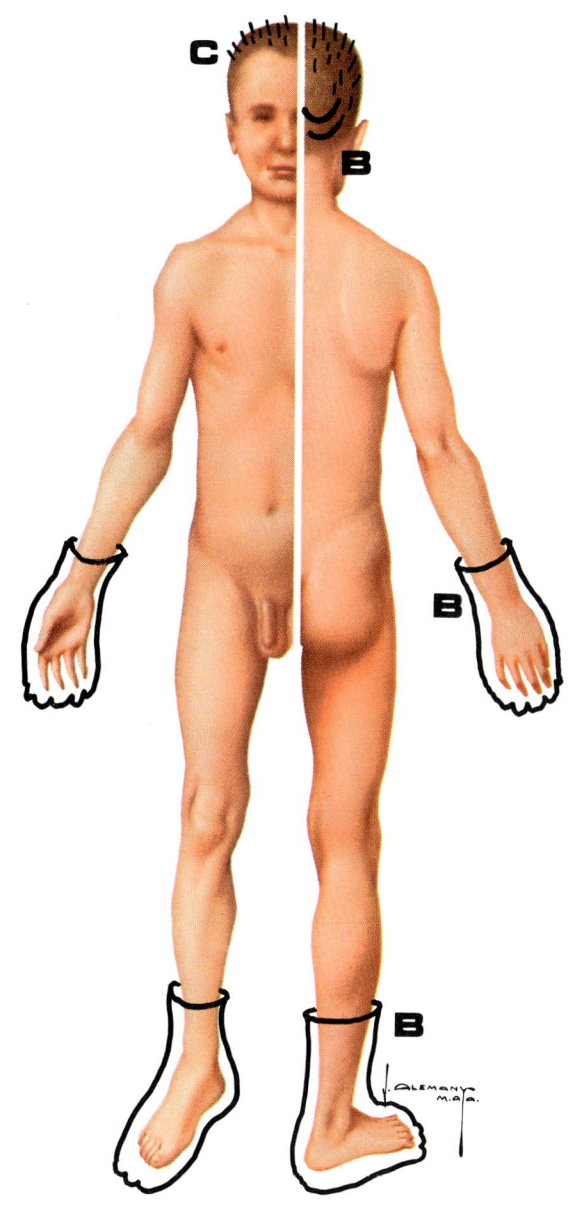

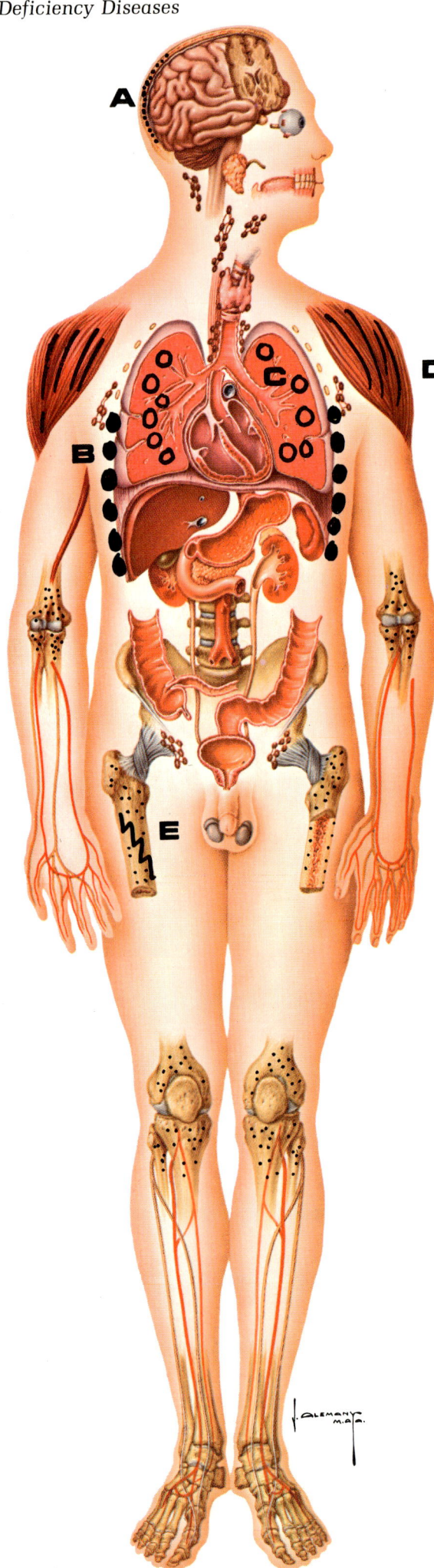

Rickets

An 11-month-old Negro child was brought to the pediatric clinic because it cried frequently and had poor growth and development.

Physical examination revealed abdominal distention, hypotonia of all muscles, softening of the occipital and parietal bones (craniotabes) (A), enlargement of the costochondral junctions (rachetic rosary) (B), hyperresonance of the thorax and prolonged expiration as evidence of pulmonary emphysema (C), and bowing of the legs. Positive Chvostek's and Trousseau's signs were elicited as evidence of neuromuscular involvement (D).

Laboratory examination revealed a serum calcium of 8.2 mg. per cent, phosphorus of 2.9 mg. per cent, and an alkaline phosphatase of 17.5 King-Armstrong units.

X-ray examination revealed irregularity (fraying), blurring and cupping of the distal ends of the radius and ulna, and multiple fractures of the ribs and long bones (E).

Treatment with vitamin D and calcium brought about marked improvement and confirmed the diagnosis.

Differential Diagnosis:
1. Malabsorption syndrome
2. Renal tubular acidosis
3. Fanconi syndrome
4. Renal osteodystrophy
5. Hypoparathyroidism
6. Hypophosphatasia
7. Metaphyseal dysostosis

Clinical Note. This is a disease of infancy and childhood involving the skeleton and neuromuscular system. Simple rickets may be distinguished from rickets of chronic nephritis by the BUN and phosphorus in the latter. The Fanconi syndrome is distinguished by a low blood phosphorus and a high urine calcium and phosphorus. Amino aciduria may occur in simple rickets as well as Fanconi syndrome. Both chronic nephritis and the Fanconi syndrome are relatively vitamin-D-resistant. Rachetic infants may also present with generalized convulsions or tetany. This child did not receive enough eggs, butter, or vitamin-D-enriched milk.

Pathology. Bone fails to calcify and therefore softens. An excess amount of new but uncalcified bone is formed at the junctions between bone and cartilage. Gravity and muscle contraction pull the soft bones out of shape, and fractures result from slight injuries.

Chapter 6

Endocrine Diseases

Since individual hormones are vital to the metabolism of not one but many organs of the body, it is to be expected that a deficiency of one of them would result in a systemic disease. The clinical picture of a deficiency of one hormone may also suggest a relative excess of another. Thus hypopituitarism may manifest as insulin shock. Or Addison's disease may manifest with weight loss, diarrhea, and the skin changes of hyperthyroidism. In most of these conditions not one or two but numerous organs manifest with clinical signs or symptoms simultaneously. Thus Cushing's disease affects the skin (acne, etc.), the bones (osteoporosis), the blood vessels (hypertension), sex organs, etc. Hypothyroidism affects the skin (myxedema), heart (cardiomegaly), nervous system (peripheral neuropathy, depression), etc.

However, since patients contact their doctors earlier in the course of an illness today, the diagnosis will more often be based on laboratory tests and history than on physical signs. The modern laboratory has saved many of these people from an otherwise useless or miserable existence.

Diagnosis of these disorders is absolutely essential because in most cases replacement therapy or surgery is easily accomplished.

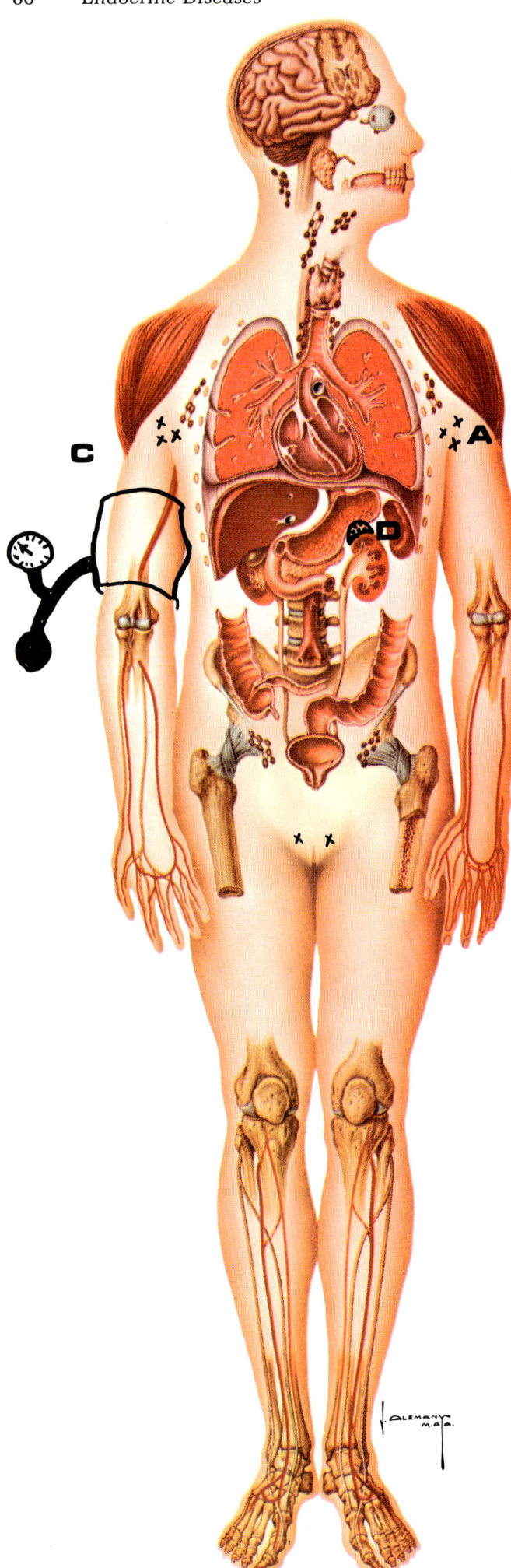

Addison's Disease

A 19-year-old white female was admitted to the hospital because of weakness and weight loss of 1 year's duration. Careful inquiry revealed she used a full salt shaker at each meal, that she was periodically irritable and jittery, and she required frequent naps during the day. Four months prior to admission she was in a state of collapse for 3 days, when all that could be diagnosed was an upper respiratory infection.

Physical examination revealed moderate emaciation, diminished axillary and pubic hair (A), and increased pigmentation of the knuckles, palmar creases, elbows, knees, and buccal mucosa (B). Her blood pressure was 82/60 mm. Hg (C).

Laboratory examination revealed decreased 24-hour urine 17-ketosteroid and 17-hydroxysteroid levels which failed to increase after exogenous ACTH stimulation. The serum sodium was 124 mEq./L., and the serum potassium was 5.4 mEq./L.

Treatment with 15 mg. of cortisol and 0.1 mg. of 9α-fluorohydrocortisone daily led to a remarkable remission.

Differential Diagnosis:
1. Pernicious anemia
2. Hypopituitarism
3. Anorexia nervosa
4. Sprue
5. Hyperparathyroidism
6. Thyrotoxicosis
7. Peutz-Jegher's syndrome
8. Albright's syndrome
9. Hemochromatosis
10. Chronic nephritis

Clinical Note. Tuberculosis used to account for the majority of these cases, but now bilateral adrenocortical atrophy (D) is more commonly responsible. It was strange that this girl did not complain of muscle cramps with such a low sodium. The jitteriness and nervousness could have been due to a low blood sugar periodically. Gastrointestinal complaints of nausea, vomiting, and diarrhea are common but were not observed here. This condition is frequently missed because of failure to look for hyperpigmentation in patients complaining of fatigue. Now that direct measurement of adrenal function is possible, the more dangerous salt withdrawal and potassium loading tests are unnecessary.

Pathology. There is bilateral adrenocortical atrophy grossly, and on microscopic examination there is diffuse loss of cortical cells in all layers with cytoplasmic vacuolization or hyperplasia of those remaining. The stroma is infiltrated with round cells and fibrous tissue.

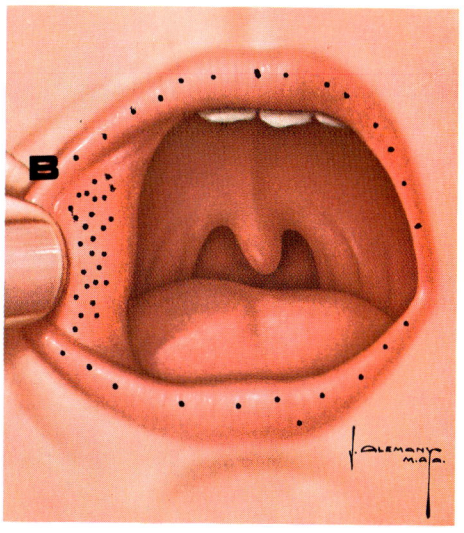

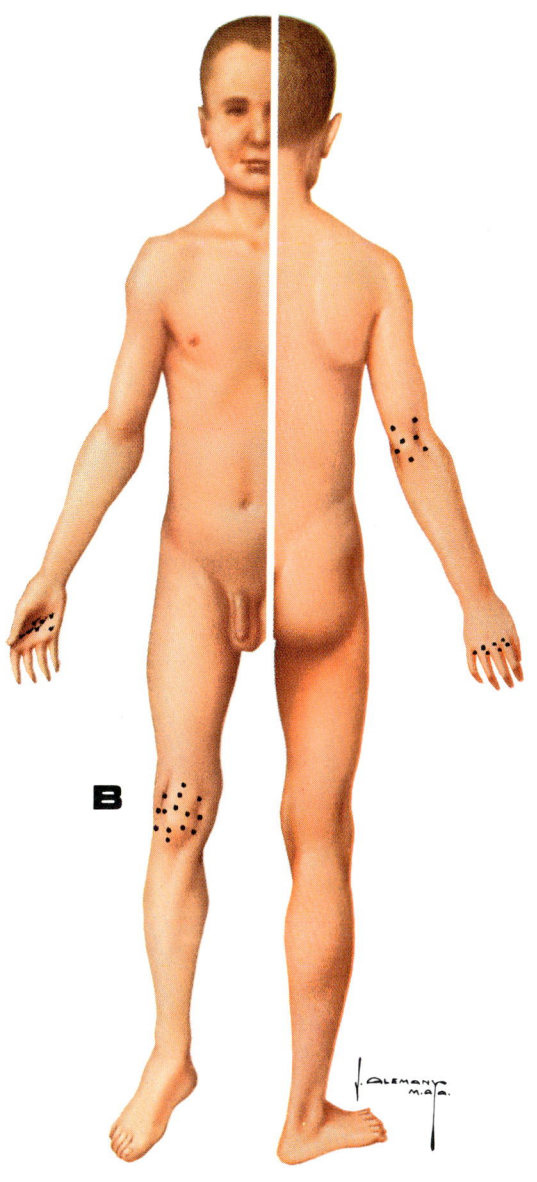

82 · Endocrine Diseases

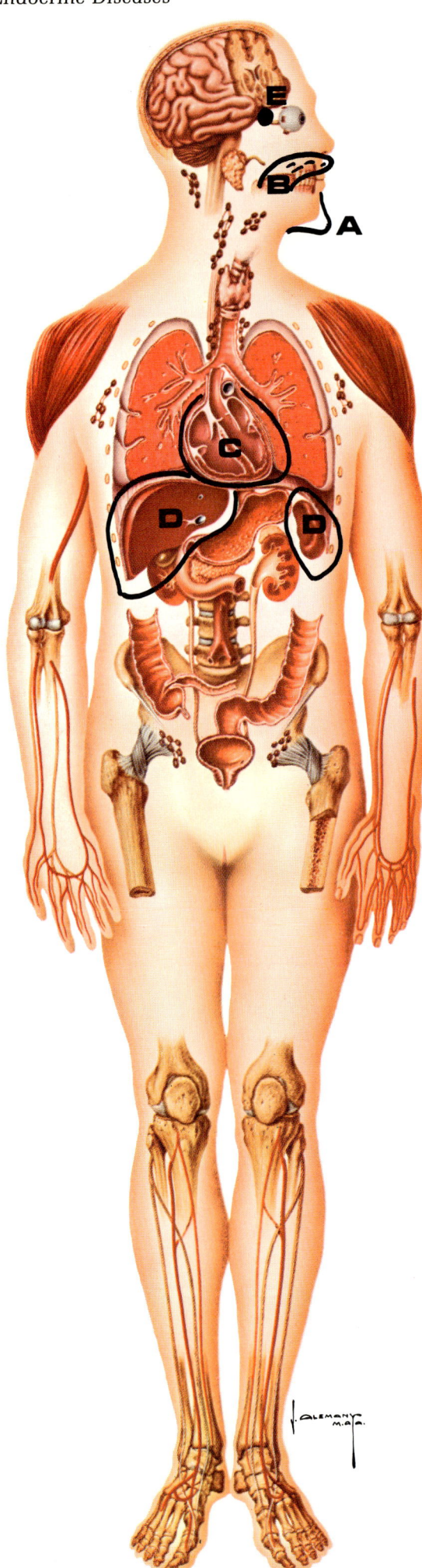

Acromegaly

A 36-year-old white female complained of severe retro-orbital headache and blurred vision.

Physical examination revealed a bitemporal hemianopia, coarse facial features, a protruding jaw (A), enlarged tongue (B), hands and feet, and tough leathery xanthochromic skin. There were cardiomegaly (C) and hepatosplenomegaly (D).

Laboratory examination revealed an FBS of 215 mg. per cent, a serum phosphorus of 5.7 mg. per cent, and an increased serum level of growth hormone.

X-ray examination of the skull revealed erosion and ballooning out of the sella turcica (E), and enlarged sinuses. The jaw bone was elongated. X-rays of the hands revealed tufting of the distal phalanges.

Treatment with radiotherapy was helpful.

Differential Diagnosis:
1. Chromophobe adenoma
2. Craniopharyngioma
3. Diabetes mellitus
4. Gargoylism
5. Gaucher's disease
6. Adrenogenital syndrome

Clinical Note. Headache and joint pain are early complaints in this disorder. Blurred vision and visual-field changes usually develop later. It is important to obtain past photographs to spot the disease early. Almost every organ in the body increases in size, including the thyroid. Acromegaly should be considered in the differential diagnosis of diabetes mellitus though only 25 per cent of acromegalic patients develop glucose intolerance. The direct assay of serum growth hormone may now be done.

Pathology. The eosinophilic cells of the pituitary may be hyperplastic, but there is usually an eosinophilic adenoma. Rarely is the tumor malignant, as are tumors of other endocrine glands.

Adrenogenital Syndrome

A 35-year-old white female complained of amenorrhea and increasing hair on her face for 4 months prior to admission.

Physical examination revealed intense hirsutism with a beard and mustache (A), increase in muscle mass (B), atrophy of breasts, diamond-type distribution of pubic hair and enlarged clitoris (C).

Laboratory examination revealed a blood sugar of 145 mg. per cent and increased 24-hour urine 17-ketosteroids, which did not change significantly after ACTH administration or dexamethasone suppression.

X-ray examination by perirenal air insufflation revealed a tumor mass in the right adrenal gland (D).

At surgery an adenocarcinoma of the adrenal cortex was removed.

Differential Diagnosis:
1. Polycystic ovaries
2. Constitutional hirsutism
3. Arrhenoblastoma of the ovary
4. Precocious puberty

Clinical Note. The picture of masculinization of the female due to excessive androgen production is also seen in the Stein-Leventhal syndrome (polycystic ovaries), but it is not nearly as intense. Like Cushing's syndrome, the adrenogenital syndrome may be produced by hyperplasia or adenoma of the cortex. There is frequently a mild diabetes, as in Cushing's syndrome. Congenital forms of adrenogenital syndrome may be found due to deficiency of 21-hydroxylase and 11-hydroxylase. These are often associated with pseudohermaphroditism. If the enzymatic block is complete in 21-hydroxylase deficiency, there may be no hydrocortisone produced, and acute and chronic adrenal insufficiency develop. In contrast, there may be hypertension in 11-hydroxylase deficiency, in which excess desoxycorticosterone (a mineralocorticoid) is produced.

Pathology. There may be adrenocortical hyperplasia, adenoma, or adenocarcinoma.

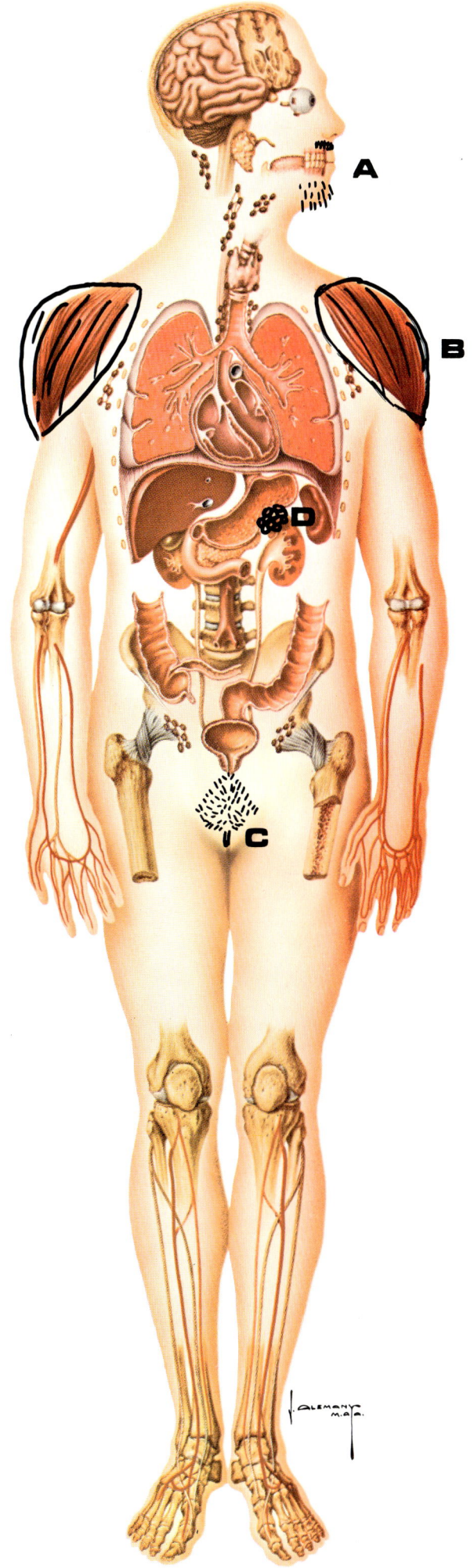

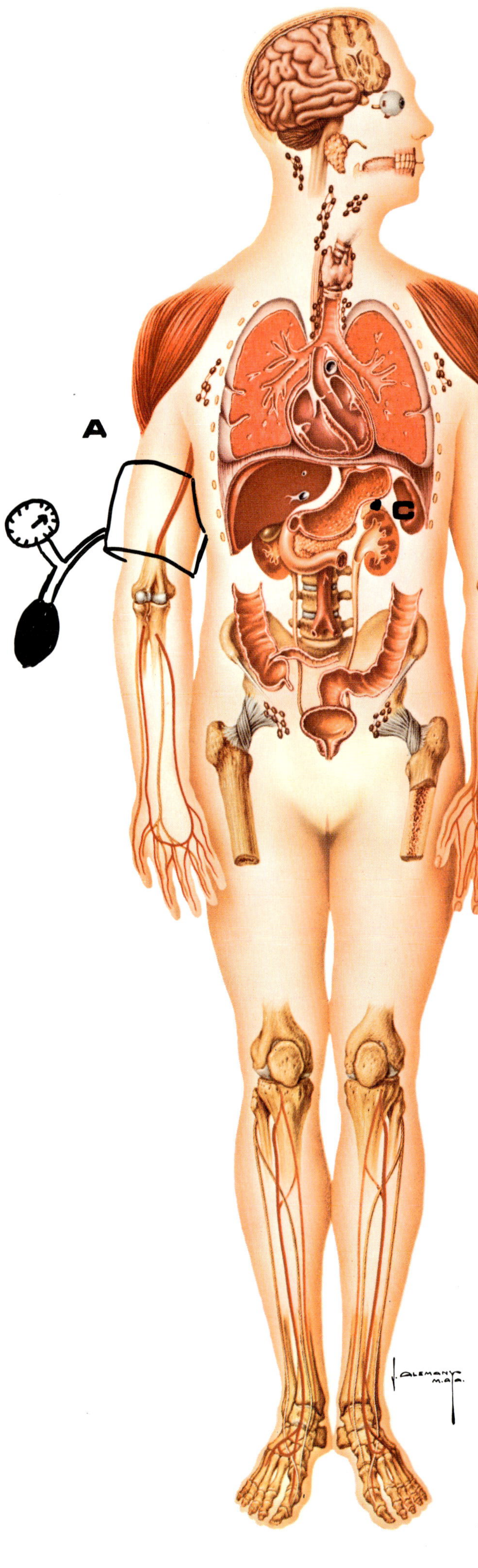

84 · Endocrine Diseases

Aldosteronism

A 35-year-old white female was discovered to have hypertension on a routine physical. Review of systems revealed that she had felt weak and suffered from leg cramps periodically. She also had experienced frequency of urination without burning.

Physical examination revealed a blood pressure of 190/110 mm. Hg (A), diminished deep tendon reflexes throughout, and a positive Trousseau's sign (B).

Laboratory examination revealed a serum potassium repeatedly below 3.0 mEq./L. and a CO^2 of 33 mEq./L. A 24-hour urine aldosterone was 170 mcg./L. Repeated plasma renin determinations were low.

X-ray examination of the adrenal glands with perirenal air was unremarkable.

Bilateral adrenal gland exploration revealed a small adrenocortical adenoma on the left (C).

Differential Diagnosis:
1. Essential hypertension
2. Cushing's syndrome
3. Chronic unilateral or bilateral renal disease
4. Pheochromocytoma
5. Coarctation of the aorta
6. Licorice addiction
7. Hypoparathyroidism

Clinical Note. Although most of these patients have low serum potassiums, as in this case, some have normal serum potassiums. Some authorities believe that as many as 20 per cent of cases of hypertension are caused by aldosterone-secreting adenomas of the adrenal cortex. The plasma renin determination has become an extremely useful method of differentiating this disorder from other causes of increased urinary aldosterone level, such as liver and heart disease and essential hypertension. Since these tumors are small, perirenal air insufflation is not so useful in diagnosis, and exploratory surgery with biopsy is the only way to be sure of the diagnosis.

Pathology. The most common lesion associated with primary aldosteronism is a glomerulosa cell adenoma of the adrenal cortex, but adrenocortical hyperplasia may be the lesion. There may be hydropic degeneration of the renal tubules and skeletal muscle degeneration as well.

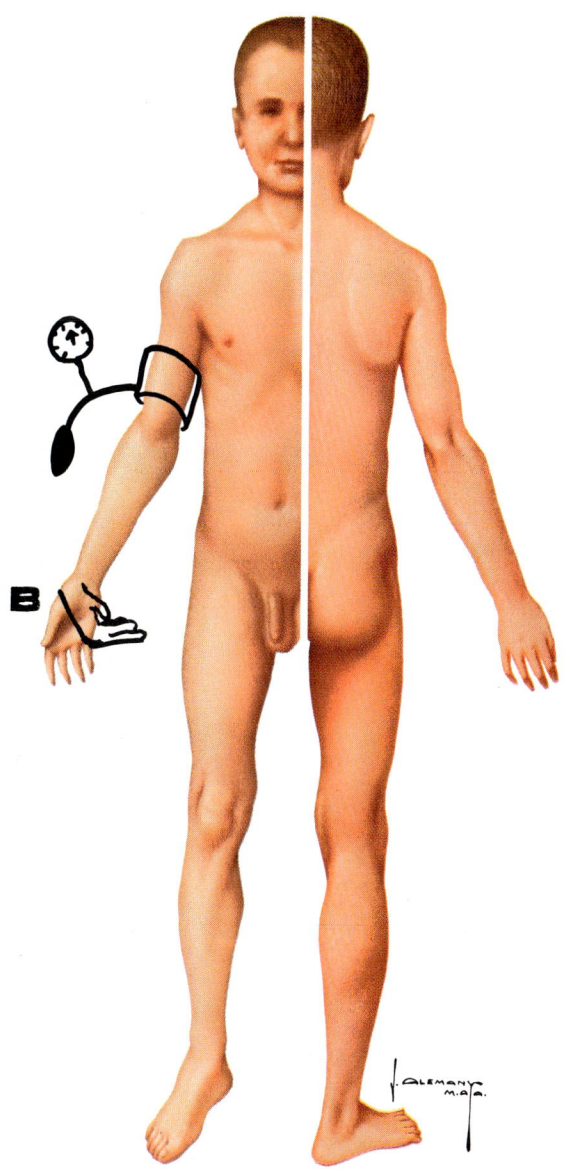

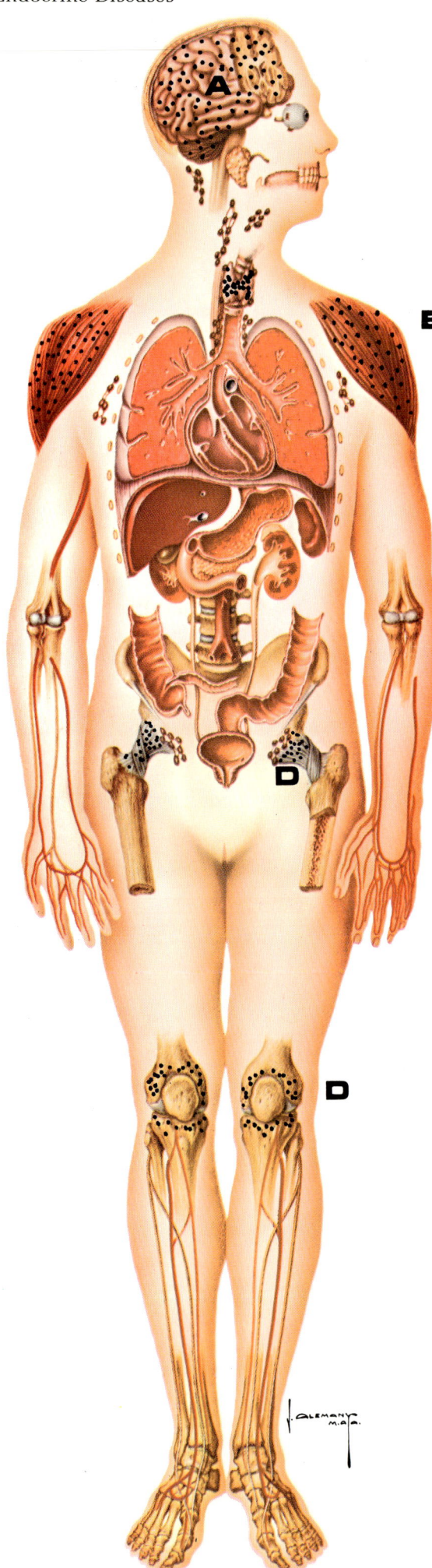

Cretinism

A 9-year-old mentally retarded female was brought to the neurology clinic for evaluation of ataxia. Her growth and development had been abnormally slow, but this was attributed to mongolism.

Physical examination revealed an I.Q. of an idiot, slow mentation, and poor attention span, indicating cerebral involvement (A); but in addition there was a wide-based ataxic gait and symmetrical muscular atrophy (B). The child was short for her age, had a broad nose, puffy eyes which were wide apart, a large tongue, and a husky voice. The skin of the hands and feet was puffy and xanthochromic (C). There was thinning of the hair on her head, and what was left was brittle. The abdomen was protrudent.

Laboratory examination revealed a PBI of 1.5 mcg. per cent and an RAI of 4.1 per cent.

X-ray examination of the bones revealed absence of some ossification centers and punctate epiphyseal dysgenesis (D).

Treatment with ¼ to 1 grain of desiccated thyroid brought about remission.

Differential Diagnosis:
1. Mongolism
2. Hypertelorism
3. Hypopituitarism
4. Osteogenesis imperfecta
5. Amyotonia congenita
6. Hurler's disease
7. Glycogen storage disease

Clinical Note. This case illustrates the unfortunate circumstance in which cretinism was mistaken for mongolism. Every mongol child should be considered a cretin until proven otherwise. The reason is that cretinism can be cured if discovered early enough. The puffy rough and dry skin and large tongue make cretinism easy to distinguish. X-rays will reveal retarded epiphyseal growth in every untreated cretin. Some of these cases are due to congenital absence of the thyroid, some are due to lack of maternal dietary iodine, and some are due to maternal ingestion of goitrogens. This case also illustrates hypothyroid myopathy.

Pathology. There may be a nodular goiter or the thyroid may be entirely absent. Sexual organs fail to develop properly. Other changes are similar to those in myxedema. Changes in the nervous system are nonspecific.

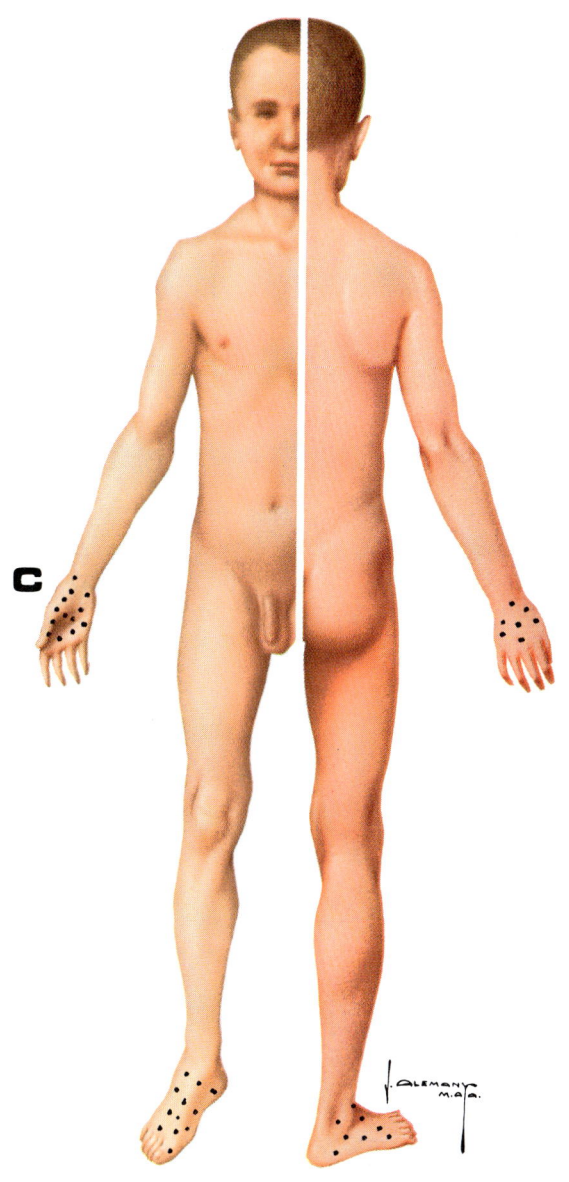

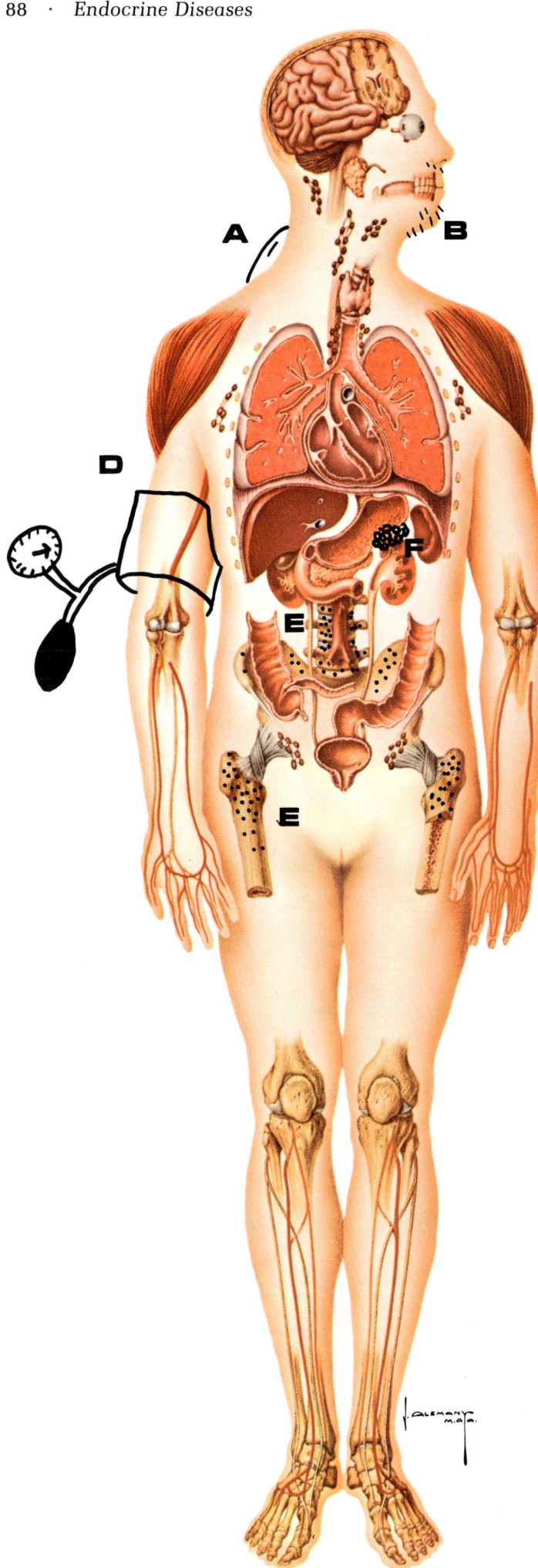

Cushing's Syndrome

This 32-year-old white female complained of gaining 100 pounds in the past 4 years and asked to be put on a diet. There had been irregularity in her periods and increased growth of hair in various areas of her body.

Physical examination revealed proximal obesity with a moon face and a buffalo hump (A), acne and generalized hirsutism (B), purple abdominal striae (C), and a blood pressure of 180/110 mm. Hg (D). Her clitoris was enlarged.

Laboratory examination revealed a blood sugar of 153 mg. per cent, neutrophilic leukocytosis with an eosinopenia, and a potassium of 3.3 mEq./L. The 24-hour urinary ketogenic steroids were elevated, but the 17-ketosteroids were normal. ACTH stimulation caused a significant rise in the urinary corticosteroids, whereas the administration of dexamethasone in doses of 2 mg. every 6 hours caused a reduction in urinary corticosteroids.

X-ray examination of the lumbosacral spine and long bones revealed osteoporosis (E), and presacral air insufflation revealed bilateral enlargement of the adrenal glands.

At surgery bilateral adrenal cortical hyperplasia (F) was found, and a bilateral subtotal adrenalectomy was performed.

Differential Diagnosis:
1. Basophilic adenoma of the pituitary
2. Adrenocortical adenoma or carcinoma
3. Diabetes mellitus
4. Acromegaly
5. Aldosteronism, primary
6. Pheochromocytoma

Clinical Note. The involvement of the skin, subcutaneous tissue, bone, and blood vessels in this case is rather typical. Unusual weight gain is rarely due to an endocrine disorder, but such conditions as Cushing's syndrome, hypothyroidism, and Fröhlich's syndrome must be considered. The laboratory findings here are typical of adrenal cortical hyperplasia. Adenomas are only slightly stimulated by ACTH and minimally depressed by dexamethasone in large doses. Adrenocortical carcinomas do not respond at all to either test. Cushing's syndrome should be considered in the differential diagnosis of hypertension and diabetes mellitus.

Pathology. In adrenalcortical hyperplasia there is hyperplasia of the zona fasciculata bilaterally. The basophilic cells of the pituitary are hyalinized or vacuolated (as described by Crooke).

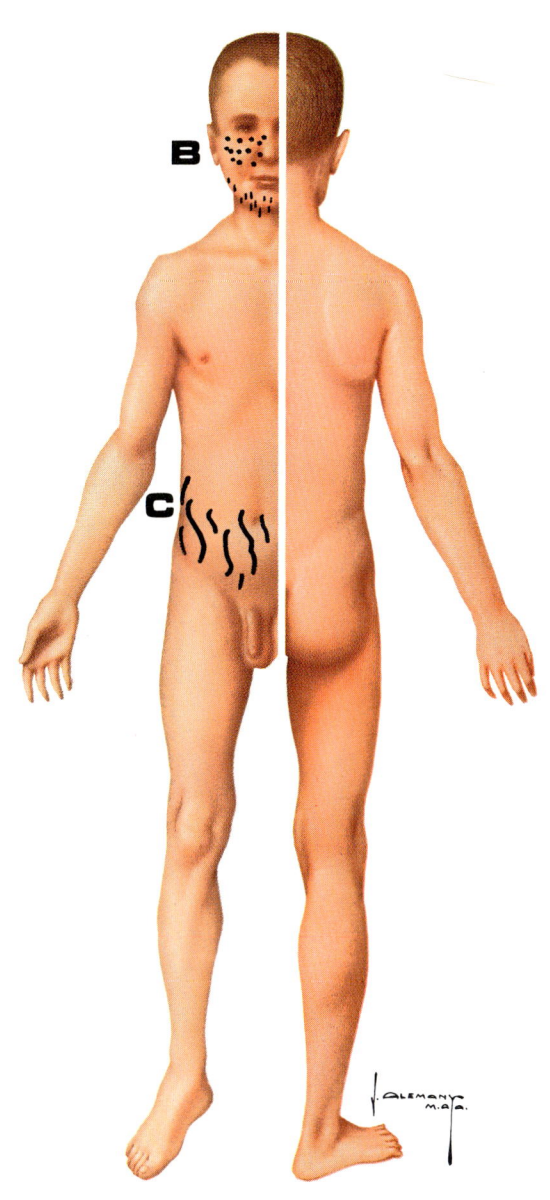

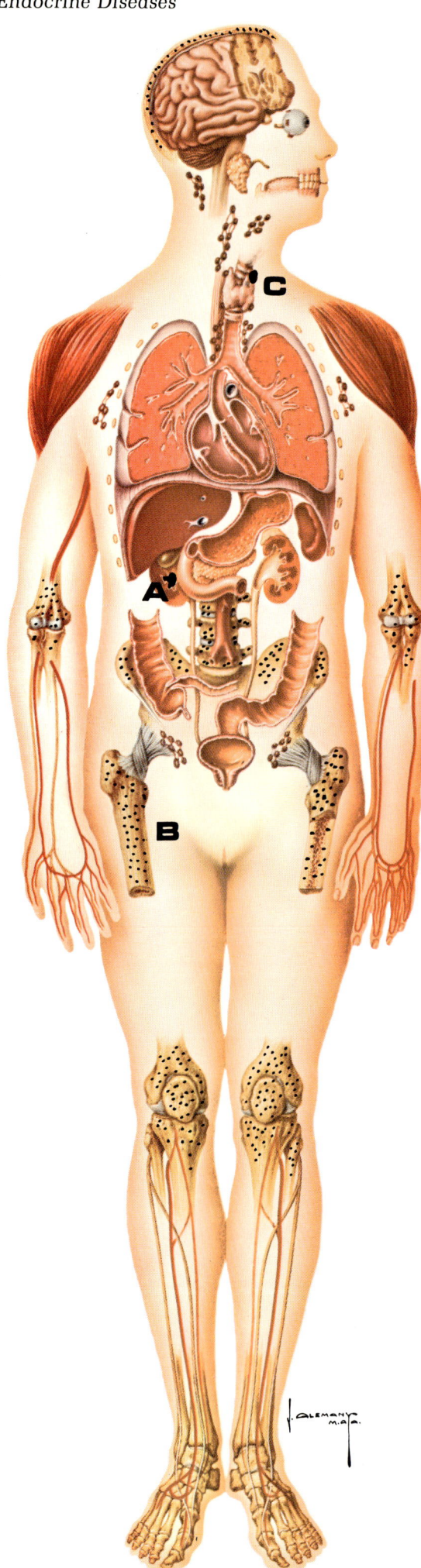

Primary Hyperparathyroidism

A 43-year-old white female complained of severe intermittent right flank pain radiating into the groin and associated with bloody urine. A review of systems revealed that for the past year she had suffered from chronic anorexia, constipation, excessive thirst, polyuria, and muscular aches and pains, which she attributed to the menopause. She had also noted confusion and irritability on many occasions.

Physical examination revealed right flank tenderness, thick dry fingernails, hypotonicity of muscles, and hyperextensibility of joints.

Laboratory examination confirmed the presence of hematuria. In addition, there were an elevated blood calcium, a low blood phosphate, and a high alkaline phosphatase. X-ray studies disclosed a stone in the right renal pelvis (A) and a generalized radiolucency of bone (B) with localized "punched out" areas, in this case most obvious in the skull.

A benign adenoma (C) was found at operation.

Differential Diagnosis:
1. Hyperthyroidism
2. Menopausal syndrome
3. Diabetes mellitus
4. Hypervitaminosis D
5. Multiple myeloma
6. Metastatic carcinoma of the bone
7. Myasthenia gravis

Clinical Note. This case again emphasizes how often endocrinopathies are passed off as functional disorders. All patients with calcified renal stones should have a blood calcium, phosphate, and alkaline phosphatase performed.

Pathology. The adenoma was composed of chief cells. Oxyphil and "wasserhelle" cell adenomas have been reported. The stones are usually composed of calcium oxalate or phosphate. Inspection of the bones reveals demineralization and destruction, with many osteoclasts and osteoblasts. The architecture of the trabeculae is fairly well preserved.

Hyperthyroidism

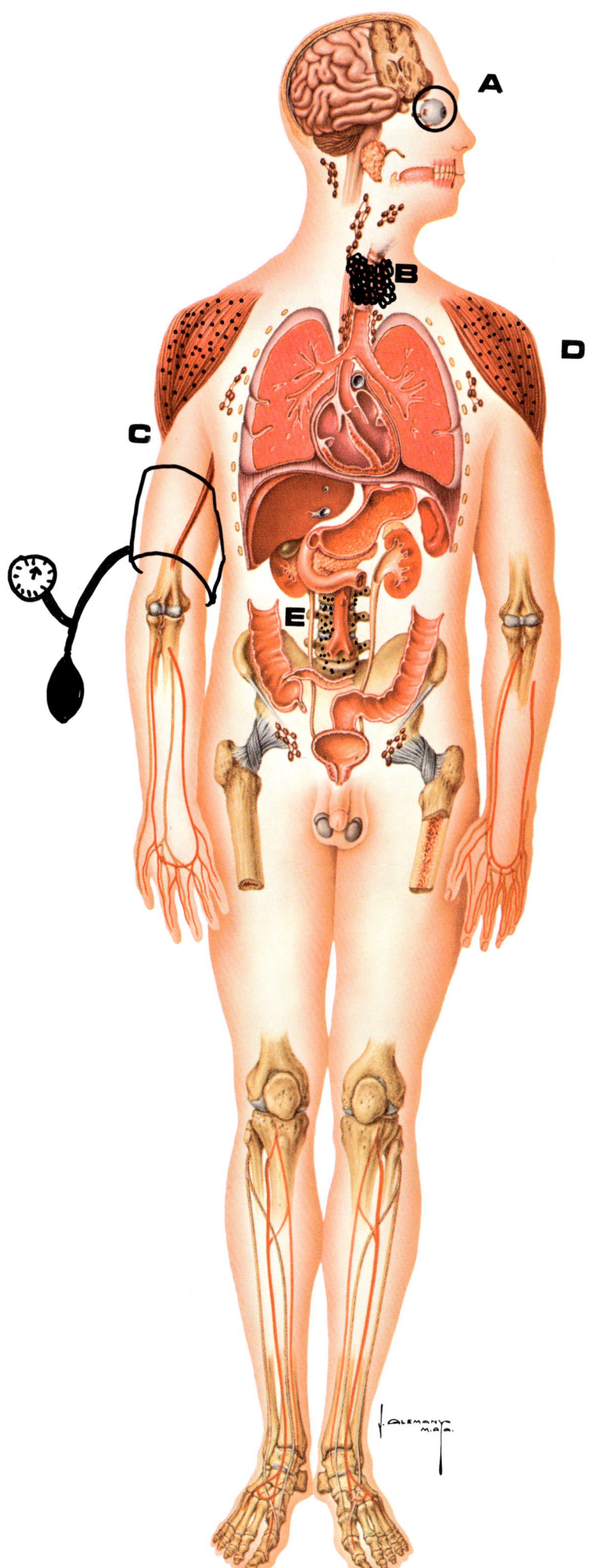

A 28-year-old white male pilot developed weakness, nervousness, and weight loss 3 months prior to admission. This was followed shortly by excessive thirst, ravenous appetite, and frequency of urination (polydypsia, polyphagia, polyuria).

Physical examination revealed exophthalmos (A), a diffusely enlarged thyroid (B), tension tremor, a blood pressure of 170/80 mm. Hg (C), and tachycardia. His skin was smooth (baby skin) and moist. There were symmetrical wasting of the shoulder and pelvic muscles (D) and longitudinal ridging of the nails.

Laboratory examination revealed a PBI of 11.2 mcg., a T_3 uptake of 42 per cent, and a radioactive iodine uptake of 54 per cent in 24 hours.

X-ray examination of the thoracolumbar spine revealed moderate osteoporosis (E).

Treatment with propylthiouracil brought about remission, but a subtotal thyroidectomy was ultimately necessary to bring about permanent remission.

Differential Diagnosis:
1. Pheochromocytoma
2. Wilson's disease
3. Myasthenia gravis
4. Diabetes mellitus
5. Hyperparathyroidism
6. Diabetes insipidus
7. Chronic glomerulonephritis
8. Iron-deficiency anemia
9. Rheumatic fever
10. Congestive heart failure
11. Parkinson's disease
12. Chronic anxiety neurosis

Clinical Note. The combination of polyuria, polyphagia, polydypsia, weakness, and weight loss is also seen in diabetes mellitus, but rarely is so typical. Hyperparathyroidism may produce polyuria, polydypsia, and weakness, but the appetite is depressed. The combination of ocular, neurologic, thyroid, muscle, cardiovascular, skin, and bone involvement makes the diagnosis easy. This condition must be considered in the differential diagnosis of diabetes mellitus and hypertension as well as congestive heart failure.

Pathology. Grossly the thyroid gland is firm and vascular with a finely lobulated appearance. Microscopically, the follicular cells have become tall and columnar, with closely packed basilar nuclei, and papillary epithelial proliferation evidenced by lace-like projection of the epithelium into the follicular lumina. Colloid is decreased. There is an increase in the number of lymphocytes with distinct germinal centers, and there may be fatty infiltration of the liver and cirrhosis in a quarter of the cases. Retro-orbital fat is increased, leading to exophthalmos.

92 · *Endocrine Diseases*

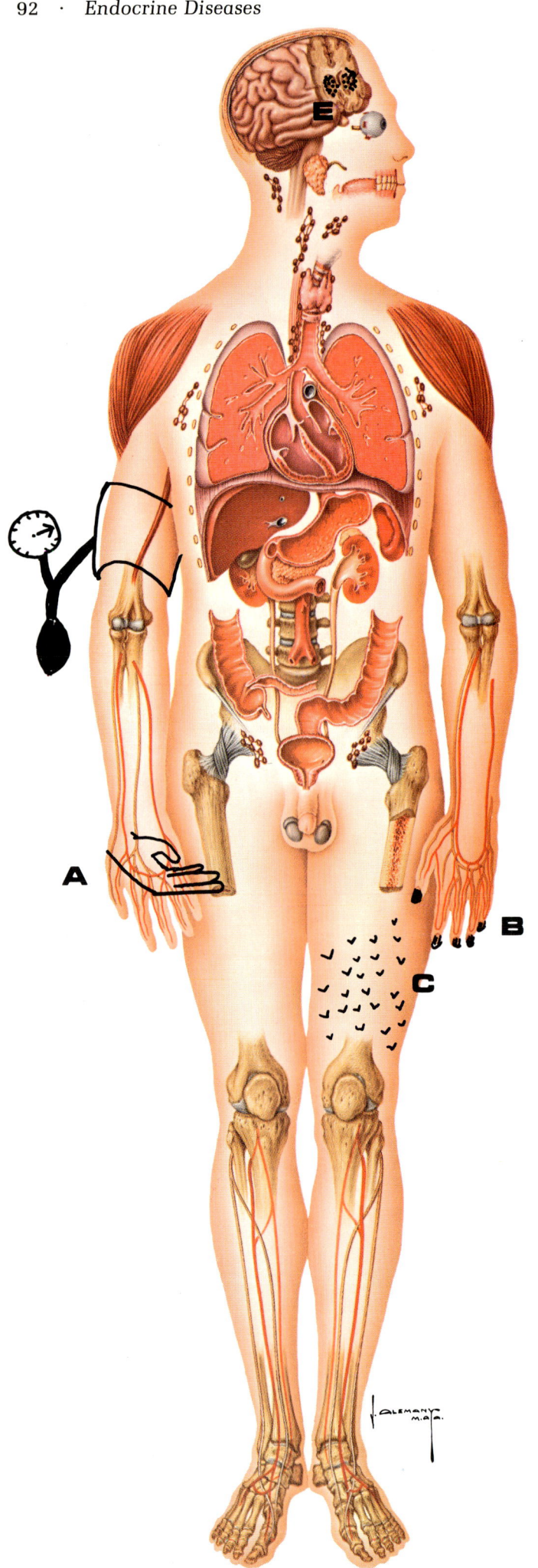

Hypoparathyroidism

This 35-year-old white male was admitted to the hospital because of a recent grand mal convulsion. A careful history revealed that for the past 2 years he had suffered from intermittent numbness, tingling, and fasciculations of the extremities, especially when he happened to lie on them at night. Occasionally, these were accompanied by cramping in the hands, calves, and feet. In the past 4 months he had lost interest in his business and was frequently depressed and irritable.

Physical examination revealed the presence of Chvostek's and Trousseau's signs (A), atrophic brittle fingernails (B), and coarse, scaly skin (C). Slit-lamp examination showed opaque granules in the lens (D). An x-ray of the skull revealed symmetrical punctate calcifications in the region of the basal ganglia (E).

Laboratory examination disclosed a calcium of 7.2 mg. per cent, an inorganic phosphate of 6.8 mg. per cent, and an alkaline phosphatase of 6 King-Armstrong units. The 24-hour urine calcium after a 3-day fast was 30 mg. per cent.

Treatment with calcium lactate and vitamin D in large doses brought relief of symptoms, and the blood calcium returned to normal.

Differential Diagnosis:
1. Pseudohypoparathyroidism
2. Hyperventilation syndrome
3. Hypovitaminosis D
4. Malabsorption syndrome
5. Fanconi syndrome
6. Aldosteronism
7. Chronic renal insufficiency

Clinical Note. This is a rare disorder when not secondary to thyroid surgery (85 cases in the literature). Other than documented seizures, most of the symptoms suggest psychoneurosis, and the physical examination is negative. Examination for a Trousseau's sign and a Sulkowitch test on all psychiatric problems and convulsive disorders may prove rewarding.

Pathology. Microscopically, the parathyroid tissue has been completely replaced by fat.

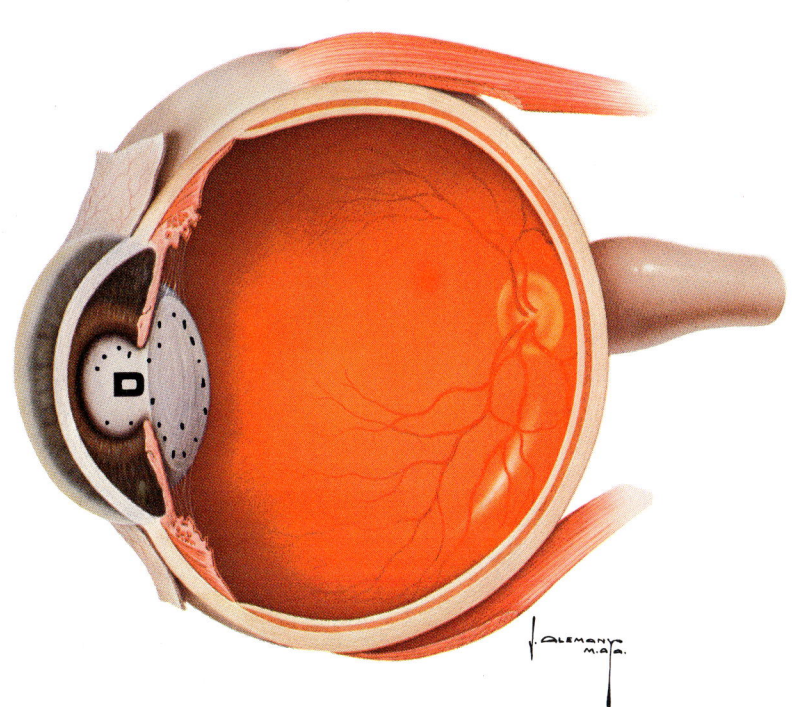

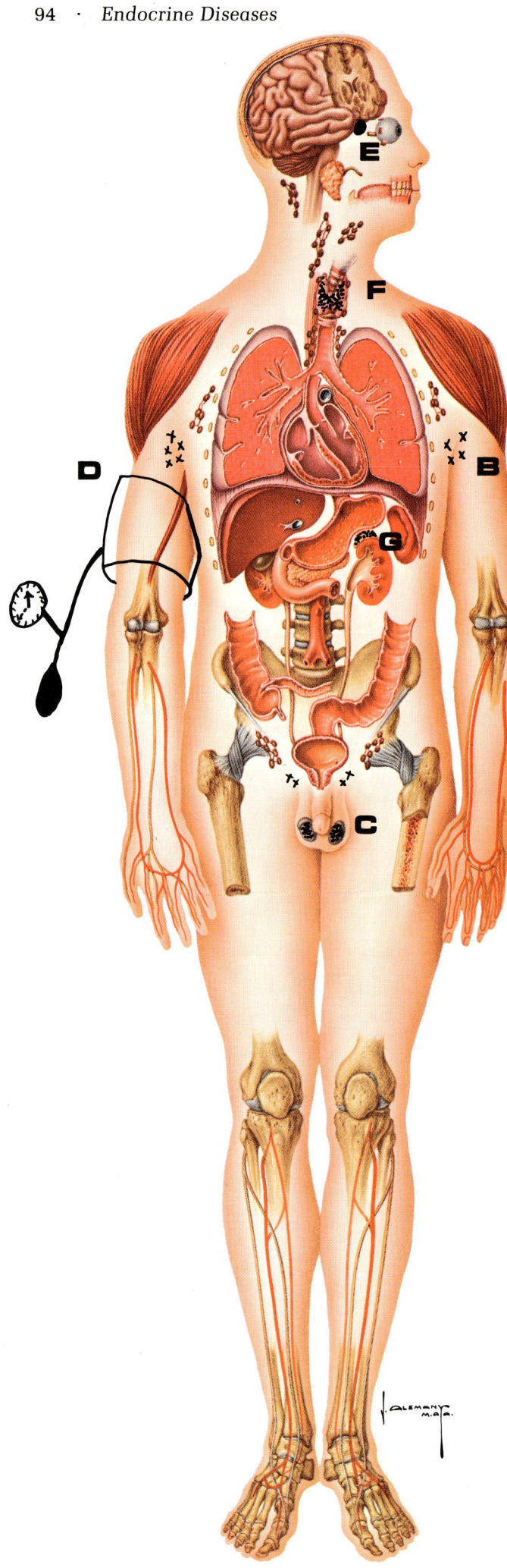

Hypopituitarism

A 62-year-old white male complained of progressive loss of peripheral vision for 3 years prior to admission. He had also noted fatigue, loss of libido (impotence), and lack of appetite.

Physical examination revealed a bitemporal hemianopia, bilateral early optic atrophy (A), thin, smooth hairless skin over most of the body, and loss of axillary and pubic hair (B). There was no hyperpigmentation. The testicles were atrophied (C). Blood pressure was 90/70 mm. Hg and fell to 75/55 mm. Hg on rising abruptly (D).

Laboratory examination revealed a PBI of 3.5 mcg. per cent and decreased 24-hour urinary 17-ketosteroids and 17-hydroxysteroids, which increased after exogenous ACTH but not following the metyrapone test.

X-ray examination revealed a ballooned-out sella turcica (E).

Surgical excision of a chromophobe adenoma was successful.

Differential Diagnosis:
1. Anorexia nervosa
2. Klinefelter's syndrome

3. Fröhlich's syndrome
4. Hypothyroidism
5. Adrenal insufficiency
6. Craniopharyngioma
7. Menopausal syndrome
8. Turner's syndrome
9. Hand-Schüller-Christian disease
10. Lawrence-Moon-Biedl syndrome

Clinical Note. Most forms of pituitary insufficiency present with this slow onset, but occasionally, particularly in Sheehan's syndrome, the onset is acute. There may be a drop in the blood sugar, precipitating convulsions, or there may be an adrenal crisis. The lack of hyperpigmentation distinguishes this from Addison's disease, and the thin skin distinguishes it from myxedema. Differentiation from other conditions is more difficult. Sheehan's syndrome is responsible for most cases of hypopituitarism seen today, and in this disorder the onset is usually gradual. Hypogonadism occurs first, as in this case, followed by thyroid or adrenal insufficiency. Diabetes insipidus may occur early or late.

Pathology. The tumor is composed of chromophobe cells with small dense nuclei and abundant pale grayish cytoplasm compressing the optic chiasm and hypothalamus (E). There is atrophy of the thyroid (F) and adrenal glands (G).

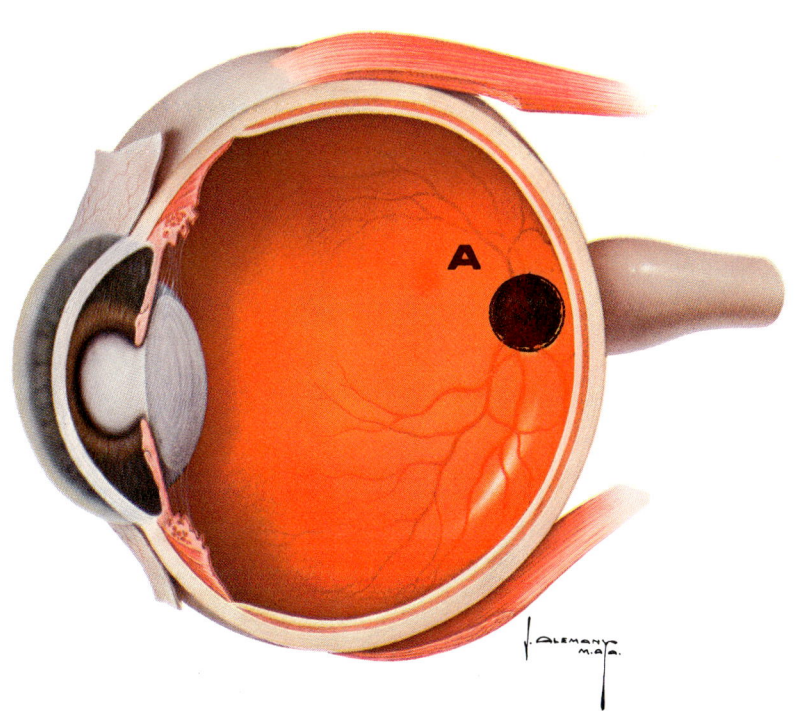

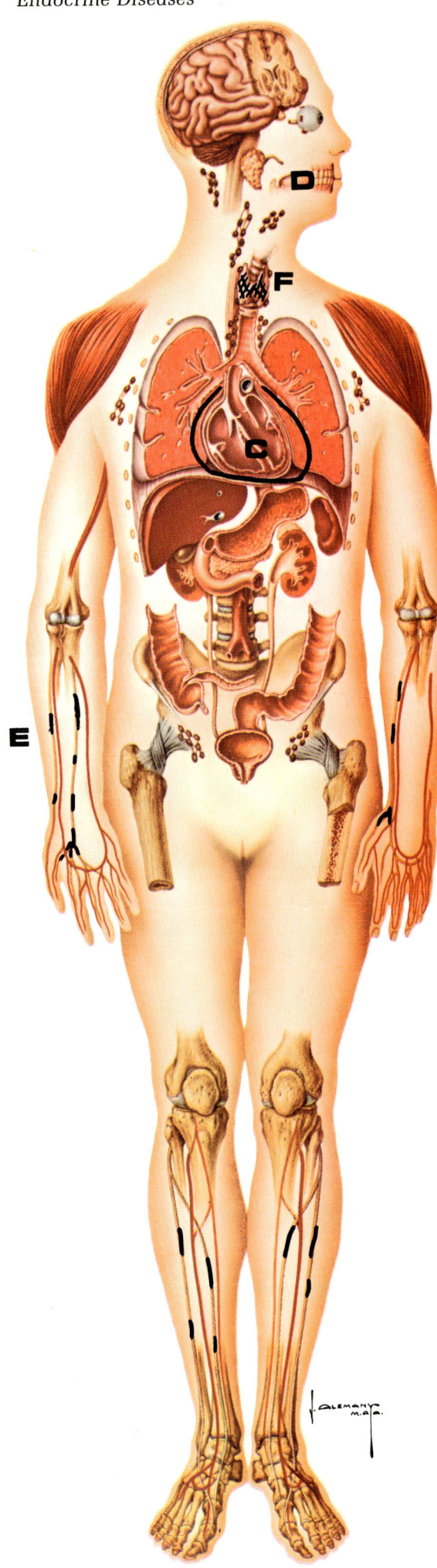

Hypothyroidism

A 46-year-old white female consulted her family physician because of increasing fatigue and weight gain. Her friends noted that her facial features had become coarse. For at least 6 months her voice had been husky. She insisted on keeping the temperature of her home at 80° F. She had become irritable and forgetful. Her periods were irregular, and she had a great deal of bleeding with each one. Her hair broke easily.

Physical examination revealed pale, xanthochromic, thick puffy skin which did not pit on pressure (A). Her hair was coarse and broken in places (B). There was loss of hair in the outer third of the eyebrows. The heart was enlarged to percussion (C), she had a large tongue (D), and there was loss of vibratory, touch and pain sensation in the distal portion of all 4 extremities, indicating a peripheral neuropathy (E). There was prolonged relaxation time in the Achilles and knee jerks bilaterally.

Laboratory examination revealed a cholesterol of 420 mg. per cent, a PBI of 1.7 mcg./100 ml., and a 24-hour RAI uptake of just 4.5 per cent. She had a macrocytic anemia. An electrocardiogram revealed low voltage QRS's and flat T-waves in the anterior wall leads.

Treatment with desiccated thyroid brought about a complete remission.

Differential Diagnosis:
1. Hypopituitarism
2. Nephrotic syndrome

3. Pernicious anemia
4. Chronic congestive heart failure
5. Menopause syndrome
6. Addison's disease
7. Scleredema
8. Beriberi

Clinical Note. The clinical picture here is the result of the slowing down of all body systems. Not one system of the body is unaffected in some way. Here is another condition that must be considered in the diagnosis of fatigue and in the differential diagnosis of every organ involvement. If the patient presents with headache, or with ringing in the ear, or with shortness of breath, the condition may be myxedema. These are only a few examples. The laboratory diagnosis has been difficult in the past because no test was 100 percent accurate. The PBI is subject to modification by organic and inorganic iodides and numerous laboratory errors. Now with the development of the free thyroxine test we are approaching 100 per cent accuracy in testing.

Pathology. The thyroid tissue is most frequently replaced by a fibrous stroma (F). In Hashimoto's disease lymphocytes are abundant. Occasionally replacement of the thyroid tissue by an invasive carcinoma is responsible for the pathology. A mucoid substance accumulates in the subcutaneous tissues, causing the myxedematous appearance. This material may be found also in the skeletal and heart muscle and blood vessels.

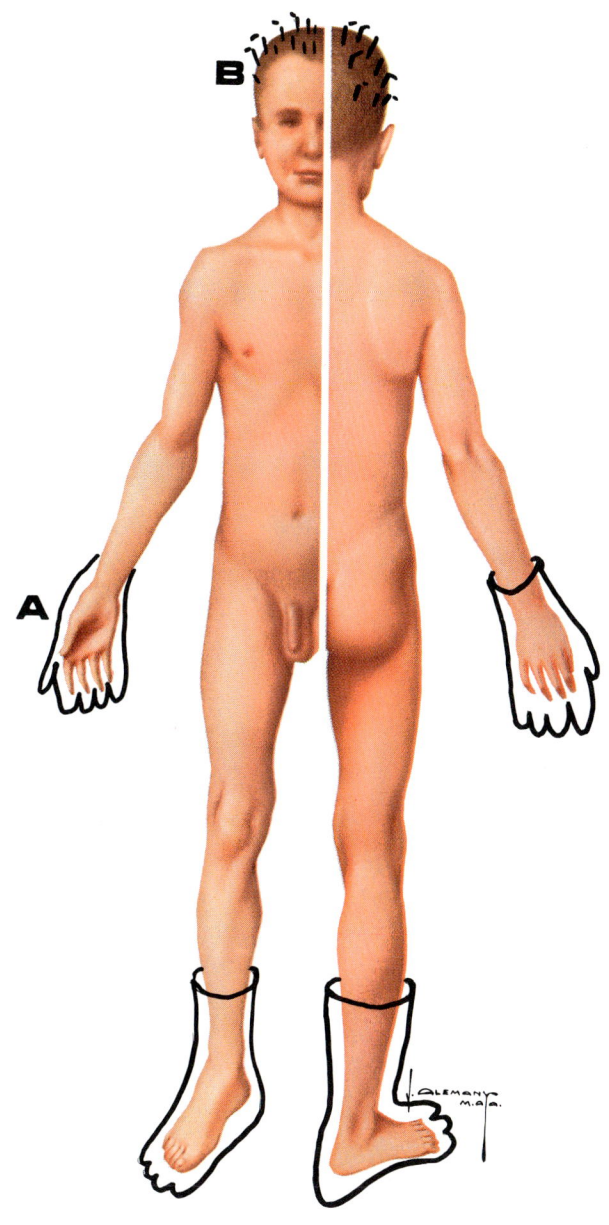

Klinefelter's Syndrome

(Seminiferous Tubule Dysgenesis)

A 17-year-old white male was brought to the endocrine clinic for evaluation of enlarging breasts.

Physical examination revealed a tall white male with gynecomastia (A), atrophic testicles (B), small genitalia, and little axillary and pubic hair (C). The extremities were long (D).

Laboratory examination revealed increased 24-hour urinary gonadotropins and normal 24-hour urinary 17-ketosteroids. A buccal smear revealed sex chromatin bodies (Barr bodies).

Differential Diagnosis:
1. Primary hypogonadism
2. Hypopituitarism
3. Addison's disease
4. Arachnodactyly
5. Gigantism

Clinical Note. As in Turner's syndrome, there are skeletal anomalies; but instead of being short in stature, these patients are tall. In contrast to Turner's syndrome, cardiovascular and renal anomalies are rare. Mental retardation is more common. Although the urinary gonadotropins are high in both Turner's syndrome and Klinefelter's syndrome, the output of sex hormones (17-ketosteroids) is usually normal in Klinefelter's syndrome, whereas both estrogen and progesterone production are low in Turner's syndrome. This is not usually a hereditary disorder.

Pathology. The atrophic testicles show hyalinization and sclerosis of the seminiferous tubules, but the Leydig cells and some Sertoli cells are usually presented. The Leydig cells are present in clumps. While the XXY chromosomal constitution is the most common finding, phenotypes of XXYY, XXXY, and XXXXY have been found, as well as various patterns of mosaicism.

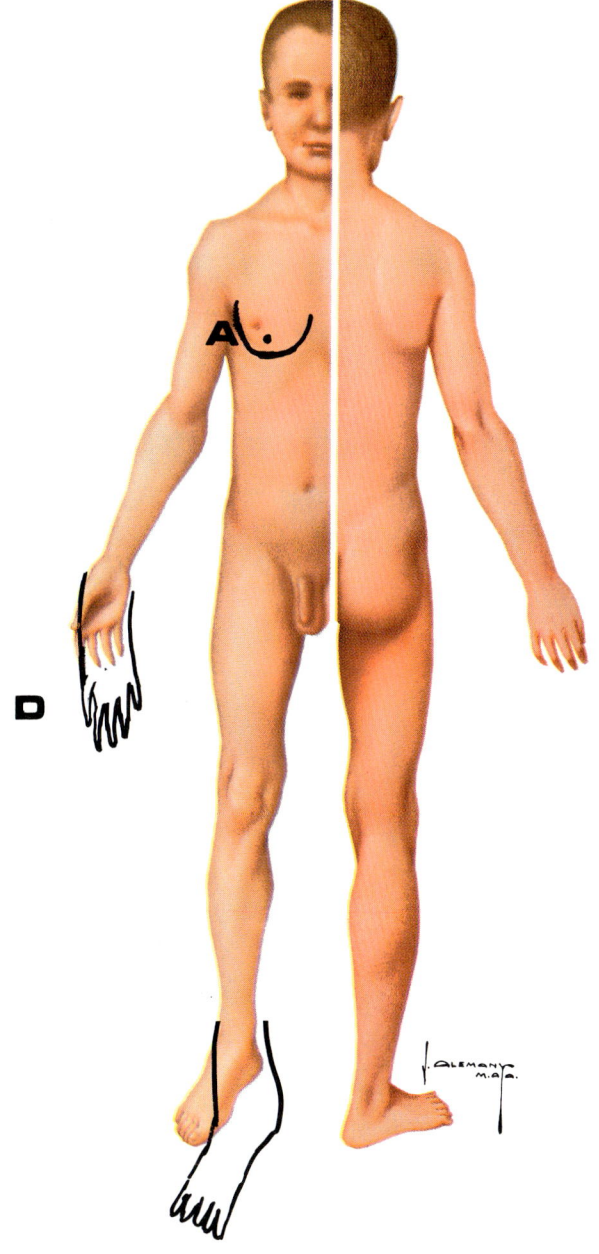

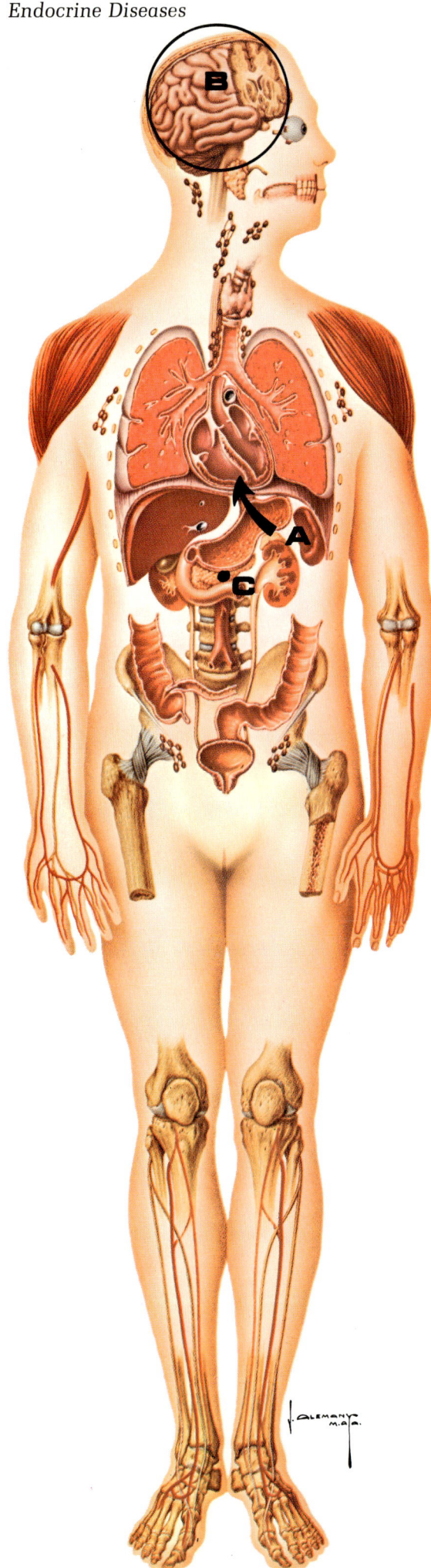

Islet Cell Adenoma

A 38-year-old white female was brought to the emergency room in a comatose state shortly after a grand mal convulsion. Discussion with her husband revealed that she had been having episodes of dizziness associated with hunger for the past 2 years. She was also frequently nervous and irritable. Her father was diabetic.

Physical examination revealed a comatose female with tachycardia (A), sweaty hands, hypoactive reflexes on all 4 extremities, and positive Babinski signs, indicating cerebral involvement (B).

Laboratory examination revealed a blood sugar of 38 mg. per cent. She recovered from the coma after administration of glucose. Later a tolbutamide tolerance test was positive.

Surgical exploration of the pancreas revealed an islet cell adenoma (C), which was removed.

Differential Diagnosis:
1. Hypoparathyroidism
2. Diabetes mellitus
3. Idiopathic epilepsy
4. Meningitis
5. Toxic encephalopathy
6. Pheochromocytoma
7. Hypopituitarism
8. Addison's disease
9. Space-occupying lesion of cerebral hemispheres
10. Functional hypoglycemia

Clinical Note. This condition must be considered in all cases with onset of epilepsy in adulthood. It is rare before the age of 18. Convulsions occur in only one third of the cases. Many of these patients are labeled psychoneurotic because of the lack of physical and laboratory findings in the conscious states. But think of the many ulcers and myocardial infarctions that present no physical findings! We can no longer pass off the patient with a normal physical examination as psychoneurotic. A 36-hour fast and the tolbutamide tolerance test differentiate insulinomas from functional hypoglycemia.

Pathology. Approximately 90 per cent of these cases are due to a benign adenoma of the beta cells. The other 10 per cent of cases are malignant or exhibit islet cell hyperplasia.

Laurence-Moon-Biedl Syndrome

A 7-year-old white male was brought to the neurology clinic for evaluation of severe mental and growth retardation since birth.

Physical examination revealed marked obesity, bilateral cataracts (A), bilateral retinitis pigmentosa (B), mongoloid facies, syndactyly of the 2nd and 3rd digits of both hands (C), and testicular atrophy (D).

Laboratory examination revealed a slight lowering of the BMR, but other tests of endocrine function were normal.

Differential Diagnosis:
1. Fröhlich's syndrome
2. Hypopituitarism
3. Klinefelter's syndrome
4. Cretinism
5. Mongolism

Clinical Note. This is a rare disease but may cause confusion in cases of mental retardation, dwarfism, or suspected hypopituitarism. This is inherited as a recessive gene.

Pathology. The microscopic pathology is insignificant.

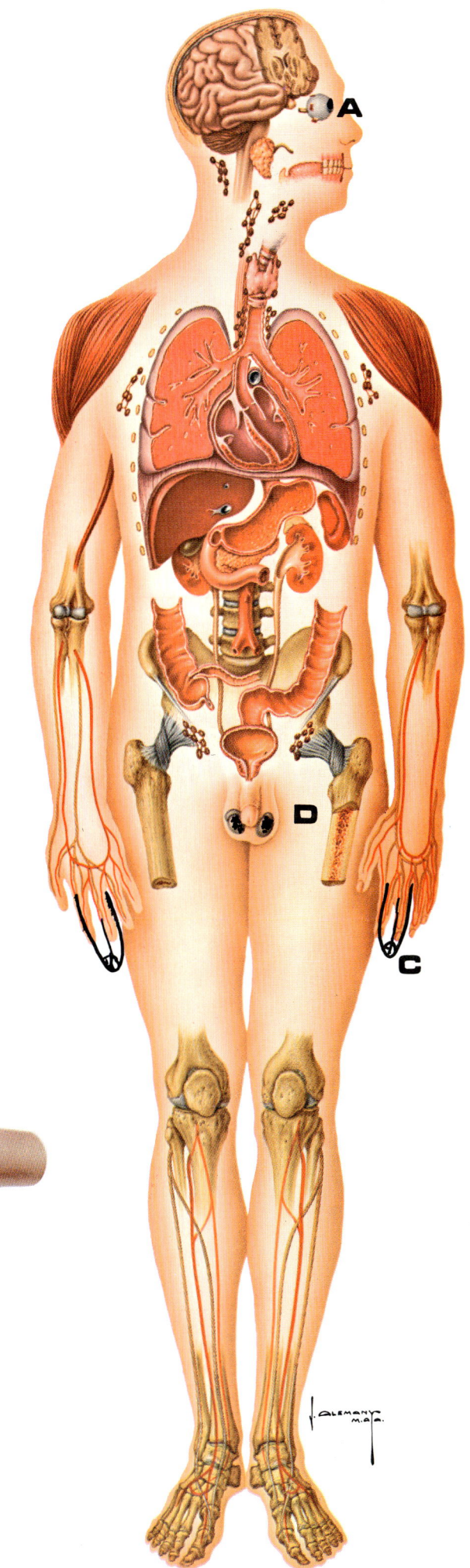

102 · *Endocrine Diseases*

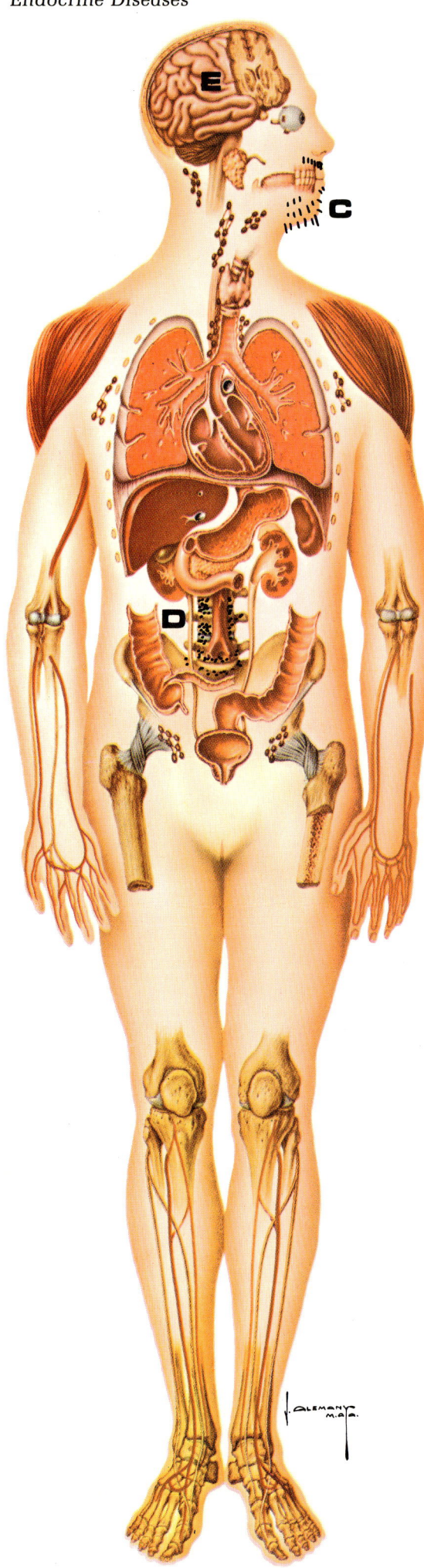

Menopause

A 47-year-old white female complained of increasing fatigue, insomnia, and depression. For the past 6 months she had had episodes during which her face and neck became hot and red (A). She had missed her last 2 periods, and prior to that her periods had been scanty.

Physical examination revealed thinning of the skin (B), hirsutism (C), and atrophic vaginal mucosa.

Laboratory examination revealed increased 24-hour urinary gonadotropins and, on vaginal smear, round or ovoid basophilic cells with hyperchromatic nuclei.

X-ray examination revealed marked osteoporosis (D) of the thoracolumbar spine.

Treatment with estrogen led to a remarkable remission.

Differential Diagnosis:
1. Pregnancy
2. Hypopituitarism
3. Stein-Leventhal syndrome

4. Turner's syndrome
5. Hyperthyroidism
6. Addison's disease
7. Hyperparathyroidism
8. Hypothyroidism

Clinical Note. Should this be considered a systemic disease? The vascular, dermatologic, and skeletal involvement should answer that question. When there is fatigue in middle-aged females, this condition must *always* be and usually is thought of; but lest we develop tunnel vision, the other disorders in the differential diagnosis must also be considered. The insomnia and depression indicate nervous system involvement (E), which may be associated with loss of memory. Some authorities still believe that most of these symptoms are due to psychologic factors. Yet 80 per cent of patients presenting in this fashion are relieved by estrogen replacement therapy. The secretion of estrogen by the ovaries drops to zero in this age group. There may be arthralgias and arthritis.

Pathology. Atrophy of the ovaries, which are replaced by fibrous stroma, is attended by absence of graafian follicles and of corpus luteum.

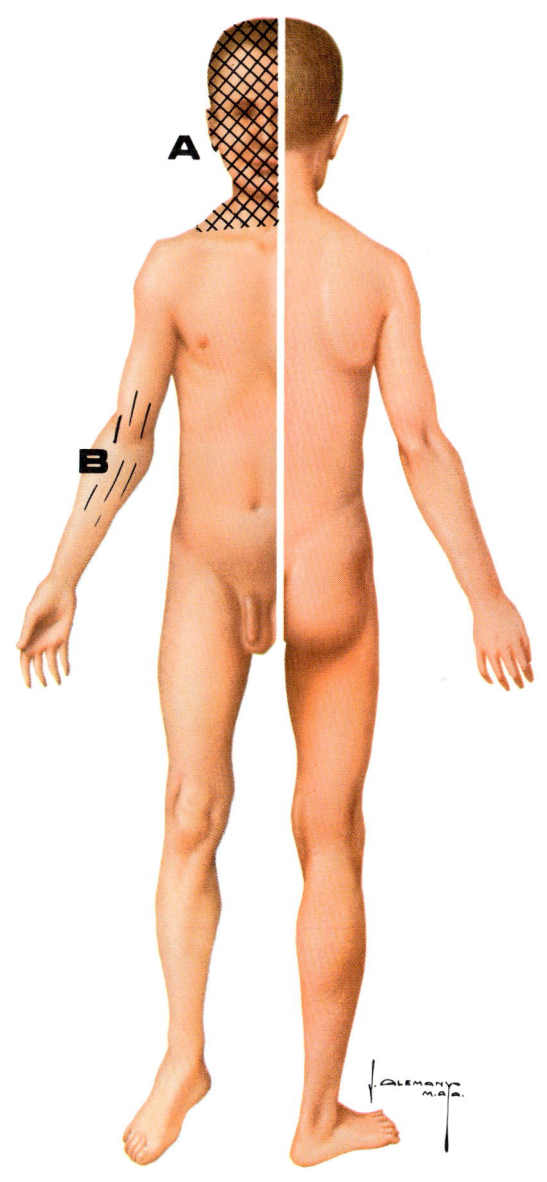

104 · *Endocrine Diseases*

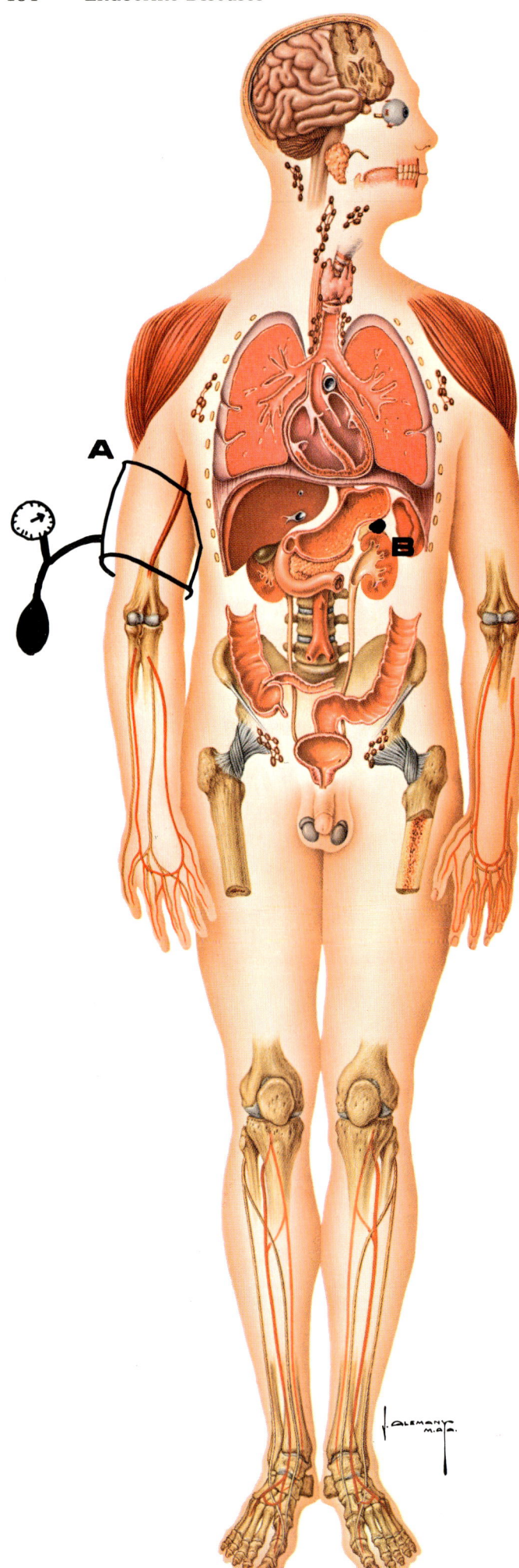

Pheochromocytoma

A 49-year-old white male complained of frequent pounding headaches associated with sweating, palpitations, nausea, and vomiting. His blood pressure was found to be very high during one such attack, and he was therefore admitted for a work-up.

Physical examination revealed a blood pressure of 170/100 mm. Hg (A), tachycardia, and a rather apprehensive individual.

Laboratory examination revealed a blood sugar of 165 mg. per cent, a BMR of +32, and a 24-hour urine vanillylmandelic acid of 26 mg.; administration of 0.05 mg. of histamine IV caused the blood pressure to rise to 250/125 mm. Hg, but Regitine, 5 mg. IV produced a gradual return to normal.

X-ray examination of the adrenal glands by presacral air insufflation revealed an enlarged left adrenal gland (B).

Treatment with surgery was successful.

Differential Diagnosis:
1. Diabetes mellitus
2. Hyperthyroidism
3. Islet cell adenoma
4. Migraine
5. Renovascular hypertension
6. Cushing's syndrome
7. Primary aldosteronism
8. Chronic glomerulonephritis
9. Chronic pyelonephritis
10. Coarctation of the aorta
11. Carcinoid syndrome

Clinical Note. Almost half of these cases have a sustained elevation of blood pressure, whereas the rest have a "labile" hypertension. Only 80 per cent of these tumors are located in the adrenal medulla. The rest are in the sympathetic chain in the neck, thorax, or abdomen. The excess epinephrine stimulates liver glycogenolysis and gluconeogenesis, causing hyperglycemia, and also accounts for the high BMR without an elevated PBI. All cases of sustained and severe labile hypertension should be screened for this disease.

Pathology. Microscopic examination shows the tumor to be composed of polyhedral cells which stain brown after fixation in bichromate. There are frequent necrotic or hemorrhagic areas in the tumor. About 10 per cent of the tumors are malignant, but this is hard to determine by microscopic examination alone.

Zollinger-Ellison Syndrome

A 47-year-old white male complained of chronic, intermittent diarrhea of 3 years' duration. During that time he had had episodes of midepigastric pain lasting 2 to 3 weeks and usually appearing 2 to 3 hours after meals. For 2 weeks prior to admission he had had a similar bout of burning midepigastric pain, this time associated with a tarry stool.

Physical examination revealed pale conjunctiva, focal tenderness in the midepigastrium, and tarry stool on rectal examination.

Laboratory examination revealed 3,500 ml. of fluid abundant in free hydrochloric acid in an overnight gastric analysis.

X-ray examination revealed multiple ulcerations of the stomach and 1st and 2nd portions of the duodenum (A).

At laparotomy a small adenoma of the pancreas (B) was found and removed. A gastrectomy was also performed.

Differential Diagnosis:
1. Hyperparathyroidism
2. Ulcerative colitis
3. Adrenal insufficiency
4. Intestinal parasites
5. Carcinoid syndrome
6. Malabsorption syndrome
7. Chronic pancreatitis
8. Regional ileitis
9. Neoplasms of the colon

Clinical Note. Most cases of chronic diarrhea are painless (intestinal parasites, carcinoid syndrome, ulcerative colitis, malabsorption syndrome), but this condition is usually associated with pain. The ulcers frequently occur in the esophagus and in the jejunum as well. The diarrhea is due to the tremendous output of gastric juice under the influence of a hormone resembling gastrin secreted by the adenoma. In some cases there are functioning adenomas of the other endocrine glands (C) (parathyroids, etc.).

Pathology. There is no uniform histologic cell type (alpha, gamma, etc.) in the islet cell adenoma. Frequently they are malignant and may metastasize to the liver. Aberrant adenomas secreting a gastrin-like substance may be found in other abdominal organs, and so surgical exploration must be carefully performed.

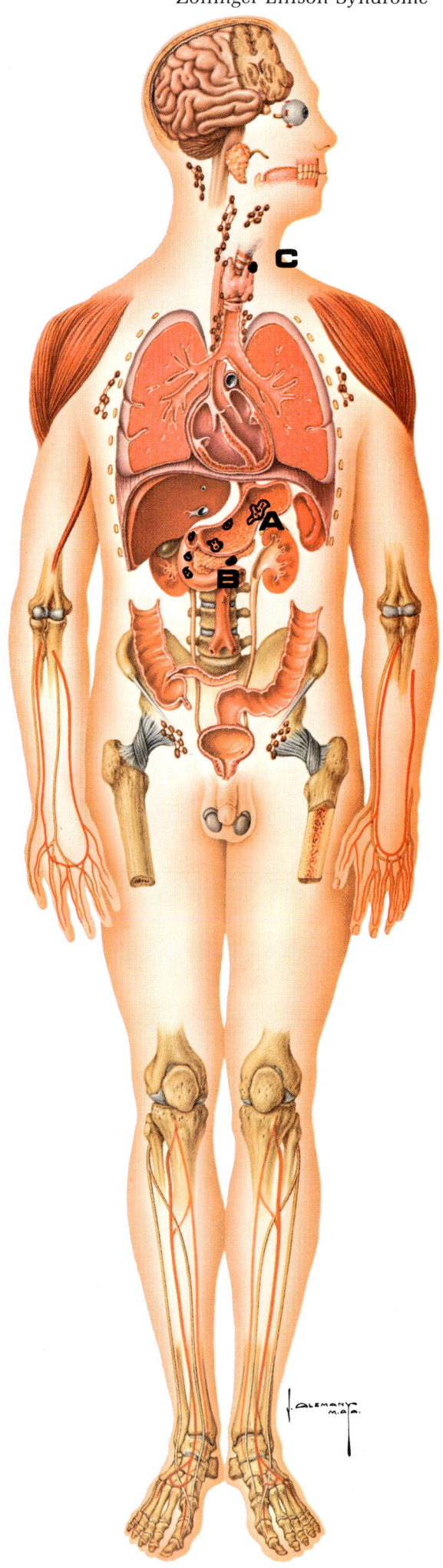

106 · *Endocrine Diseases*

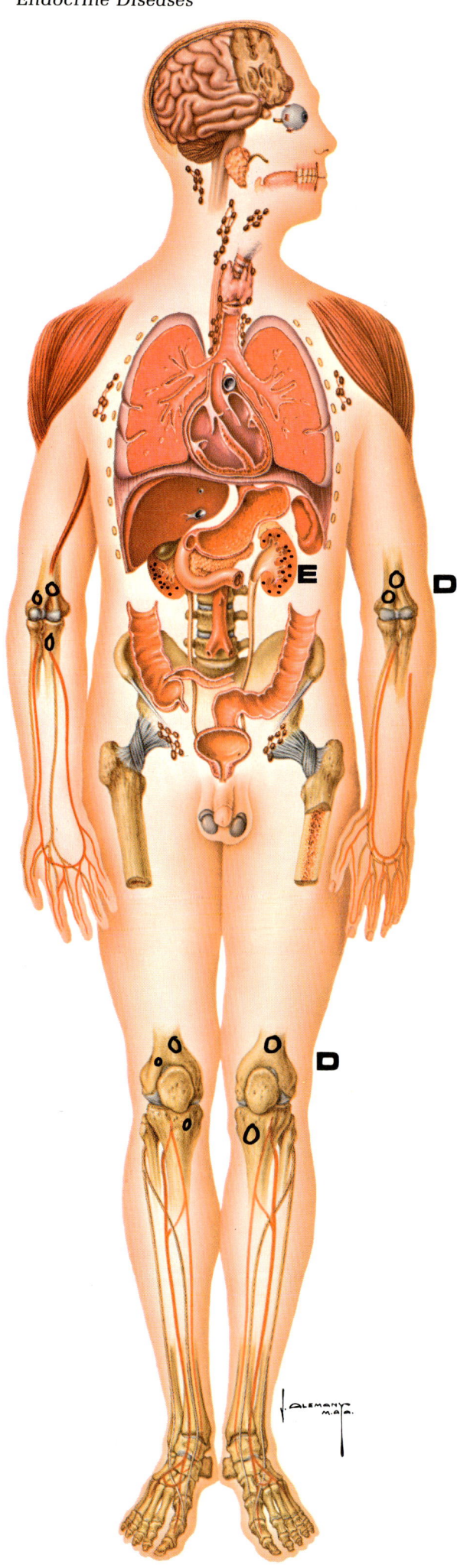

Pseudohypoparathyroidism

A mother presented her 4-year-old child at the pediatric clinic with the chief complaint that he was "too short" for his age. A review of systems revealed that he had often complained of cramps in his arms, legs, and feet, which were passed off as "growing pains."

Physical examination was significant in that he had a round face (A), short stubby build, and shortening of all but the index fingers (B). A Trousseau's sign was elicited (C). Examination of a younger sister revealed similar findings.

Laboratory examination revealed a low calcium, high phosphate, and high alkaline phosphatase. Injection of parathyroid hormone caused a 6-fold increase in urinary phosphate excretion (Ellsworth-Howard test).

X-rays of the long bones revealed cystic radiolucencies (D) not unlike those seen in hyperparathyroidism.

Differential Diagnosis: See Hypoparathyroidism.

Clinical Note. This case emphasizes the congenital malformations of this disorder, its familial nature, and the fact that overt tetany is rarely a complaint of these patients. Although soft-tissue calcifications are more prevalent than in hypoparathyroidism, cataracts are rare. The Ellsworth-Howard test is not always so definitive as in this case.

Pathology. Aside from the bony and soft-tissue changes already noted, there is hyperplasia of the parathyroid glands rather than atrophy. A genetically determined defect in the renal tubules (E) is assumed to prevent them from responding to parathyroid hormone, and reabsorption of phosphate goes uninhibited. The short stature is probably due to premature epiphyseal closure.

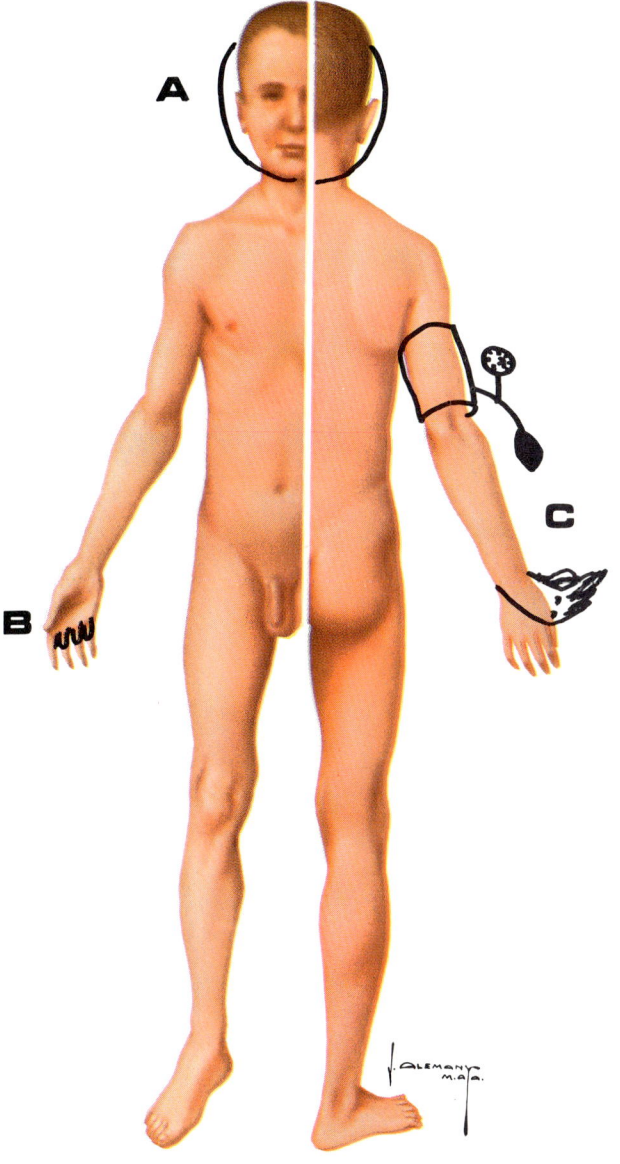

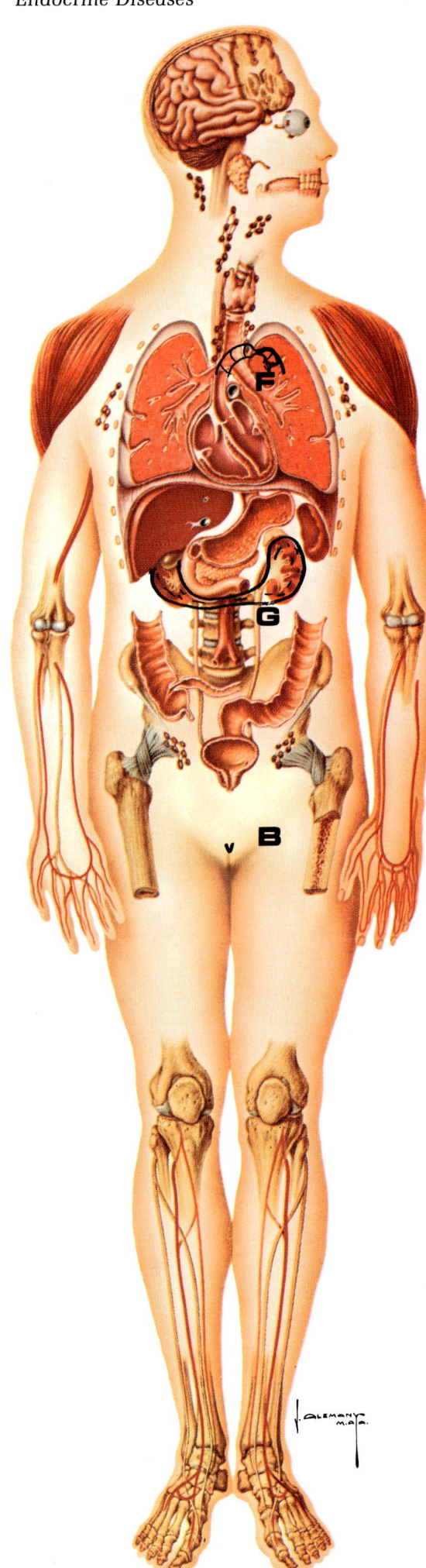

Turner's Syndrome

(Gonadal Dysgenesis)

A 10-year-old white female was brought to the pediatric clinic because her parents were worried about her short stature.

Physical examination revealed dwarfism, a webbed neck (A), absence of pubic and axillary hair, a small clitoris and uterus (B), and no palpable ovaries, widely spaced inverted nipples (C), a high arched palate (D), and cubitus valgus (increased angulation of the elbows) (E). The blood pressure in her right arm was 180/100 mm. Hg but was 90/60 mm. Hg in both legs, suggesting a coarctation of the aorta (F).

Laboratory examination revealed a high 24-hour urine gonadotropin, and a buccal smear revealed absence of the sex chromatin body (Barr body).

X-ray examination revealed a horseshoe kidney (G).

Differential Diagnosis:
1. Hypopituitarism
2. Constitutional dwarfism
3. Achondroplasia
4. Celiac disease
5. Cretinism
6. Hermaphroditism
7. Rickets
8. Hurler's disease

Clinical Note. Since partial forms of this disease are common, many cases are not discovered until puberty. Skeletal, renal, and cardiovascular anomalies are frequent in this disorder. Mental retardation may occur. These patients are actually like males with female sex organs, whereas in Klinefelter's syndrome patients are like females with male sex organs.

Pathology. The ovaries are reduced to fibrous streaks in the broad ligaments, and some contain Leydig cells. Although the XO sex chromosome constitution is the most typical finding, sex chromosome mosaicism has been found with XO/XY and XO/XYY patterns.

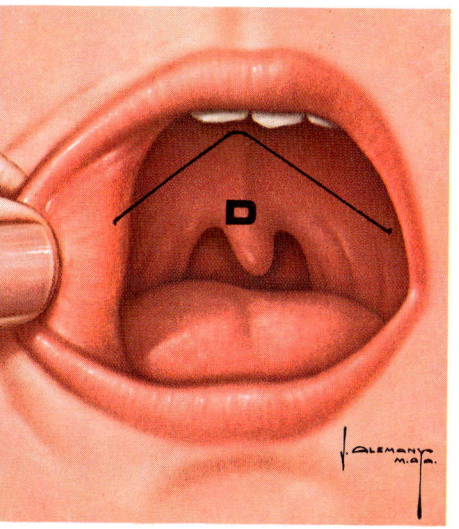

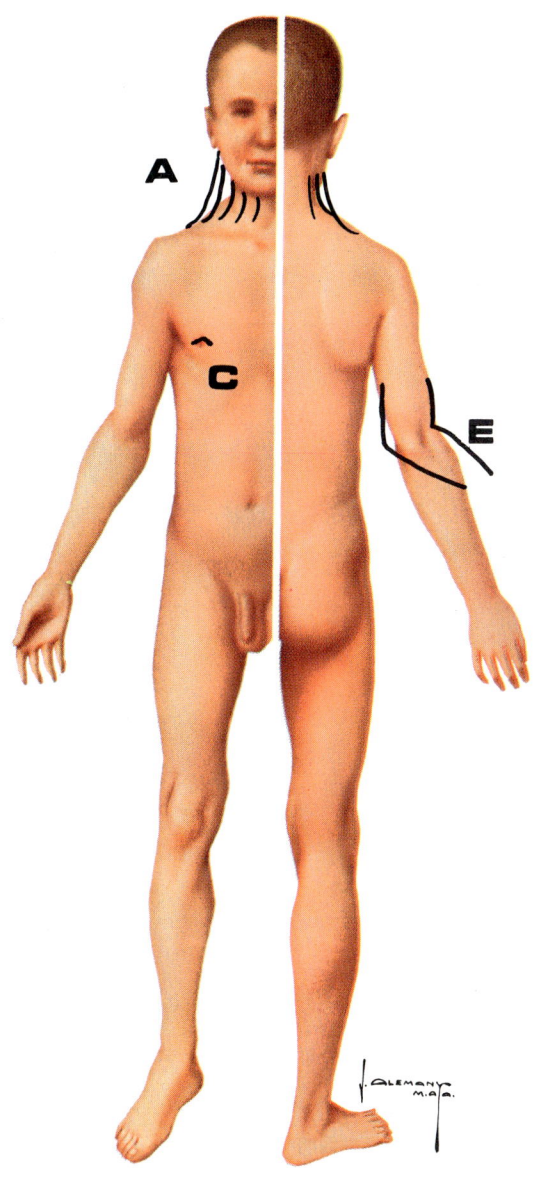

Chapter 7

Infectious Diseases

Since almost every infectious disease may involve more than one organ of the body in individual cases, all infectious diseases might be considered systemic diseases. Many of them involve a certain combination of organs. These are considered here.

Infectious diseases have certain clinical features in common. Most manifest with fever, but any of these may not show fever in individual cases. Most of them cause malaise, loss of appetite, and loss of weight if they become chronic. Physical signs of lymphadenopathy and splenomegaly often appear in chronic cases regardless of the etiology.

Chronic infectious diseases may be classified into stages similar to the stages applied to syphilis. Thus the signs produced at the site of the first invasion may be designated the *primary stage;* the invasion of the bloodstream with its clinical signs may be designated the *secondary stage;* metastasis and development of the infection in a particular organ may be designated the *tertiary stage.* For example, the primary stage of tuberculosis is usually found in the lung. The invasion of the bloodstream (secondary stage) is usually asymptomatic except in infants (miliary tuberculosis). The tertiary stage may be noted clinically in tuberculosis of the kidney or Addison's disease. This sequence can be applied to all infectious diseases.

"Culture everything" should be the byword in diagnosing infectious diseases, particularly fevers of unknown origin. Clinicians often neglect even a simple nose and throat culture and rarely get a blood culture or spinal fluid culture until the fever has progressed to the 2nd or 3rd week. Serologic and skin tests should be used more often, too.

VIRAL DISEASES

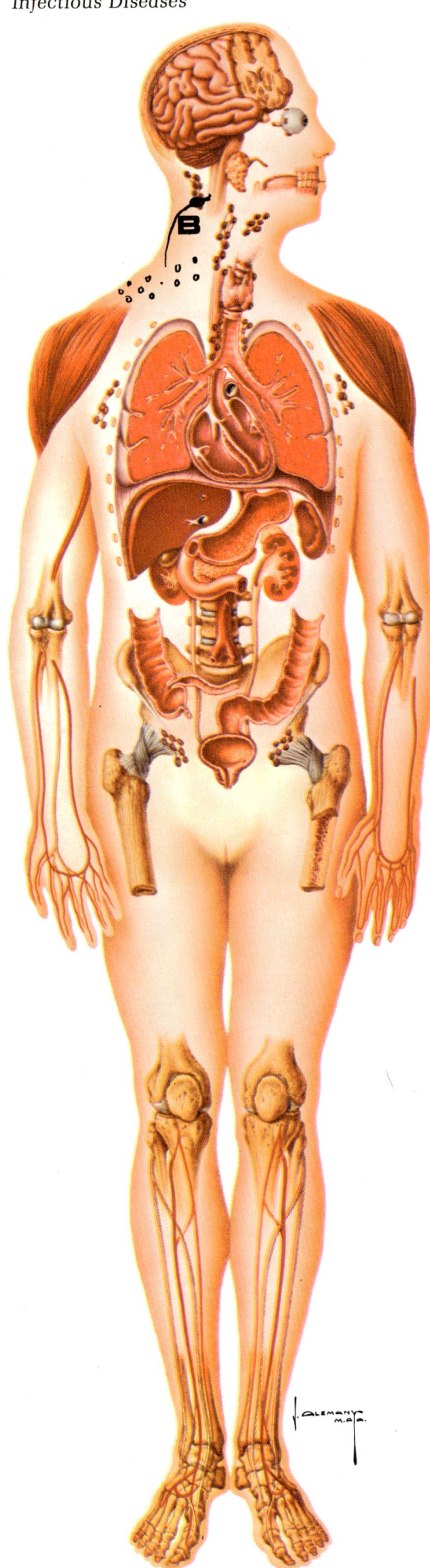

Chickenpox (Varicella)

An 8-year-old white female complained of weakness, fever, and severe pruritic rash.

Physical examination revealed a temperature of 102° F, and a few small vesicles on the face and trunk (A). Over the next 5 days these increased in number.

Laboratory examination revealed multinucleated giant cells in scrapings taken from the skin lesions.

Differential Diagnosis:
1. Measles
2. Smallpox
3. Scarlet fever
4. Rubella
5. Infectious mononucleosis

6. Meningococcemia
7. Drug eruption
8. Secondary syphilis
9. Rickettsiae

Clinical Note. If this condition characteristically affects only the skin, why include it in a book on systemic diseases? Because the virus that causes the chickenpox in children is now believed also to cause herpes zoster in adults. Herpes zoster affects the dorsal root ganglion (B) as well as the skin, and the rash presents in a dermatomal distribution (C). It may affect cranial nerves as well as the spinal nerves. There is often associated regional lymphadenopathy. Finally, a specific pneumonitis with bilateral infiltrates has been noted in leukemic children. As with the other exanthems, a post-infectious encephalomyelitis may occur, but it is rare.

Pathology. Basal and prickle cells of the skin undergo ballooning with fluid and rupture, and multinucleated giant cells appear with intranuclear inclusion bodies.

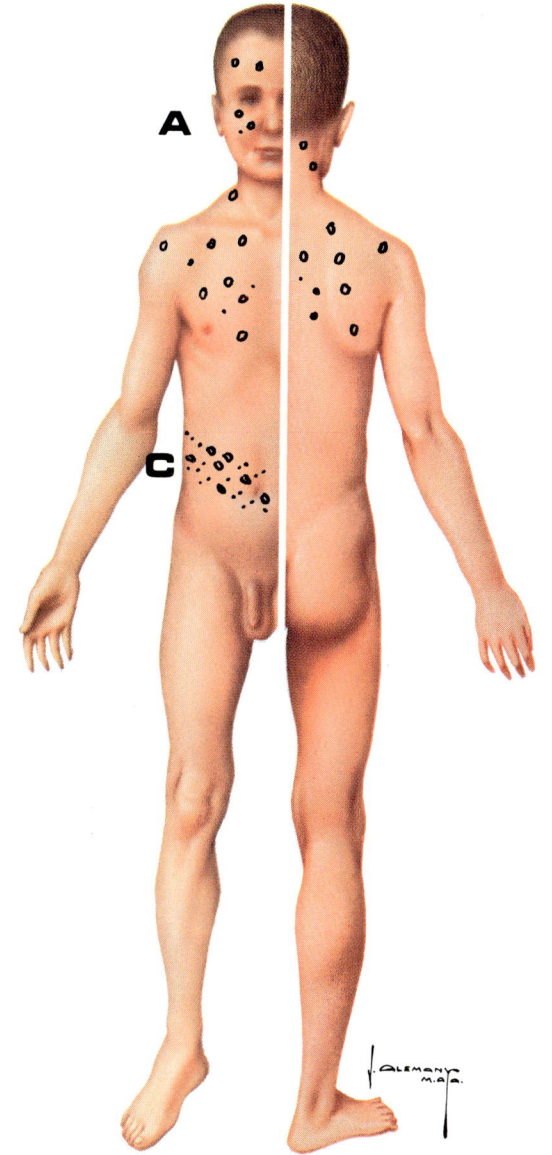

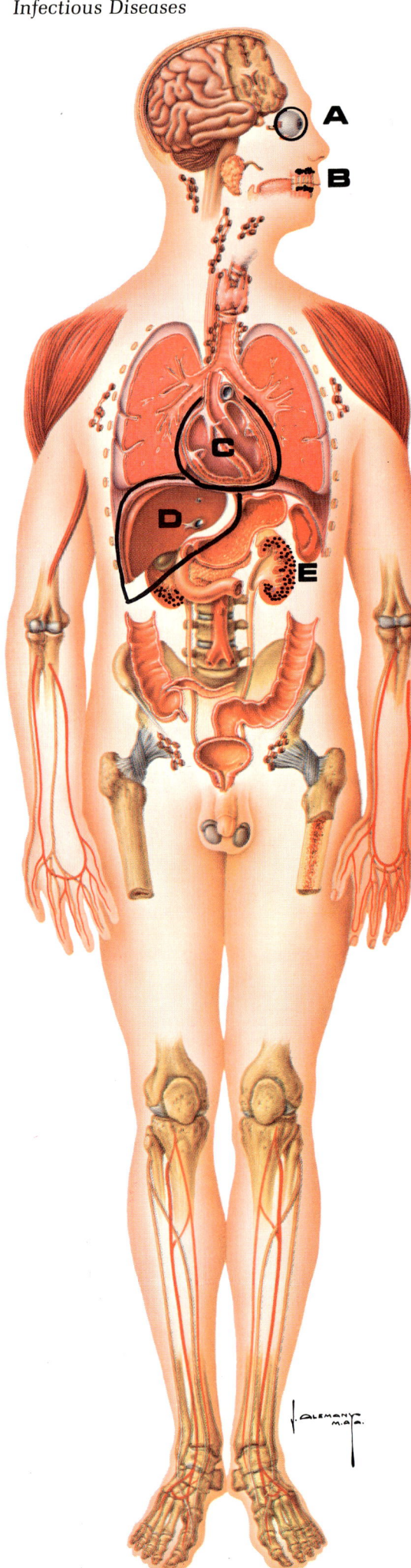

Yellow Fever

A 24-year-old white male South American developed sudden fever, chills, generalized aches and pains, and nausea and vomiting. He gradually improved, but 4 days later the fever returned, and his eyes and skin became yellow.

Physical examination revealed a temperature of 103° F., icteric sclerae and skin (A), swollen bleeding gums (B), a pulse of 65/min., cardiomegaly (C), and hepatomegaly (D).

Laboratory examination revealed marked albuminuria, indicating renal involvement (E). Liver biopsy was diagnostic.

Differential Diagnosis:
1. Infectious hepatitis
2. Cirrhosis of the liver
3. Infectious mononucleosis
4. Weil's disease
5. Schistosomiasis
6. Ascending cholangitis
7. Carcinoma of the pancreas
8. Malaria
9. Toxic hepatitis
10. Sickle cell anemia

Clinical Note. This disease has a marked similarity to both malaria and Weil's disease. In malaria the fever may drop, and the patient temporarily improves for 2 to 3 days, but yellow fever does not continue in recurrent episodes. Weil's disease involves the kidney, as does yellow fever, but is often more severe, and frequently there is nervous system involvement. Like poliomyelitis, most cases of yellow fever are mild. Since only a few develop jaundice, the name would seem to be a misnomer. There is no treatment, but an excellent vaccine is available. Mosquito control is important in prevention.

Pathology. The lobules of the liver reveal midzone necrosis, and the necrotic cells contain an eosinophilic hyaline material known as Councilman bodies. There is little cellular reaction, and no attempt is made to repair by fibrosis. The kidneys are pale and swollen; microscopically they show severe degeneration of the tubular epithelium. The heart muscle fibers are degenerated, and there are scattered petechial hemorrhages. Although the nervous system is often involved in animals, it is usually spared in humans.

Infectious Mononucleosis

A 24-year-old white male developed fever, chills, and sore throat unresponsive to antibiotics 5 days prior to admission.

Physical examination revealed an injected exudative throat and tonsils (A), petechial hemorrhages of the soft palate, enlarged, tender anterior and posterior cervical lymph nodes bilaterally (B), and hepatosplenomegaly (C) without jaundice.

Laboratory examination revealed a heterophil antibody titer of 1:896, absorbable with beef erythrocyte antigen but not guinea pig kidney; 90 per cent atypical lymphocytes on the blood smear; a transaminase of 140 units, and an alkaline phosphatase of 27.8 King-Armstrong units.

Differential Diagnosis:
1. Streptococcal pharyngitis
2. Viral pharyngitis
3. Acute leukemia
4. Agranulocytosis
5. Diphtheria
6. Infectious hepatitis
7. Typhoid fever

Clinical Note. Although most cases present in this fashion, silent cases occur frequently. Hepatic involvement is constant, but jaundice is infrequent. When the heterophil test is positive, there is no difficulty in differentiating this from other conditions; but when it is negative, an extensive laboratory investigation is required. Infrequently, infectious mononucleosis presents with a meningoencephalitis (D) or with infectious polyneuritis with root and cord involvement (E). Focal lesions of the myocardium, lungs, and kidneys, and a maculopapular rash have been described.

Pathology. The reaction is mainly in the reticuloendothelial system of the body, with proliferation of both lymphocytic and reticuloendothelial elements. Histologic changes may be found in every body tissue.

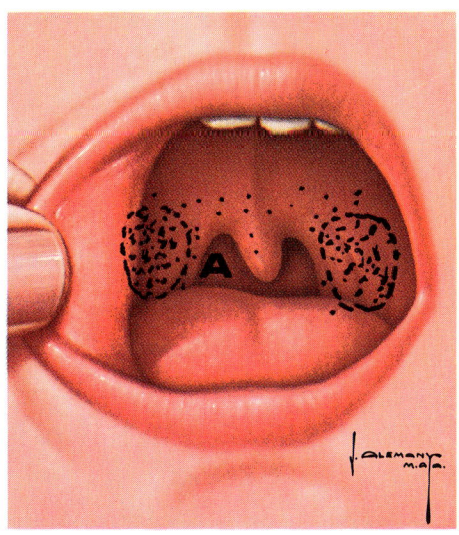

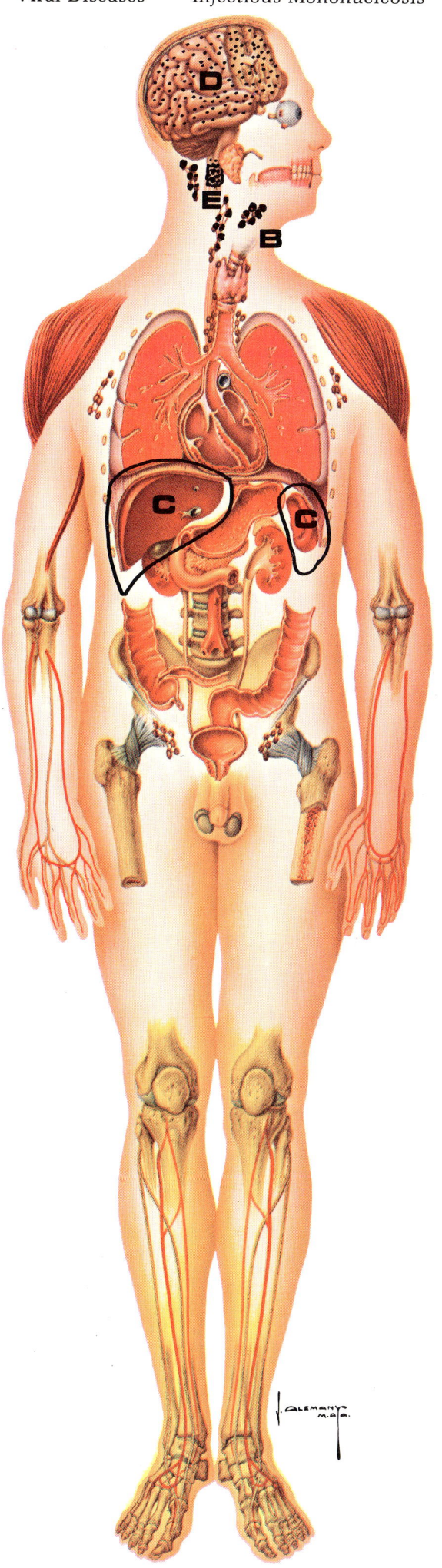

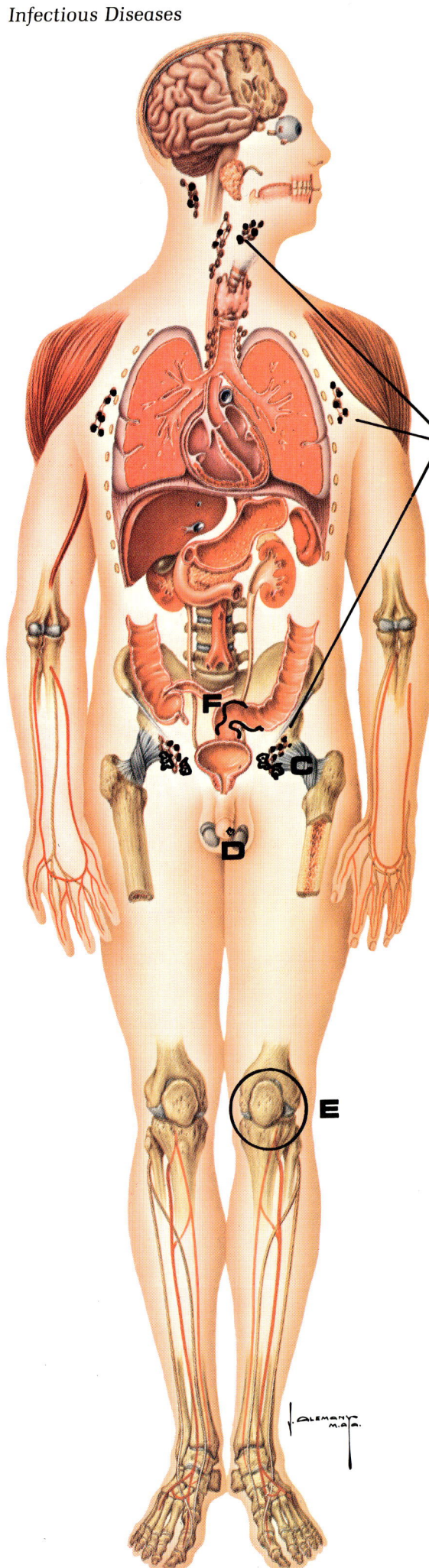

Lymphogranuloma Venereum

A 34-year-old Negro male complained of swollen tender masses draining in both groins of 1 week's duration. He also complained of pain in both ankles and the right elbow.

Physical examination revealed injection of both conjunctivae (A), generalized lymphadenopathy (B), and swollen, tender inguinal nodes bilaterally with multiple draining sinuses in both (C).

Laboratory examination revealed hyperglobulinemia, and a positive Frei test. A biopsy of the inguinal nodes was diagnostic.

Treatment with sulfonamides was successful.

Differential Diagnosis:
1. Reiter's disease
2. Gonorrhea
3. Syphilis
4. Chancroid
5. Inguinal hernia
6. Lymphoma
7. Granuloma inguinale

Clinical Note. The initial ulcer of the penis (D) is usually so small that it goes unnoticed. The joints occasionally show clinical enlargement and tenderness (E) so that there is a marked similarity to Reiter's syndrome. In rare cases there may be meningitis and pericarditis. The most common complication is rectal stricture (F) in women and homosexual males.

Pathology. Microscopic examination of the inguinal nodes reveals lymphoid hyperplasia with discrete foci of macrophages arranged in a palisade around areas of typical stellate abscesses and cellular debris.

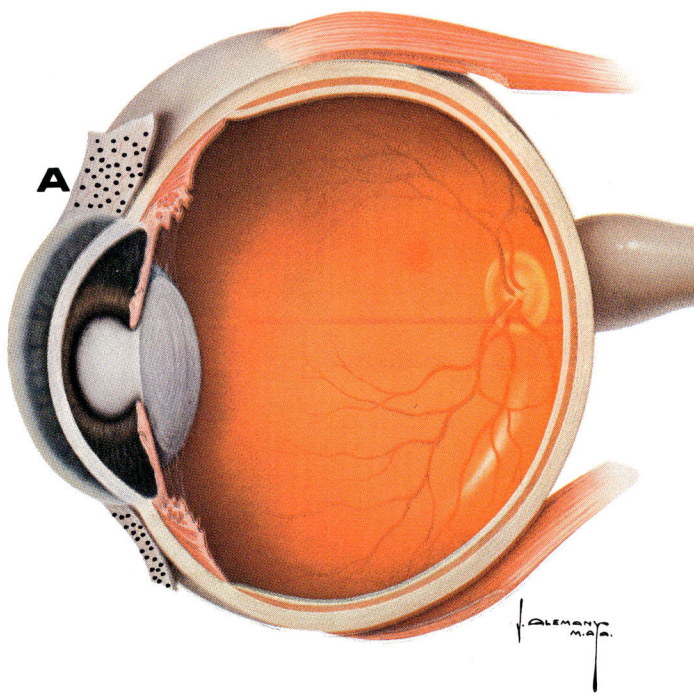

Mumps

A 17-year-old white male developed fever, chills, and swelling and pain in both jaws. Four days later he developed marked pain and swelling of the left testicle.

Physical examination revealed a temperature of 101° F., swollen tender parotid glands bilaterally (A), swelling and erythema of the openings of both Stensen's ducts (B), and swollen tender left testicle (C).

Laboratory examination revealed an elevated serum amylase and a rising titer of antibodies on the mumps complement-fixation test.

Differential Diagnosis:
1. Salivary-gland calculus
2. Sarcoidosis
3. Sjögren's disease
4. Hodgkin's disease
5. Tuberculosis

Clinical Note. Testicular involvement occurs in 20 per cent of the cases and produces sterility if there is bilateral involvement. Only a few patients have orchitis without parotitis. Less frequently there is clinical meningoencephalitis (D), but subclinical meningeal involvement may occur in a quarter of the cases. Pancreatitis (E) may occur, but does not account for the high serum amylase in most cases. Almost any organ of the body may be involved.

Pathology. There are edema and perivascular infiltration of the parotid glands with destruction of the glandular tissue and plugging of the tubules by epithelial debris.

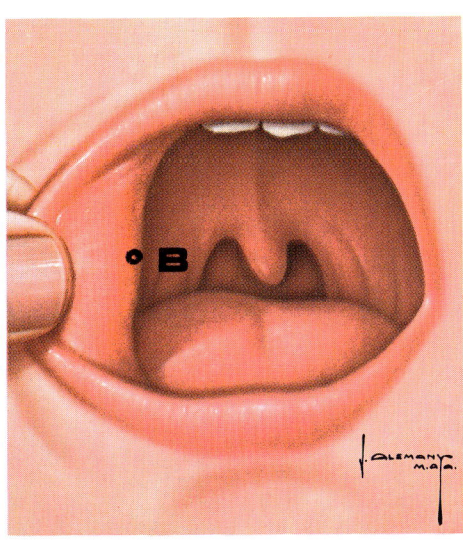

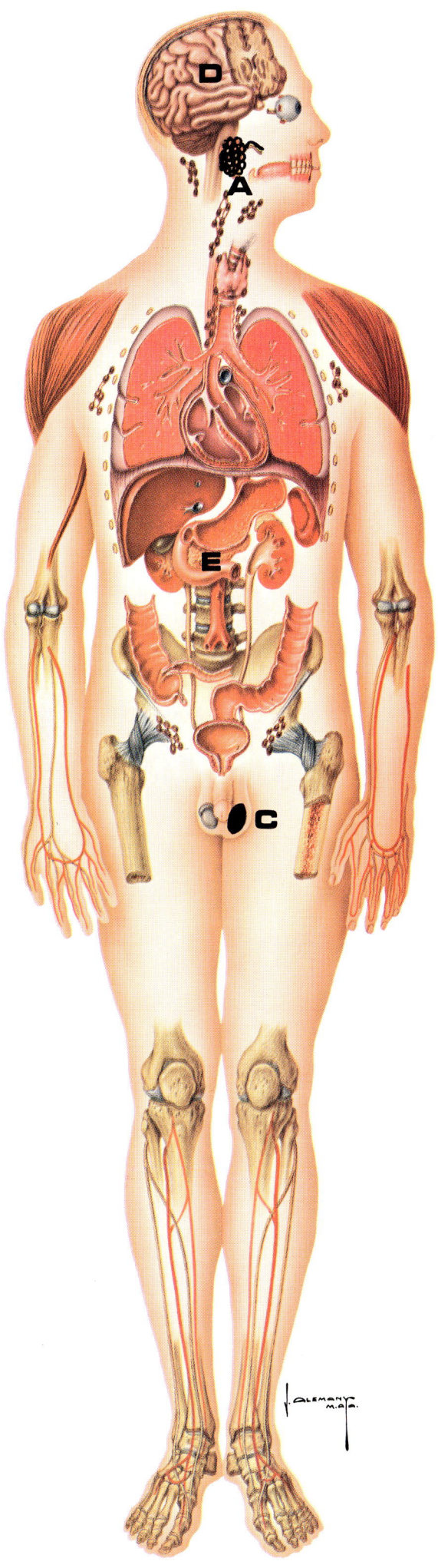

120 · Infectious Diseases

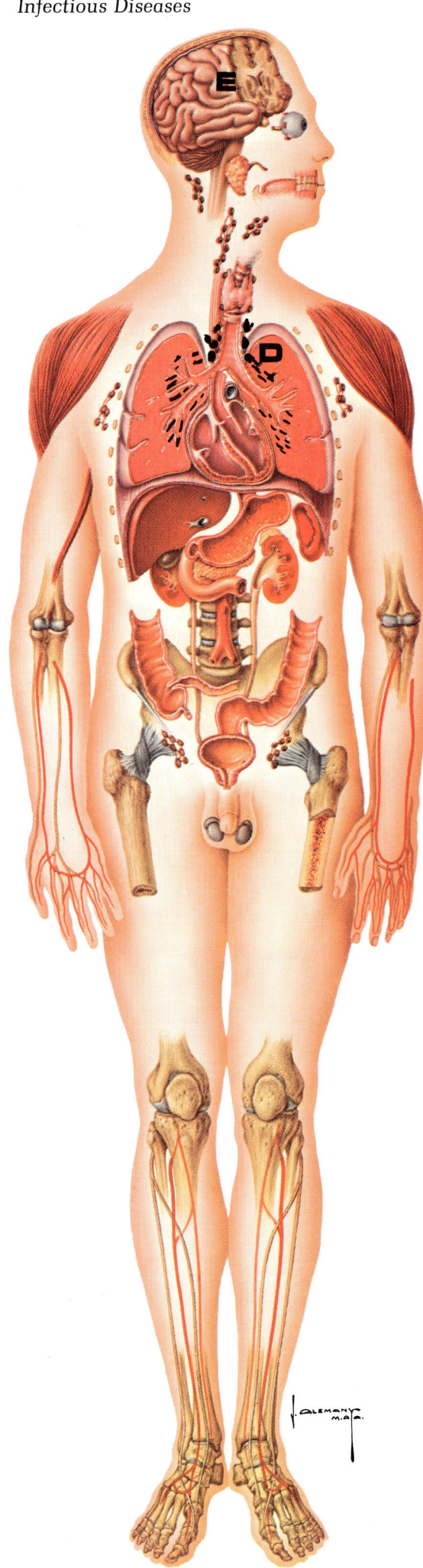

Measles (Rubeola)

A 7-year-old white male was admitted to the hospital because of fever, cough, and severe burning pain in both eyes.

Physical examination revealed injected conjunctiva (A), swollen nasal turbinates, injected throat, and sibilant and sonorous rales throughout both lung fields. Close inspection of the mouth revealed small white papules (Koplik's spots) (B) on the buccal mucosa adjacent to the molars. Two days after admission he developed a maculopapular rash (C), at first behind the ears and then spreading to face, trunk, and extremities. The bottoms of the hands and feet were not involved.

Laboratory examination revealed a moderate leukopenia, and multinucleated giant cells were detected in the nasal exudate.

X-ray examination of the chest revealed hilar adenopathy and streaky densities extending from both hila (D).

Differential Diagnosis:
1. Rubella
2. Scarlet fever

3. Enteroviral eruptions (Coxsackie, etc.)
4. Rickettsiae
5. Meningococcemia
6. Exanthema subitum
7. Penicillin allergy
8. Infectious mononucleosis
9. Leukemia

Clinical Note. This case illustrates that, both preceding and during the attack of measles, involvement of the respiratory tract is often prominent. This helps to differentiate measles from rubella and other exanthems. Superimposed bacterial infections of the ears, sinuses, and lungs are also common. Encephalitis as a complication of measles (E), not present in this case, is not so rare as was once believed. As many as 51 per cent of children with measles may have electroencephalographic changes. In children with leukemia a giant cell pneumonia has been described.

Pathology. Subepithelial round cell infiltration and multinucleated giant cells are characteristic. There may be cytoplasmic and nuclear inclusion bodies. The rash is the result of proliferation of the capillary endothelium under the skin.

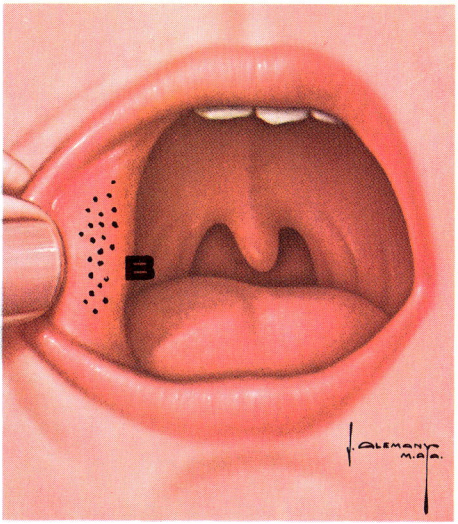

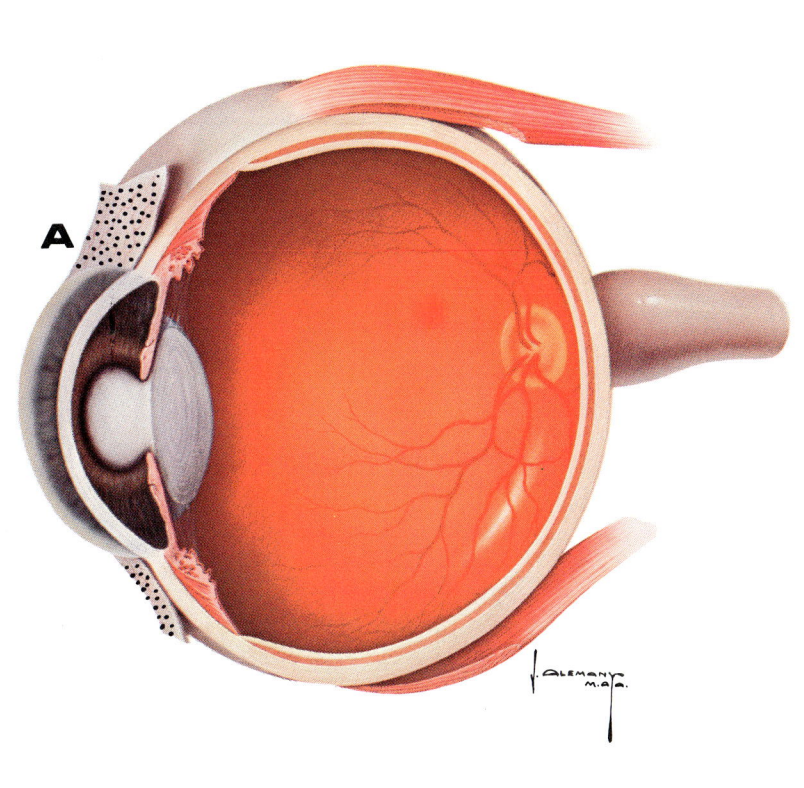

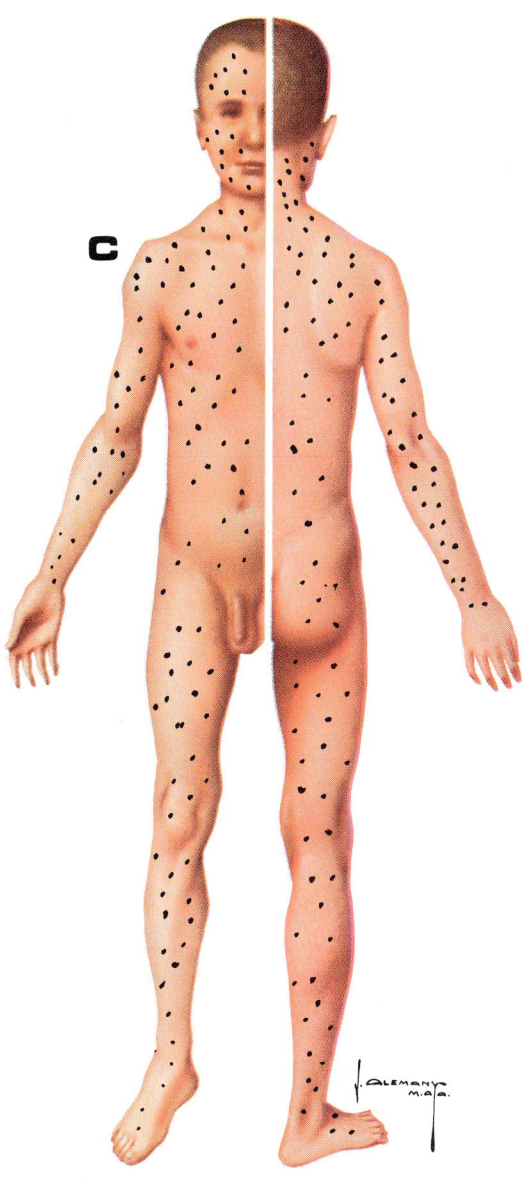

122 · Infectious Diseases

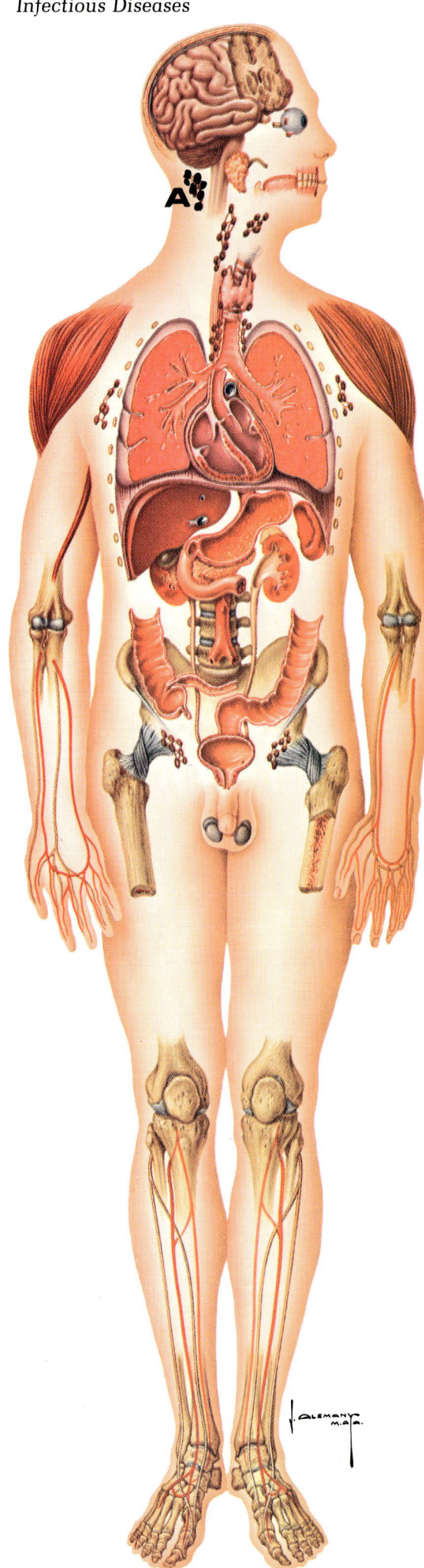

Rubella

A 6-year-old white male was brought for examination because of lumps behind his ears. One day later he developed a rash on his face, which spread to the rest of his body.

Physical examination revealed hard, tender postauricular and suboccipital lymph nodes bilaterally (A), a temperature of 100° F., and erythematous macular rash of face, neck, trunk, and upper arms (B).

Laboratory examination was unremarkable.

X-ray examination was unremarkable.

Differential Diagnosis:
1. Measles
2. Infectious mononucleosis

3. Scarlet fever
4. Enteroviral eruptions
5. Rickettsiae
6. Meningococcemia
7. Exanthema subitum
8. Drug eruption
9. Leukemia

Clinical Note. Unlike rubeola, conjunctivitis and upper respiratory symptoms are unusual. However, the lymphadenopathy is striking. Encephalitis is rare, as are other systemic complications such as neuritis and thrombocytopenic purpura. In the fetus of an infected mother this virus may involve any organ system—heart, auditory nerves, teeth, nervous system—and is a typical systemic disease.

Pathology. Because death from the uncomplicated case is unknown, no record of histologic changes in the disease has been made.

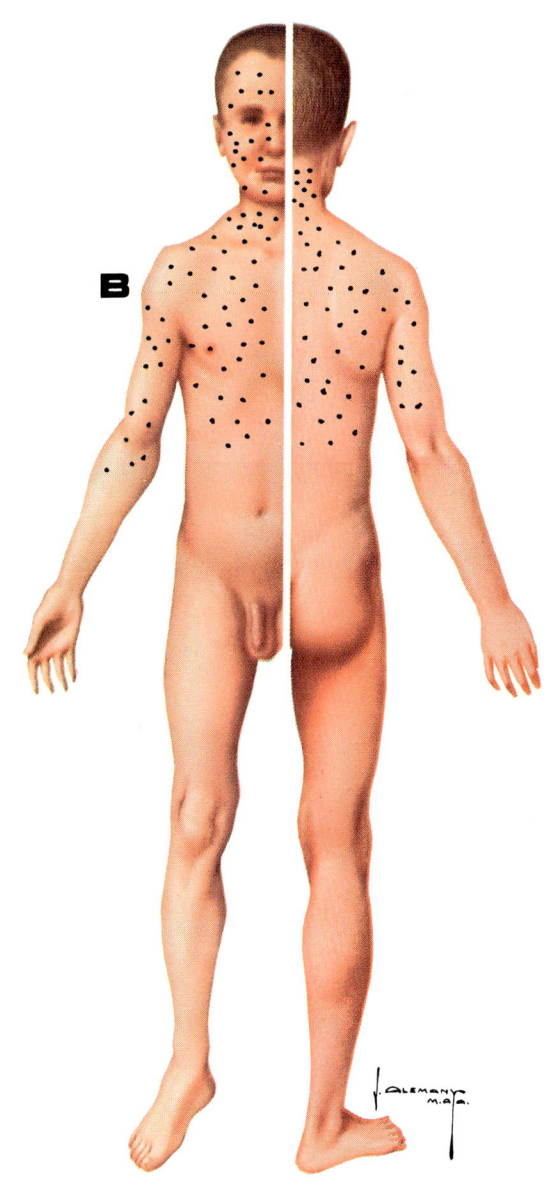

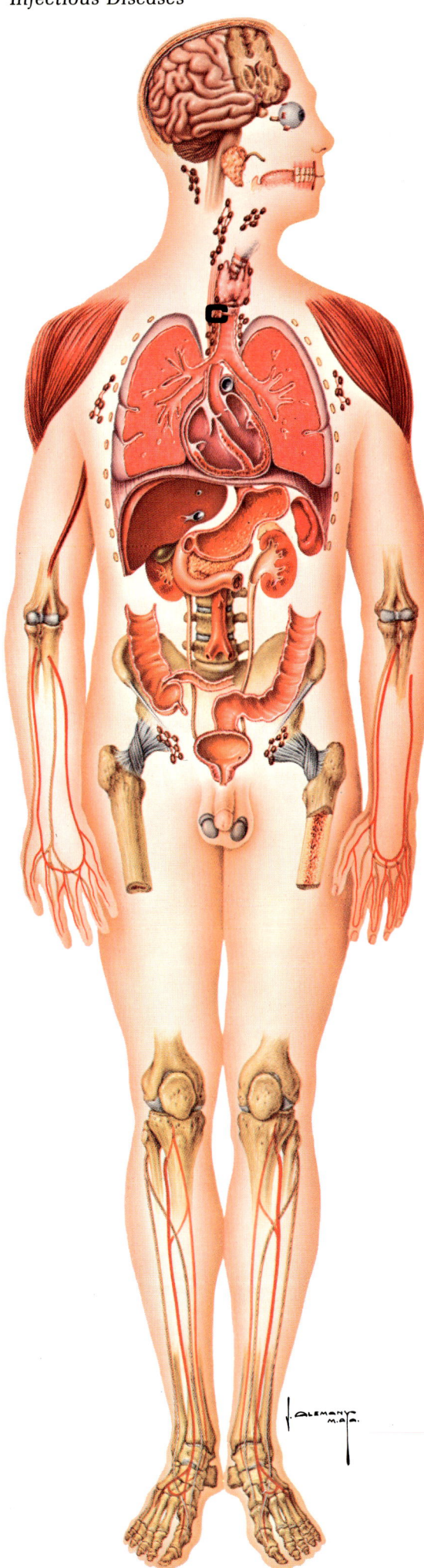

Smallpox

A 21-year-old white male developed high fever, prostration, and generalized muscular aches and pains, diagnosed as viral influenza by his local physician. A rash of his face, which developed the day of admission, spread to the rest of his body.

Physical examination revealed a temperature of 104° F., and a papular eruption of the entire body, including the palms and soles (A). Papular lesions were also noted in the mouth and throat (B). A few days later the lesions were indurated, and multilocular vesicles began to form over the papules. Still later the lesions became pustular.

Laboratory examination revealed virus particles in the vesicular fluid.

Differential Diagnosis:
1. Chickenpox
2. Measles
3. Rubella
4. Scarlet fever
5. Rickettsiae
6. Meningococcemia
7. Drug eruption

8. Secondary syphilis
9. Infectious mononucleosis

Clinical Note. Here is another condition that customarily affects only the skin, but the prodromal myalgia and severe prostration, plus the involvement of the oral mucosa, justify its consideration as a systemic disease. Mucosal lesions also occur in the trachea and esophagus (C). This disease is so fulminating as to suggest meningococcemia or rickettsiae, and yet most texts go into very great detail to distinguish smallpox from chickenpox, a disease that has very few constitutional symptoms. The rash of the two is vesicular at some time; but in chickenpox it develops rapidly, is centripedal, and there may be macules, papules, and vesicles at the same time, whereas in smallpox it is slow in development, centrifugal (more on the limbs), and rotates from crops of papules to crops of vesicles. The lesions of smallpox are deep-seated, whereas those of chickenpox are superficial and collapse if they are pricked.

Pathology. Histologically, in smallpox there is first vascular congestion with mononuclear infiltration of the skin. The epithelial cells are invaded by the organism, swell, and burst, releasing the fluid which forms the vesicles. Inclusion bodies may be found in the epithelial cells.

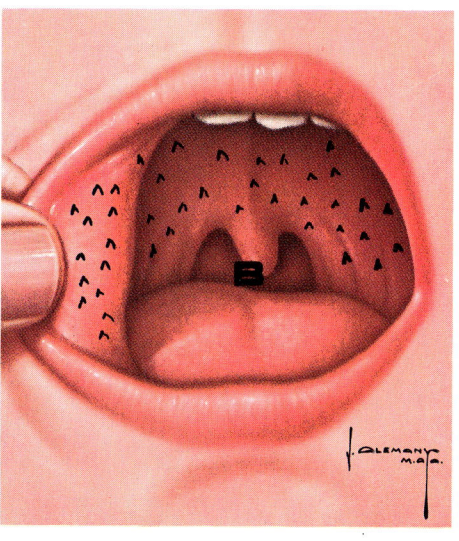

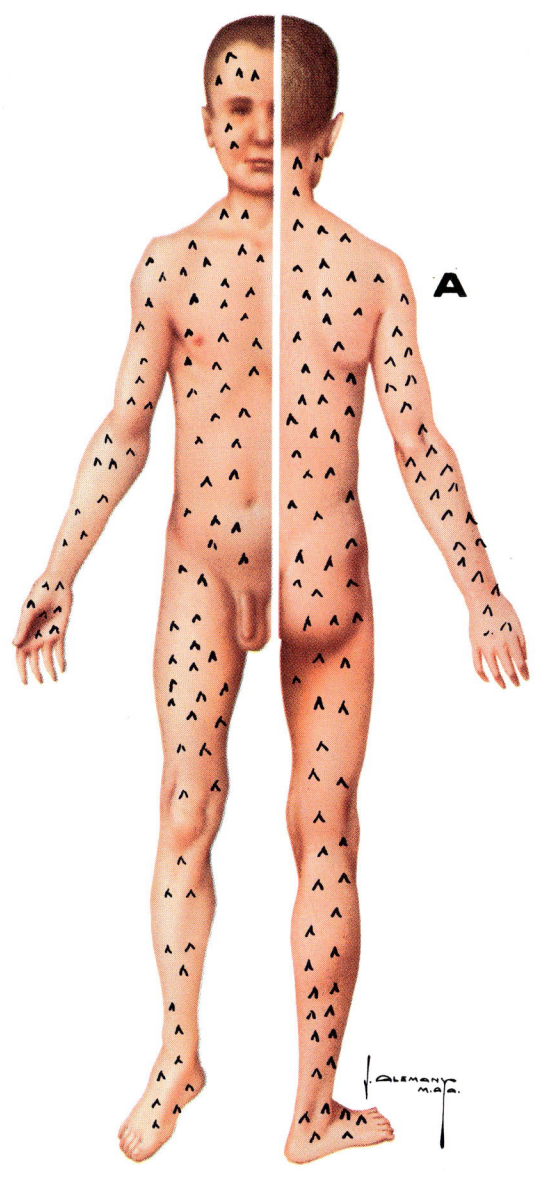

126 · Infectious Diseases

Poliomyelitis

A 14-year-old white male developed nausea, vomiting, diarrhea, and a slight fever 2 days prior to admission (indicating a gastroenteritis) (A). On the day of admission he developed severe muscle spasms in both legs.

Physical examination 48 hours later revealed paraplegia and hypoactive reflexes in both lower extremities. There were fasciculations of the muscles of the lower extremities. There was also an atonic urinary bladder. All these signs indicated anterior horn involvement of the spinal cord (B). There were no sensory changes. There were nuchal rigidity and a positive Kernig's sign.

Laboratory examination of the spinal fluid revealed 250 WBC per cu. mm., most of which were lymphocytes, and an elevated protein. Culture was negative; however, acute and convalescent sera for viral antibodies revealed a rising titer of neutralizing antibodies to polio virus.

Differential Diagnosis:
1. Aseptic meningitis
2. Bacterial meningitis
3. Tuberculous meningitis
4. Cryptococcosis
5. Spinal cord tumor
6. Epidural abscess
7. Hemophilia
8. Syphilitic meningitis
9. Trichinosis
10. Anterior spinal artery thrombosis
11. Multiple sclerosis
12. Porphyria

Clinical Note. Over 90 per cent of cases of this disease are clinically silent or manifest merely a pharyngitis or gastroenteritis. Others have purely fever and merely meningeal irritation. Paralytic poliomyelitis may be primarily monoplegic or hemiplegic, and there are bulbar and cerebral forms as well. If the sympathetic nervous system is involved, there may be tachycardia and hypotension. There may be myocarditis (C).

Pathology. The anterior horn cells and, to a lesser extent, other areas of the cord and brain reveal intense perivascular infiltration of leukocytes, small hemorrhages, and cell degeneration. Eventually glial proliferation and scar formation occur.

RICKETTSIAE

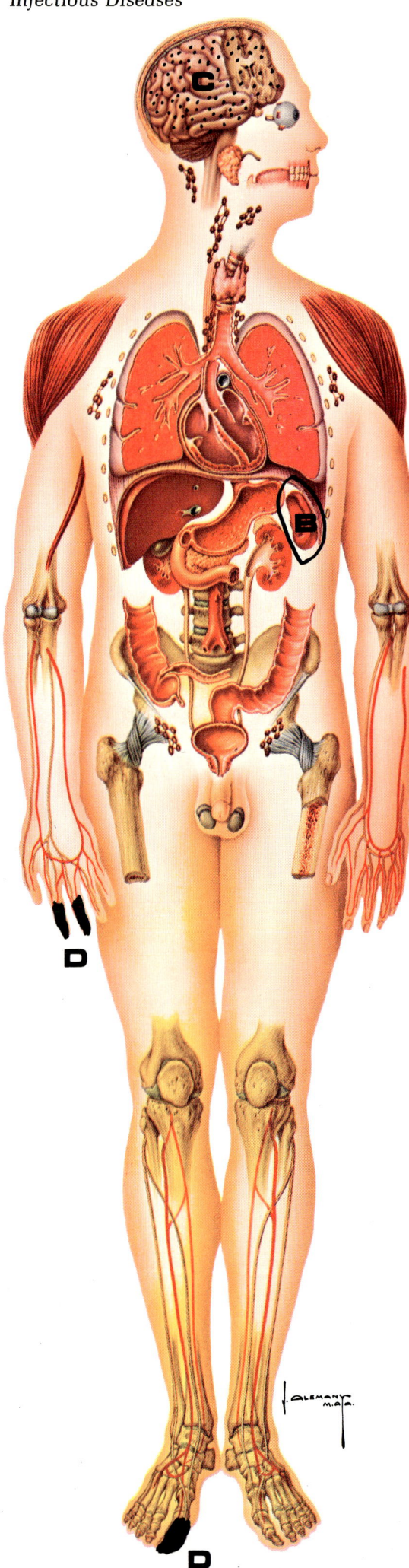

Rocky Mountain Spotted Fever

A 27-year-old white male developed fever and chills, generalized aches and pains, and a severe headache for 5 days prior to admission. He developed a rash of the wrists, ankles, and back, which gradually covered the whole body.

Physical examination revealed a generalized maculopapular rash with petechiae in places (A) and splenomegaly (B). The patient was delirious, and there was generalized hyperesthesia, indicating nervous system involvement (C).

Laboratory examination revealed a positive Weil-Felix reaction to all 3 strains of *Proteus vulgaris* (OX-19, OX-2, and OX-K), but the highest titer was with OX-19. The complement-fixation test was positive for *Rickettsia rickettsii*.

Differential Diagnosis:
1. Meningococcemia
2. Measles
3. Murine typhus

4. Periarteritis nodosa
5. Systemic lupus erythematosus
6. Thrombocytopenic purpura
7. Scurvy
8. Subacute bacterial endocarditis
9. Stevens-Johnson syndrome
10. Trench fever
11. Typhoid fever
12. Serum sickness

Clinical Note. The angiitis so typical of this disease is usually manifested in the skin and nervous system and less commonly in the spleen. It may occasionally lead to shock and renal shutdown. Often there is gangrene of the fingers and toes (D) in later stages due to thrombosis secondary to the angiitis. Deafness and visual disturbances may persist after recovery. It is easy to see why this disorder is so often confused with other conditions leading to angiitis. It is not well known that the disease frequently occurs in the Southern states, such as Virginia, and is rare in the Great Lake areas.

Pathology. Microscopic examination of the small blood vessels reveals proliferation of the endothelium, perivascular infiltration, and intravascular thrombosis.

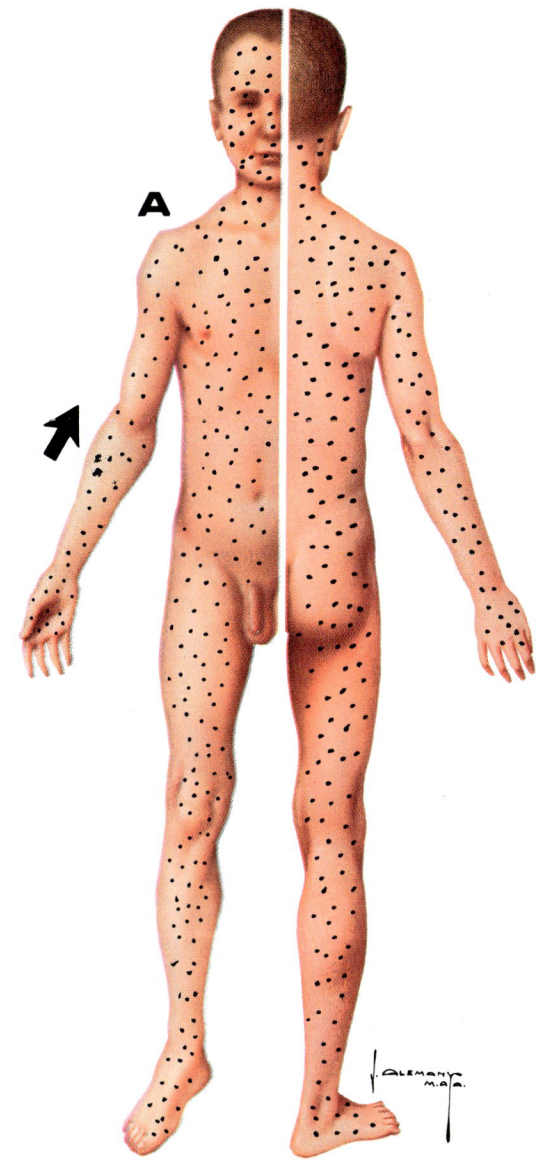

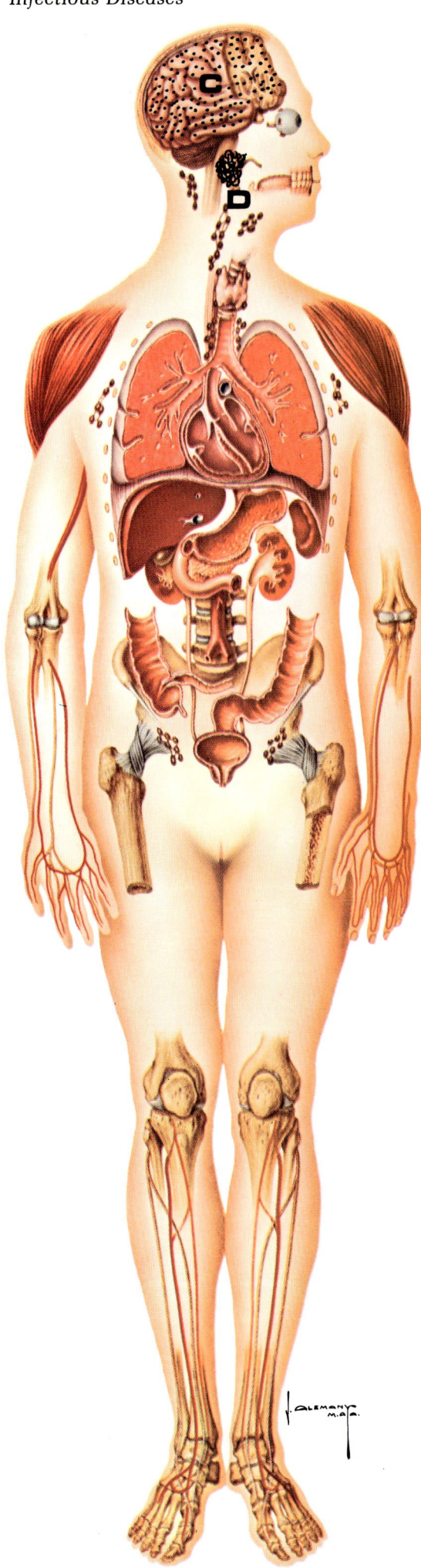

Epidemic Typhus

A 43-year-old white female complained of a severe unrelenting headache, fever, and chills for 5 days. There were also an unproductive cough and occasional loose stools. On the day of the visit to the office she developed a rash.

Physical examination revealed a temperature of 103° F., a maculopapular rash of the back and chest (A), and subconjunctival hemorrhages (B). By the 3rd hospital day the rash was generalized, sparing only the face, palms, and soles; and there were papilledema, agitation, and delirium, indicating central nervous system involvement (C). One week later there was bilateral swelling of the parotid glands (D).

Laboratory examination revealed a positive Weil-Felix reaction to OX-19 strains of *Proteus* and a rise in the complement-fixation titer for *R. Prowazekii* a few weeks after admission.

Differential Diagnosis:
1. Meningococcemia

2. Measles
3. Rocky Mountain spotted fever
4. Typhoid fever
5. Smallpox
6. Periarteritis nodosa
7. Serum sickness

Clinical Note. As in Rocky Mountain spotted fever, the skin is the major organ affected by the angiitis; but a severe purpura is less common here. Epidemic typhus, like spotted fever, causes focal and peripheral gangrene in the later stages. The 2 diseases may also be distinguished by the spread of the rash. In epidemic typhus it begins on the trunk and spreads centrifugally (E), whereas in Rocky Mountain spotted fever it begins on the wrists and ankles, spreads centripedally, and involves the palms and soles. All cases of arteritis we see in the United States may not be periarteritis nodosa.

Pathology. Microscopically, the small vessels show endothelial proliferation, thrombosis, and perivascular cuffing. These lesions are particularly common in the skin, brain, and heart muscles. An interstitial pneumonia may develop, as in Q-fever.

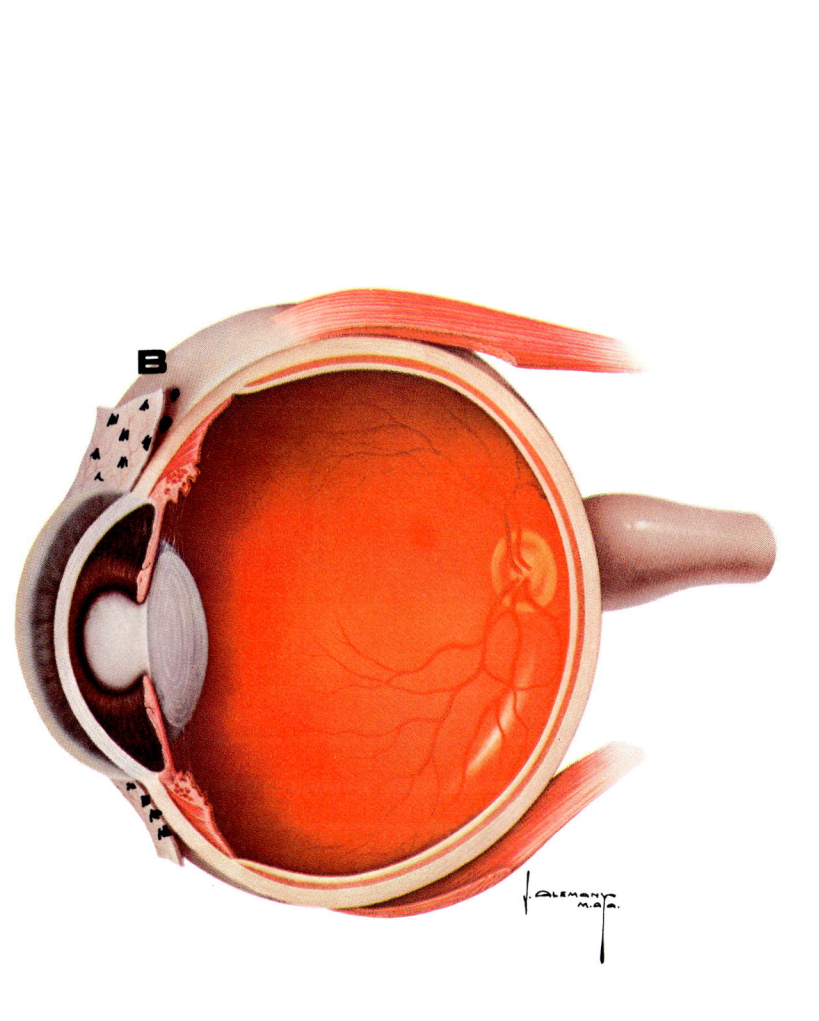

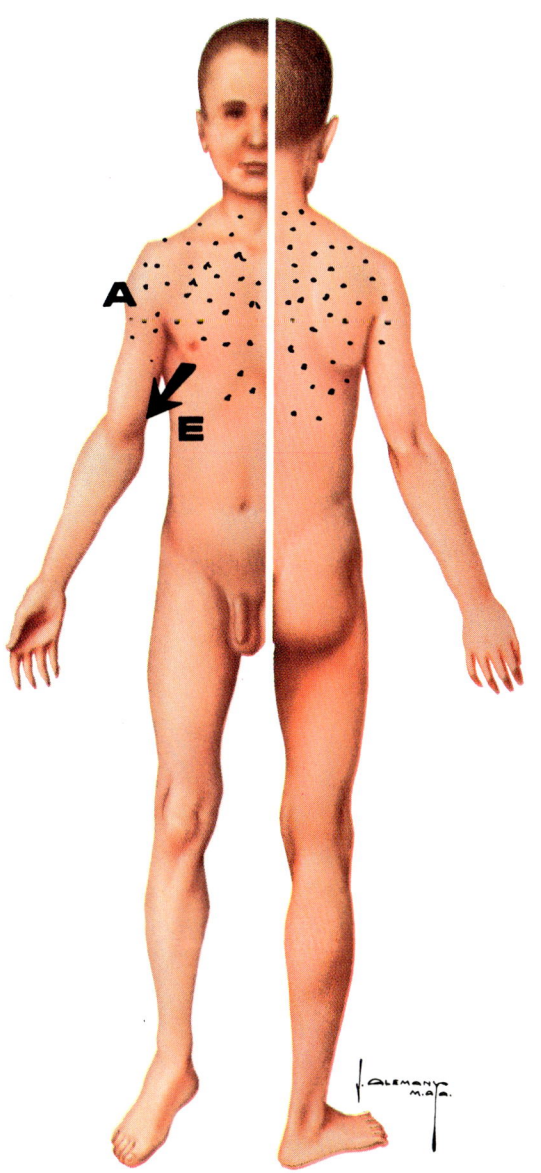

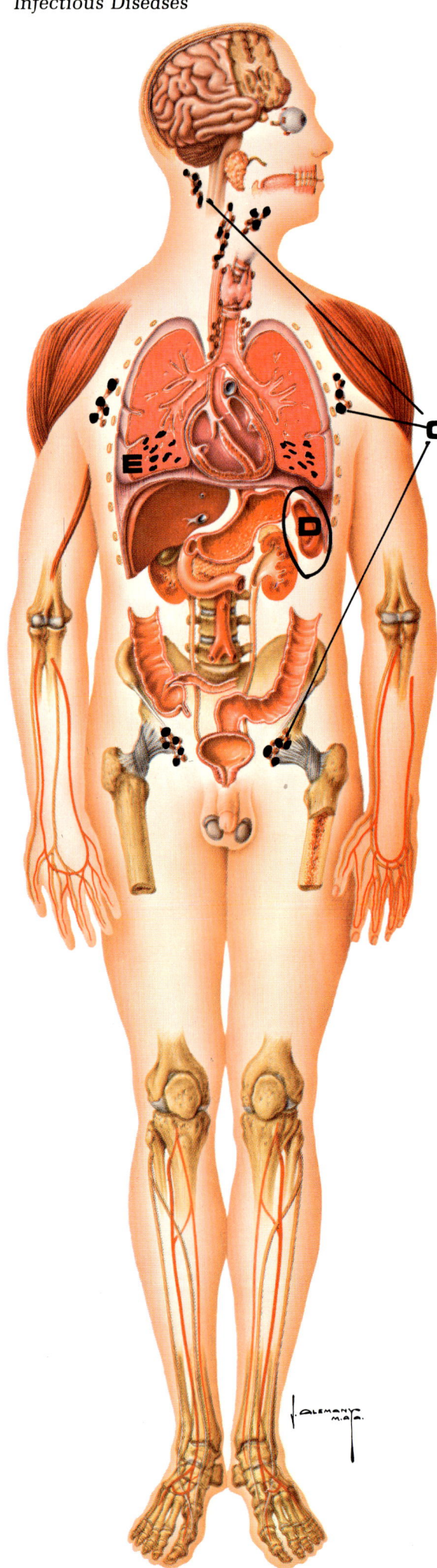

Scrub Typhus

A 36-year-old Korean farmer suddenly developed headache, fever, and chills. By the time he arrived at the physician's office 3 days later, he complained of a sore on his right arm.

Physical examination revealed a temperature of 104° F., a large eschar on the right arm (A), a macular rash of his chest and back (B), generalized lymphadenopathy (C), and splenomegaly (D).

Laboratory examination revealed a positive Weil-Felix reaction to the OX-K strains of *Proteus vulgaris* and, 3 weeks later, a positive complement-fixation test.

X-ray examination of the chest revealed patchy infiltration in both lower lobes (E).

Treatment with chloramphenicol was very effective.

Differential Diagnosis:
1. Meningococcemia
2. Rat-bite fever
3. Q-fever
4. Typhoid fever
5. Malaria
6. Leptospirosis
7. Tularemia
8. Bubonic plague
9. Periarteritis nodosa

Clinical Note. The eschar at the site of the mite bite makes this disease easy to diagnose, but unfortunately it is present in only half the cases. In addition, the rash rarely is purpuric and is hard to see on dark-skinned people, as in Rocky Mountain spotted fever and epidemic typhus. The nervous system may be involved with the angiitis. The rash spreads centrifugally, as in epidemic typhus. The geographical distribution (in the coastal regions of Asia from Korea to India and the Pacific Islands) helps to distinguish this disease from other rickettsiae.

Pathology. This is microscopically similar to other rickettsial diseases with endothelial proliferation, thrombosis, and perivascular cuffing of the small blood vessels. Myocarditis and encephalitis are found in most fatal cases.

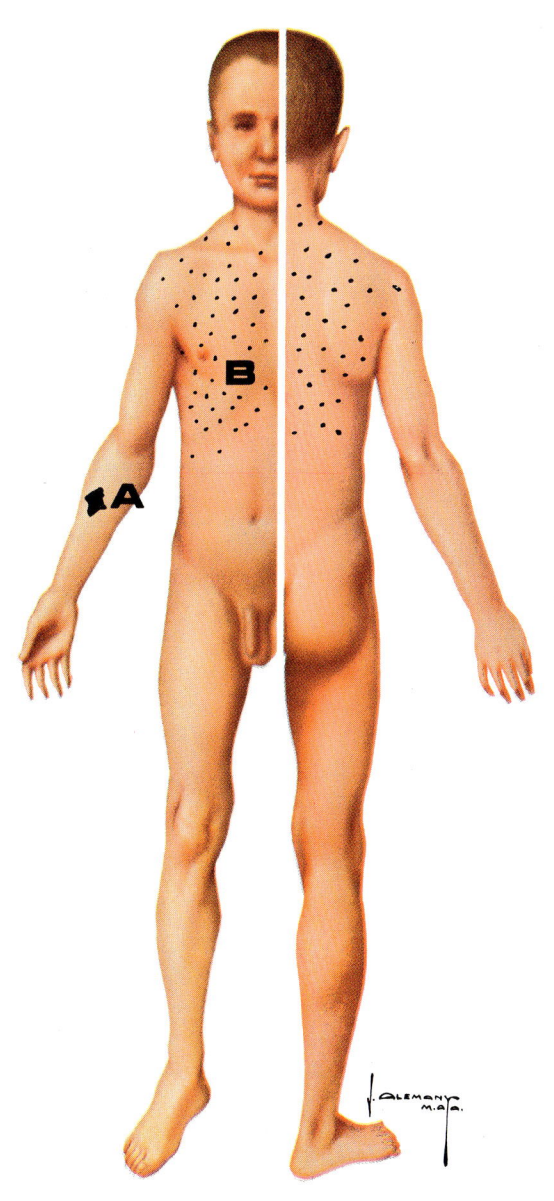

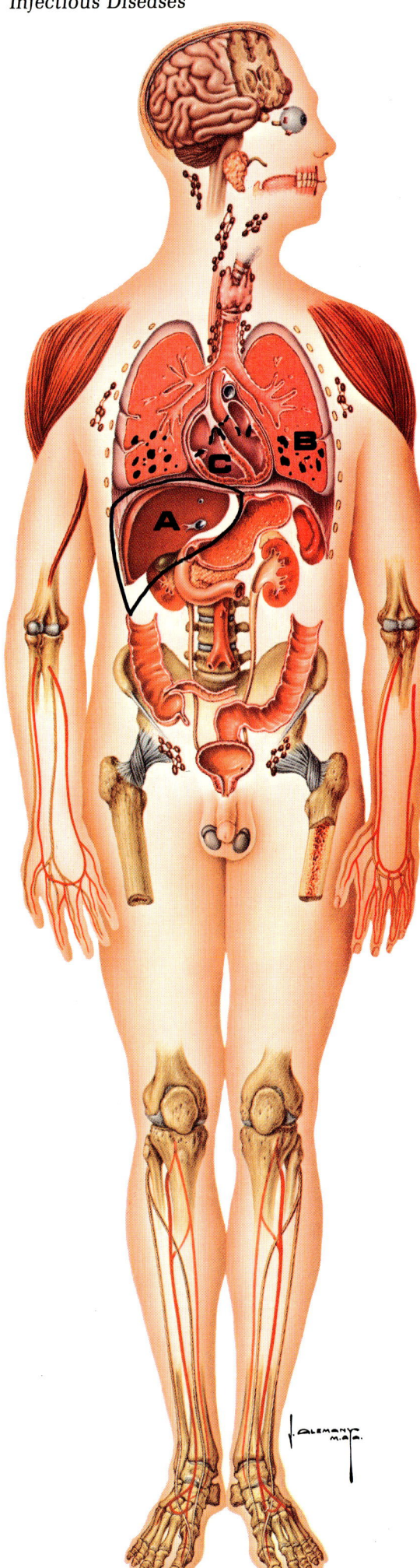

Q-Fever

A 38-year-old farmer developed a severe generalized headache, retro-orbital pain, and fever 1 week prior to admission. On the day of admission he developed a severe dry cough.

Physical examination revealed a temperature of 102° F., a few crepitant rales at both lung bases, and hepatomegaly (A).

Laboratory examination revealed a negative Weil-Felix reaction, but the complement-fixation test showed a rising titer 2 weeks later.

X-ray examination revealed patchy areas of consolidation throughout both lower lobes of the lungs (B).

Differential Diagnosis:
1. Psittacosis
2. Coccidioidomycosis
3. Histoplasmosis
4. Tuberculosis
5. Tularemia
6. Eaton agent pneumonia

Clinical Note. The lung is typically involved in this disease, and hepatomegaly is not common except in prolonged illness. Chronic infection is also associated with an endocarditis (C). The illness usually ends in complete recovery, but relapses are not unusual. Physicians encounter numerous cases of an influenza-like syndrome these days, and it is dangerous to pass them all off as viral without further investigation for not just rickettsia but for tuberculosis and fungal diseases, which are treatable.

Pathology. Microscopically, there is mononuclear infiltration of the alveolar walls and a serofibrinous exudate of the alveolar lumina. This disorder presents a close resemblance to viral pneumonia. In some cases there are miliary granulomata of the liver and vegetations of the mitral and aortic valves.

BACTERIA

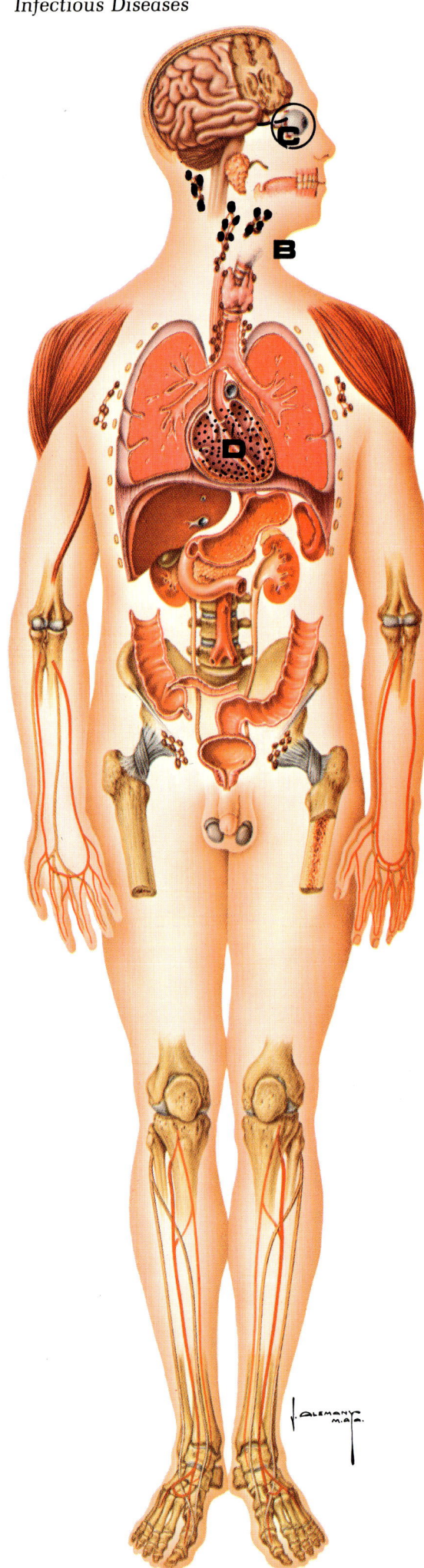

Diphtheria

A 13-year-old white male developed fever, chills, and a mild sore throat 24 hours before admission. On the day of admission he became hoarse, and his breathing became labored.

Physical examination revealed a pale, cyanotic wheezing white male with tachypnea, tachycardia, and flaring of the alae nasi. His throat, tonsils, and larynx were covered with a grayish-yellow membrane (A). There was cervical lymphadenopathy (B).

Laboratory examination revealed a positive culture for *Corynebacterium diphtheriae* and a moderate leukocytosis.

Treatment with 40,000 units of diphtheria antitoxin was begun, and a tracheostomy was performed. One week later he developed a convergent squint, and bilateral external rectus palsy (C) was observed on examination.

Differential Diagnosis:
1. Infectious mononucleosis
2. Streptococcal pharyngitis
3. Agranulocytosis
4. Leukemia
5. Viral pharyngitis

Clinical Note. Here is a disease that affects the throat, heart, and nervous system. Neuropathy appears in only 5 to 10 per cent of cases of diphtheria and usually involves the cranial nerves, particularly the 3rd, 4th, 6th, and 10th (with paralysis of the soft palate). A peripheral neuropathy has been observed as well. Myocarditis (D) may also occur as early as the 2nd week, progressing to congestive heart failure. Over half of the patients with diphtheria have EKG changes at some time during their course. Both the heart and nervous system involvement are due to injury by the toxin and not direct infection with the bacteria. Diphtheria organisms are difficult to recognize on a smear and must be confirmed on culture, which takes time. Thus treatment must often be begun before culture results are reported. The "sore" throat is often mild in this disease.

Pathology. Microscopically, the heart shows interstitial edema and hyaline degeneration in cases with myocarditis. Occasionally there is a cellular exudate. In some cases there may be an acute noncellular interstitial nephritis. The peripheral nerves show degeneration and sometimes complete destruction of the myelin sheaths. Occasionally the axis cylinders also are destroyed.

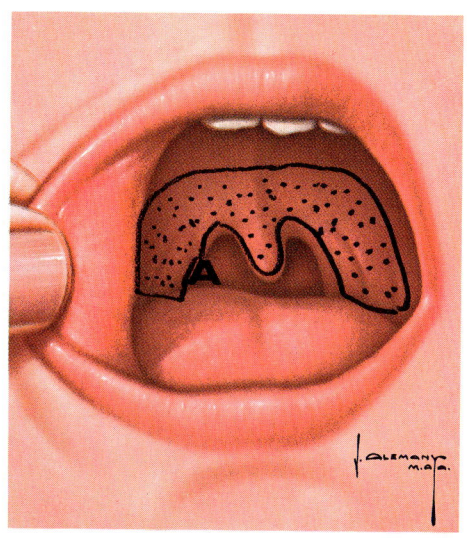

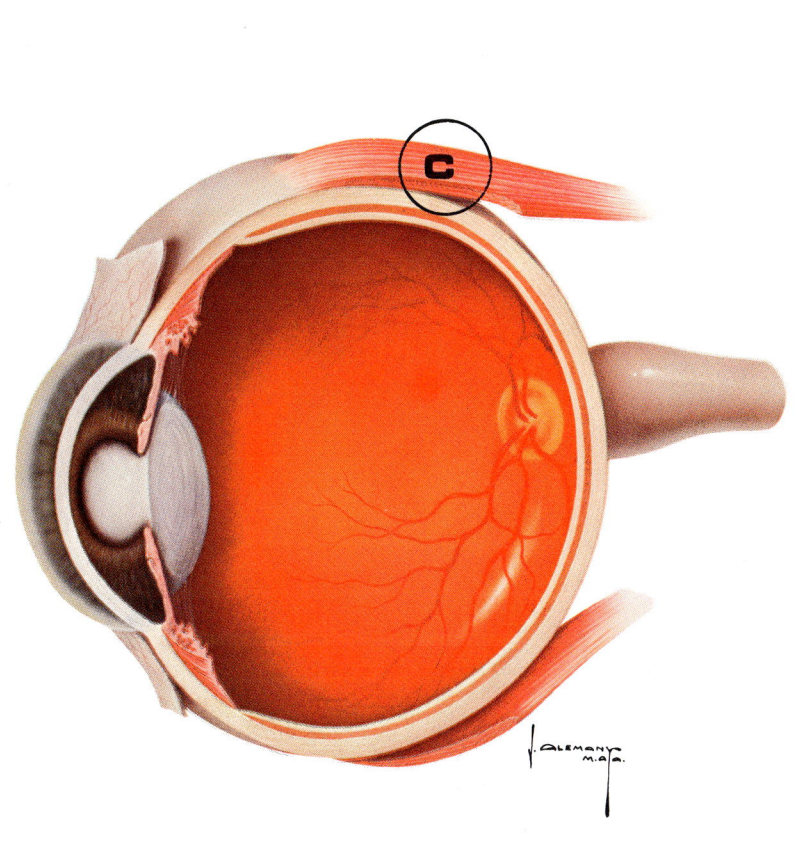

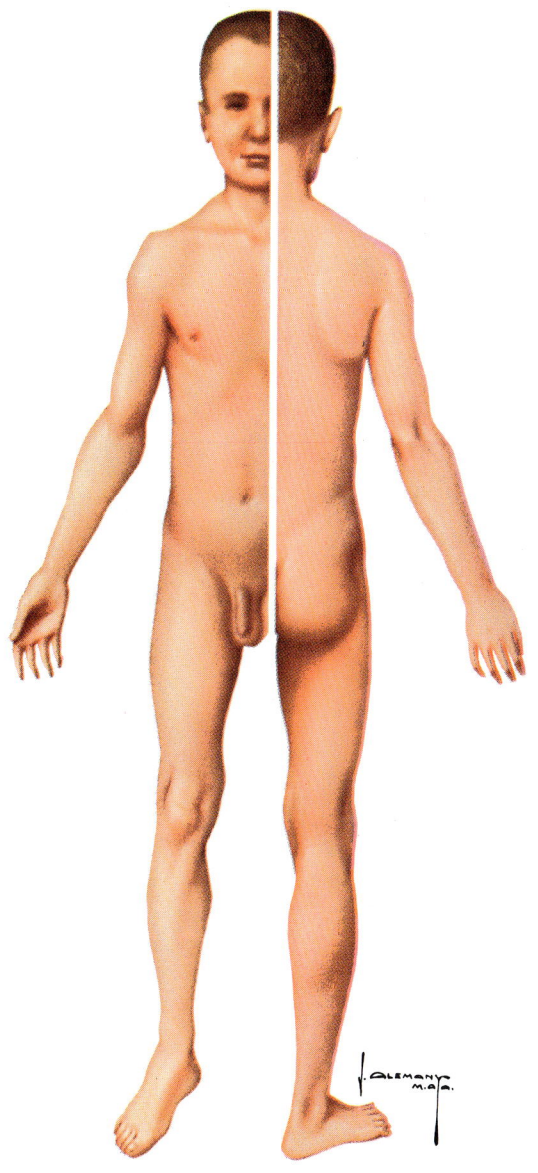

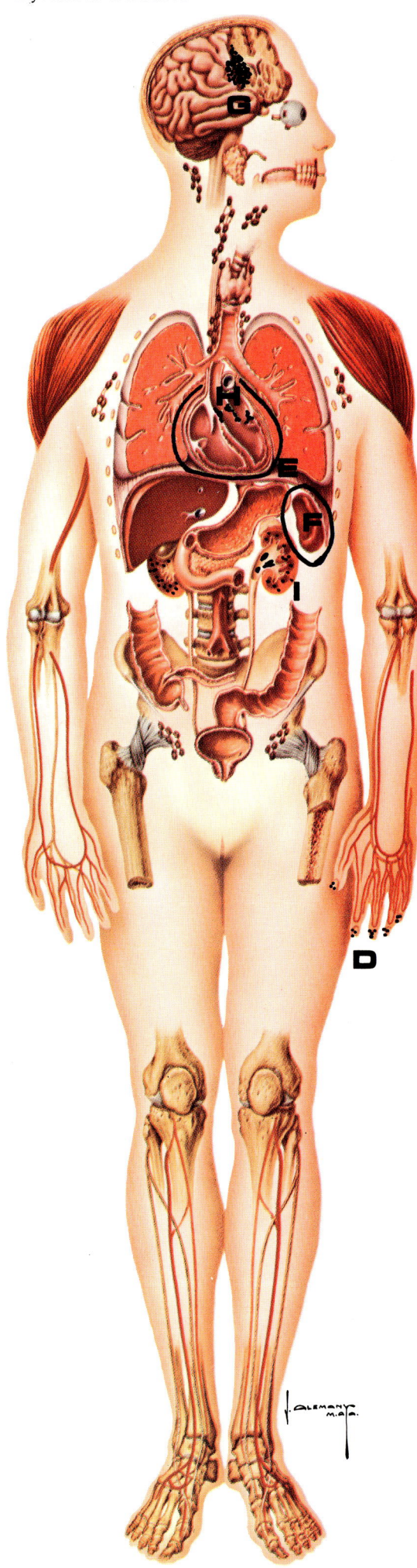

Subacute Bacterial Endocarditis

A 34-year-old white female complained of sudden left flank pain and blood in her urine. She had had rheumatic fever as a child and was left with a murmur, but was not presently on antibiotic prophylaxis.

Physical examination revealed retinal hemorrhages (A), petechial hemorrhages of the conjunctiva (B), Osler's nodes (pea-sized nodules on the pads of the fingers) (C), nail hemorrhages (D), a grade III apical systolic murmur transmitted over the precordium and axilla, cardiomegaly (E), and splenomegaly (F). Three days after admission she developed left hemiplegia (due to cerebral embolism) (G).

Laboratory examination revealed leukocytosis, gross hematuria (I), and positive blood and bone marrow cultures for *Streptococcus viridans*.

Treatment with 40 million units of crystalline penicillin daily intravenously brought about recovery.

Differential Diagnosis:
1. Lupus erythematosus
2. Periarteritis nodosa
3. Brucellosis
4. Tuberculosis
5. Metastatic carcinoma
6. Renal calculus
7. Thrombotic thrombocytopenic purpura
8. Hodgkin's disease
9. Serum sickness
10. Acute rheumatic fever
11. Auricular fibrillation
12. Acute myocardial infarction with emboli
13. Meningococcemia

Clinical Note. This is another disease that may involve virtually every organ. The blood vessels go everywhere, and so emboli can go everywhere. Hemiplegia, coma, or other neurologic manifestations may be the initial symptom. If there is embolism to the spleen, there may be left upper quadrant pain and a friction rub. Often the only complaint is persisting fever, and the only finding a heart murmur. All too frequently therapy is begun before an adequate number of blood cultures has been taken. This is the reason that there are so many negative blood cultures today. A bone marrow may be positive when the blood cultures are negative. Although *Streptococcus viridans* accounts for the majority of cases, staphylococcus, enterococcus, pneumococci, and gram-negative organisms are being found increasingly in the antibiotic era. Bacterial endocarditis may develop on congenital and atherosclerotic lesions of the heart and great vessels.

Pathology. The aortic and mitral valves are most frequently involved (H) with friable masses of fibrin, bacteria, and valve substance. There is rarely any intense cellular reaction, but fibrous organization occurs later. The aortic valve may undergo perforation, and rupture of chordae tendineae or papillary muscle may occur. All three of these may produce congestive heart failure. Emboli may be found anywhere in the body, and there may be miliary abscess formation, particularly with organisms other than *Streptococcus viridans*.

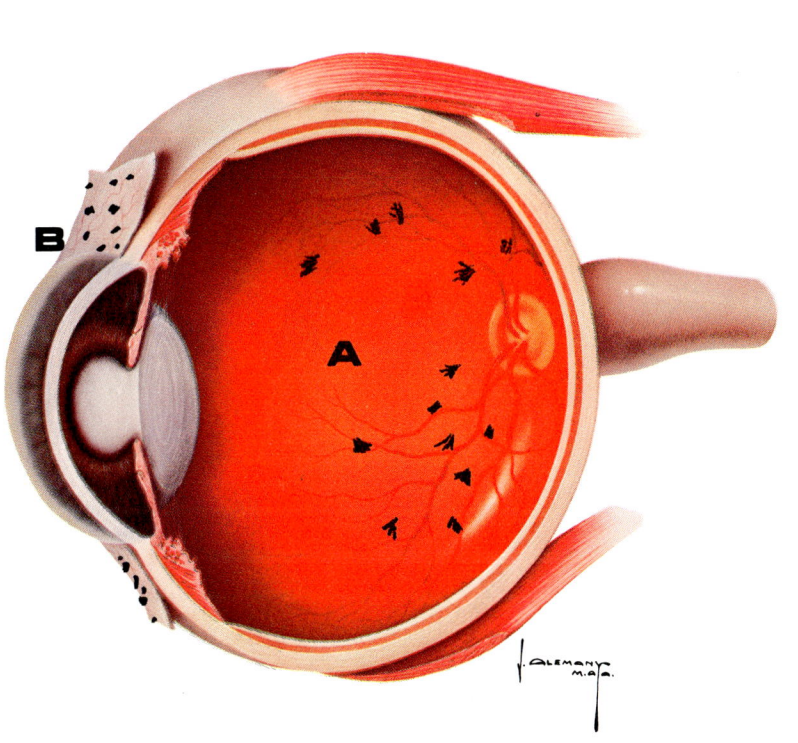
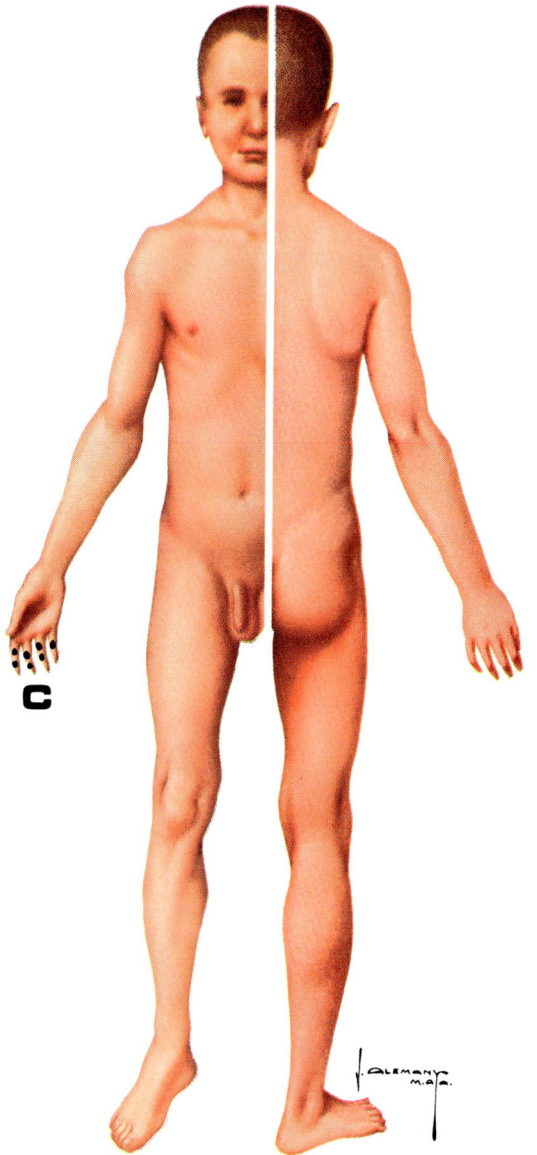

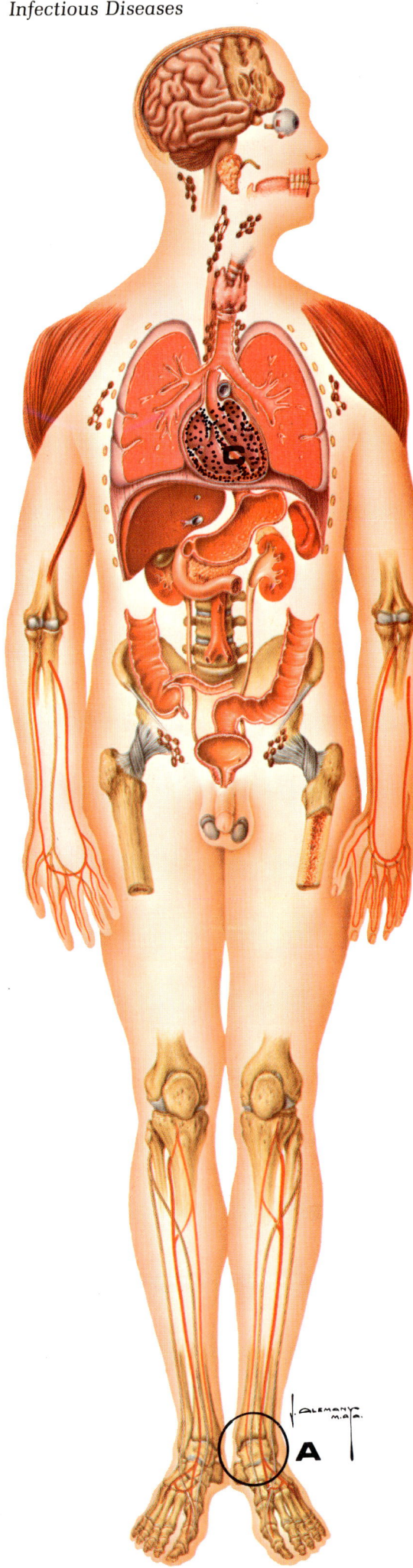

Acute Rheumatic Fever

A 15-year-old white boy was admitted to the hospital with a spiking temperature and a painful swollen left ankle. Twelve days prior to admission he had developed a sore throat and fever, which quickly subsided when treated by his local physician. He had had frequent sore throats since early childhood. His mother had had rheumatic fever as a child.

Physical examination revealed a temperature of 101° F., a red-hot swollen left ankle (A), iris-shaped lesions of the dorsum of the hands, arms, and thorax (erythema multiforme) (B), and a grade III apical holosystolic murmur (C), indicating cardiac involvement. The murmur and rash changed from day to day, and the swelling of the left ankle disappeared. Subsequently subcutaneous nodules (D) were felt over the elbows.

Laboratory examination revealed an ASO titer of 1,225 units, an elevated sedimentation rate, and the C-reactive protein was 4+. A throat culture revealed beta-hemolytic streptococci. The EKG was normal.

Treatment with salicylates was effective. A 10-day course of penicillin was also given.

Differential Diagnosis:
1. Rheumatoid arthritis
2. Lupus erythematosus
3. Infectious mononucleosis
4. Gonorrhea
5. Serum sickness
6. Subacute bacterial endocarditis
7. Wilson's disease
8. Brucellosis
9. Haverhill fever
10. Sickle cell anemia

Clinical Note. Here is a disease that involves the skin, joints, heart, and nervous system (Syndenham's chorea was not present in this case). Lupus erythematosus may do this, but other disorders in the differential list rarely affect all 4 of these. Most cases of rheumatic fever are not as typical as this one. There may be merely fever and tachycardia without clinical evidence of specific organ involvement. According to the Jones criteria, diagnosis may be established if there are 2 major manifestations present (carditis, arthritis, chorea, skin manifestations) or 1 major and 2 or more minor manifestations (fever, elevated ASO titer, prolonged PR interval, etc.). The case presented here fulfills this criteria easily (3 major manifestations: carditis, dermatitis, arthritis). The ASO titer is not always elevated, but at least one of the antibodies to streptococcus is (antistreptodornase, antihyaluronidase, etc.). The EKG changes of prolonged PR interval and prolonged QT interval were not present in this case. Adequate treatment of a streptococcal infection consists of the administration of penicillin for at least 10 days.

Pathology. Multiple areas of inflammation in the collagen tissue, particularly of the blood vessels, is seen throughout the body, especially in the heart, skin, joints, and brain. Rarely is there pulmonary involvement. The Aschoff body, which has been described as a "fibrinoid degeneration of the collagen," is the most typical pattern, just as the tubercle is the typical pattern of tuberculosis.

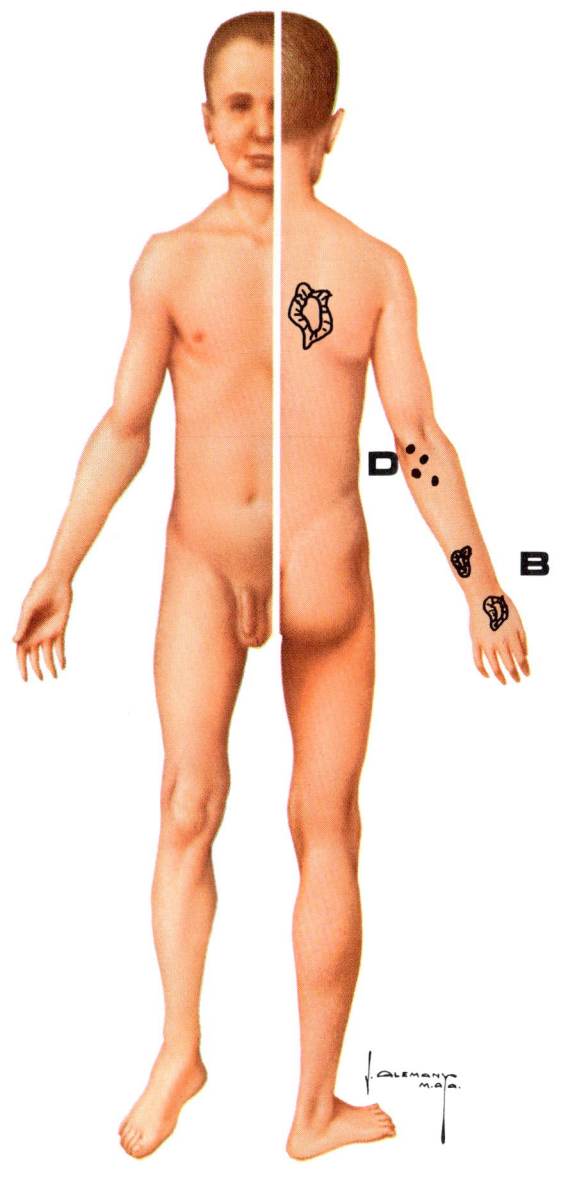

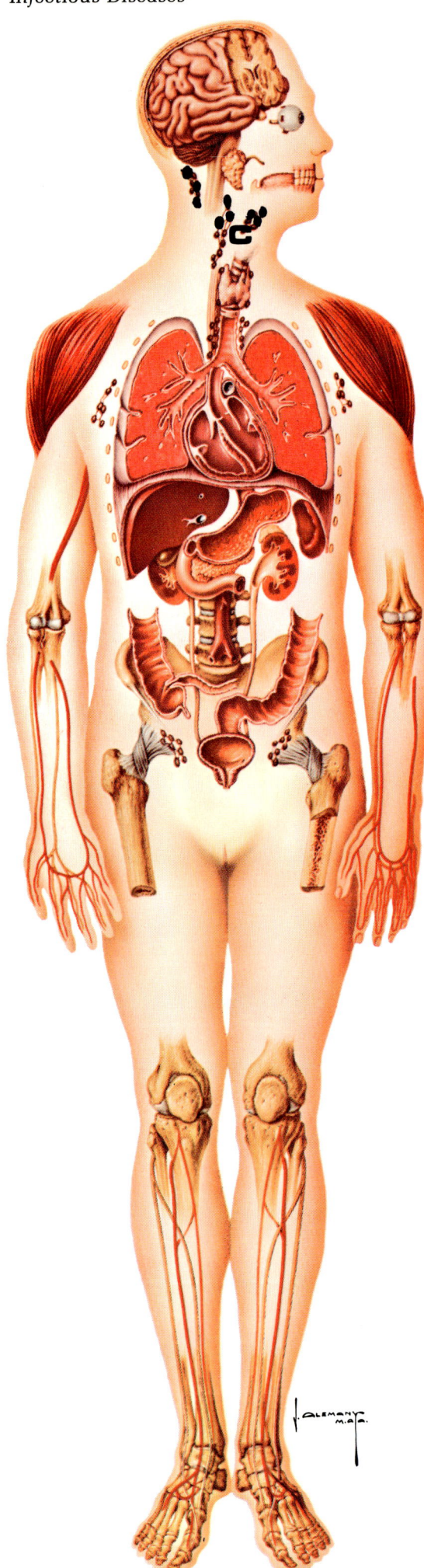

Scarlet Fever

A 4-year-old white female developed sudden fever, vomiting, and difficulty in swallowing.

Physical examination revealed swollen red exudative tonsils (A), a white strawberry tongue (B), enlarged anterior and posterior cervical lymph nodes (C), and an erythematous confluent eruption of the neck, trunk, and proximal portion of the extremities, with circumoral pallor (D).

Laboratory examination revealed group A beta-hemolytic streptococci on culture and a positive Schultz-Charlton reaction. On testing, there was a positive Rumpel-Leede phenomenon.

Treatment with a 10-day course of penicillin was effective.

Differential Diagnosis:
1. Measles
2. Rubella
3. Infectious mononucleosis

4. Diphtheria
5. Agranulocytosis
6. Leukemia
7. Meningococcemia
8. Drug eruption
9. Enteroviral eruptions
10. Viral pharyngitis

Clinical Note. Exudates are not present in all cases of streptococcal pharyngitis; nor is a "scarlet" rash present very often anymore. Occasionally there is a bacteremia with septic arthritis, as in gonorrhea. The worst complications are rheumatic fever (p. 140) and acute glomerulonephritis. It is not well recognized that hemolytic streptococci are the only significant bacterial cause of pharyngitis, exudative or nonexudative. Pneumococcus and staphylococcus do not cause this type of infection.

Pathology. There is a toxic injury to the capillary endothelium in the skin, leading to atony and dilatation of the capillaries. Edema and round cell infiltration in the skin fill out the picture.

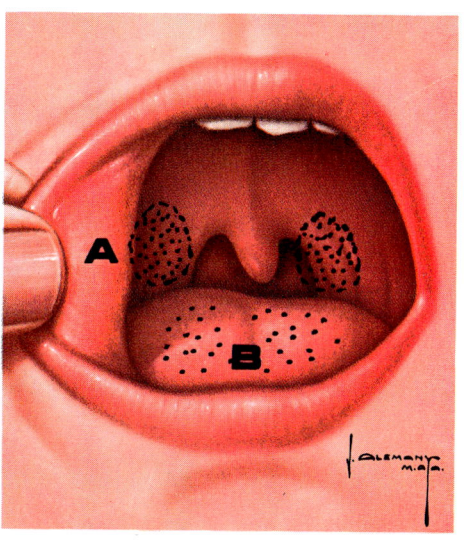

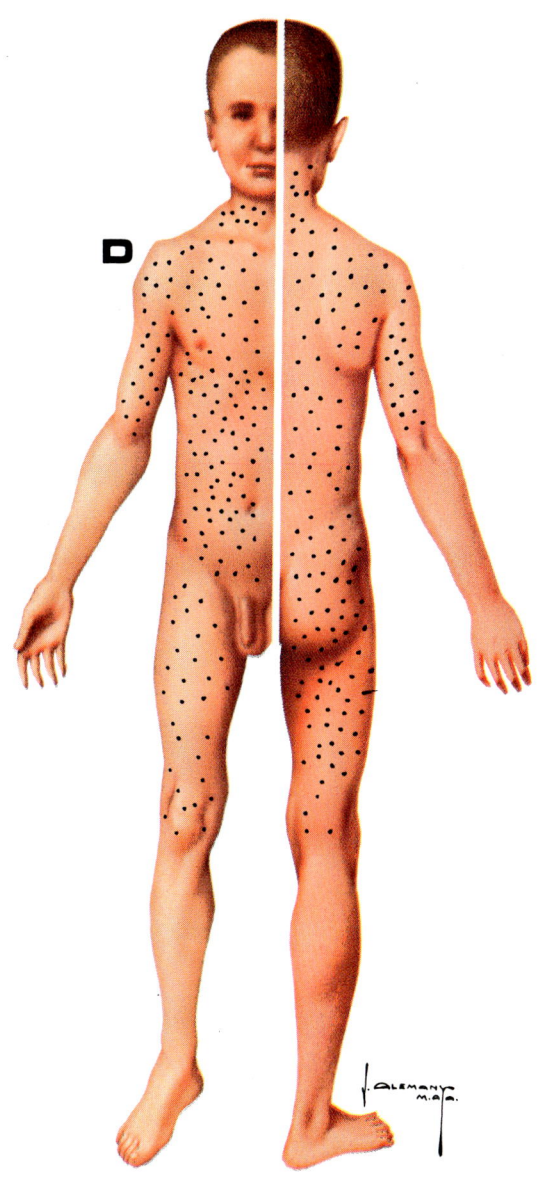

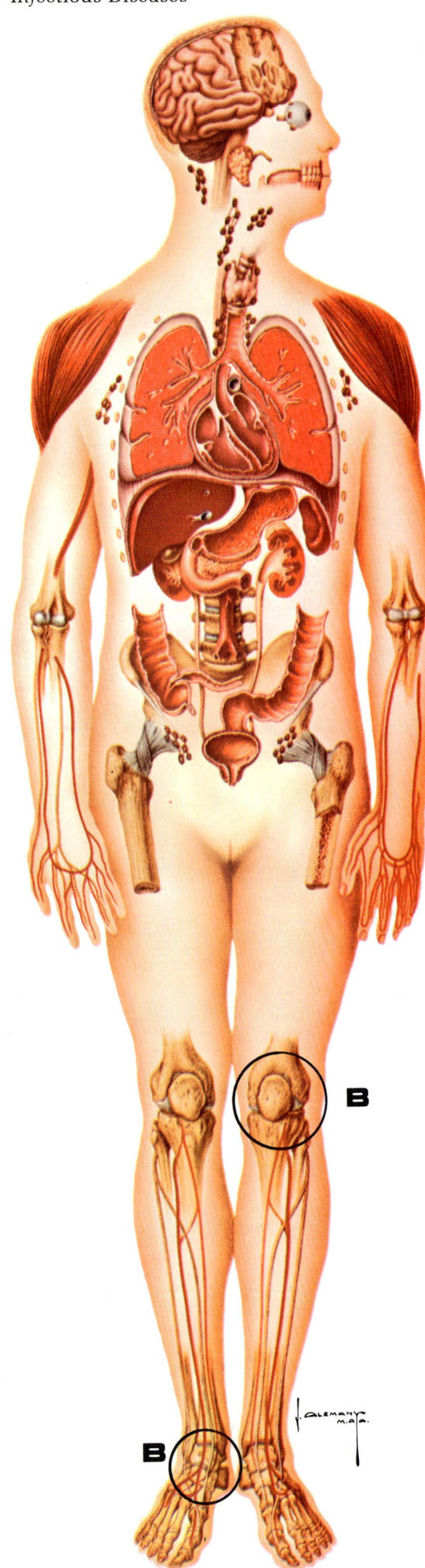

Streptobacillary Fever

An 8-year-old white female developed a sudden temperature, headache, nausea, and vomiting 4 days prior to admission. Two days later her mother noted a generalized maculopapular rash. On the day of admission her left knee and right ankle became swollen and painful.

Physical examination revealed a generalized maculopapular rash (A) and swollen, tender, red left knee and right ankle joints (B).

Laboratory examination revealed a white count of 18,500 cells/cu. mm., most of which were neutrophils. The Wassermann was nonreactive, but there was a high titer of agglutinins to *Streptobacillus moniliformis,* and a mice inoculation test was positive.

Treatment with penicillin was effective.

Differential Diagnosis:
1. Acute rheumatic fever
2. Infectious mononucleosis
3. Spirillary rat-bite fever

4. Reiter's syndrome
5. Syphilis
6. Rheumatoid arthritis
7. Scarlet fever
8. Meningococcemia
9. Brucellosis
10. Gonorrhea
11. Lupus erythematosus
12. Serum sickness

Clinical Note. It is readily apparent that this disease is different from spirillary rat-bite fever. A nonmigratory frank arthritis is present, there is rarely an inflammatory reaction at the bite-site, regional adenopathy is insignificant, and there is no false positive Wassermann. This condition greatly resembles acute rheumatic fever and, in fact, may cause an ulcerative endocarditis. The diagnostic value of a good course of penicillin is worth mention. In this way acute rheumatic fever and rheumatoid arthritis may be differentiated.

Pathology. In this condition many more organs are involved pathologically than are reflected clinically. Cloudy swelling is found in liver and kidney cells, and there is hyperplasia of the spleen.

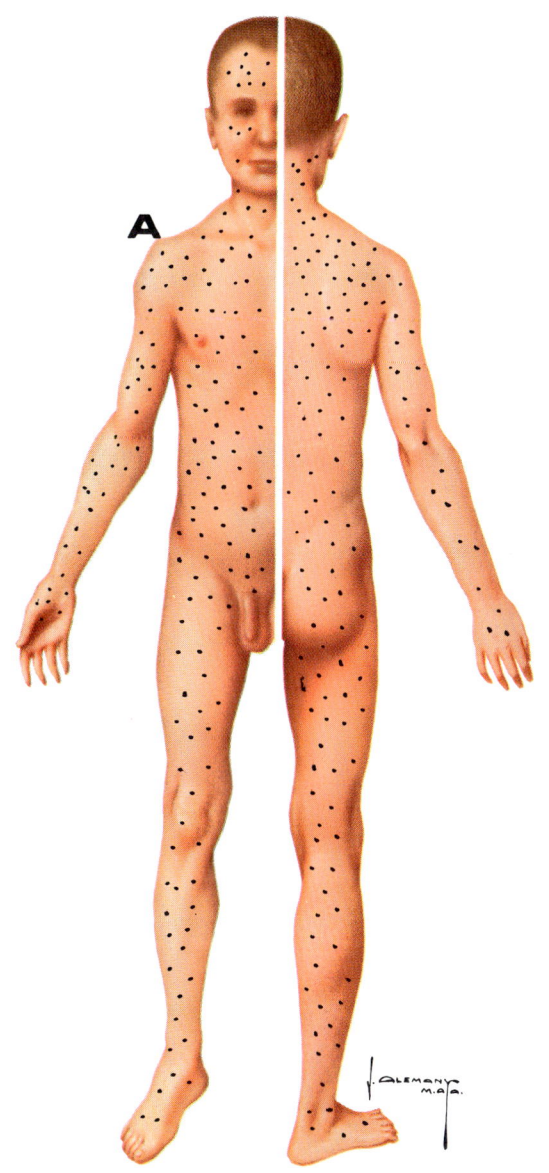

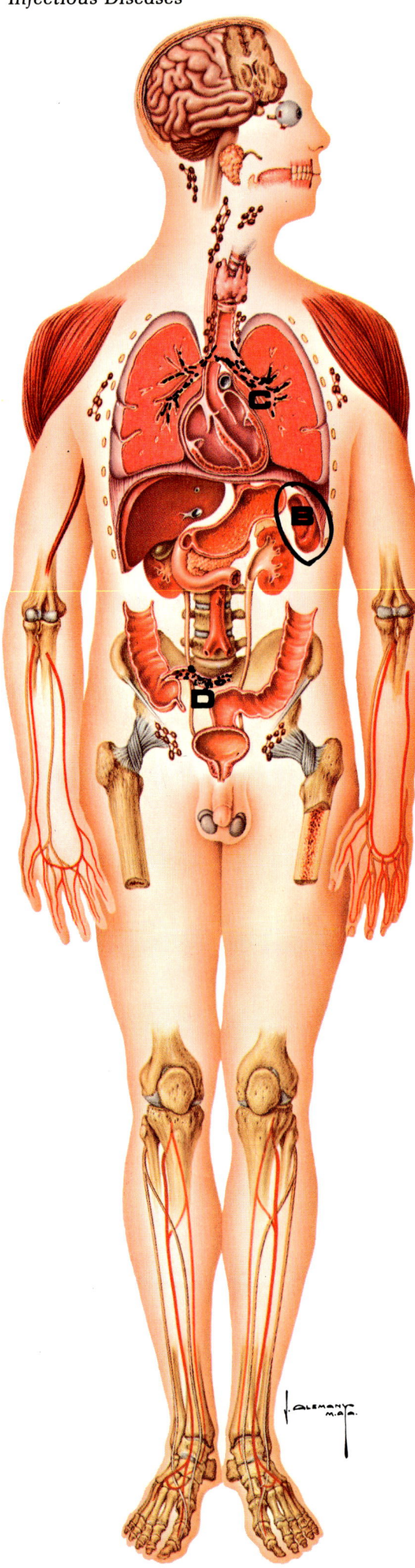

Typhoid Fever

A 26-year-old white male developed a low-grade fever, headache, and a nonproductive cough 1 week prior to admission. His local physician had diagnosed his condition as viral influenza. At home, despite bedrest and supportive measures, the temperature continued and began to spike higher each day. On the day of admission he had a nosebleed.

Physical examination on admission was unremarkable except for fever. However, 3 days after admission he developed watery greenish diarrhea. The fever continued. One week after admission he developed a macular rash (A) on the trunk and abdomen, and the spleen (B) could be palpated.

Laboratory examination disclosed a white count of 4,800 cells/cu. mm., with an absolute neutropenia. Stool culture on the 4th hospital day was positive for *Salmonella typhosa*. Febrile agglutinins revealed rising titers of both H and O typhoid antibodies.

Treatment. Chloramphenicol is an excellent drug to use in this disease.

Differential Diagnosis:
1. Atypical pneumonia (Eaton agent)
2. Murine typhus fever
3. Rocky Mountain spotted fever
4. Tuberculosis
5. Hodgkin's disease
6. Brucellosis
7. Malaria
8. Tularemia
9. Paratyphoid fever
10. Dengue

Clinical Note. This condition is frequently mistaken for a viral disease and must be thought of in any case of fever of unknown origin, especially one with a stair-step character. Although this is usually thought of as an enteric disease, diarrhea appears late. Physical examination is usually of no help in early stages. The organism can be isolated from the blood only in the 1st week, but a bone marrow puncture may be positive anytime in the first 4 weeks.

Pathology. There is inflammation of the bronchi (C), and generalized lymphoid hyperplasia, especially in Peyer's patch (D) of the terminal ileum, where necrosis and ulceration develop. These ulcers may hemorrhage or perforate. The "rose spots" are probably sites of bacterial embolization.

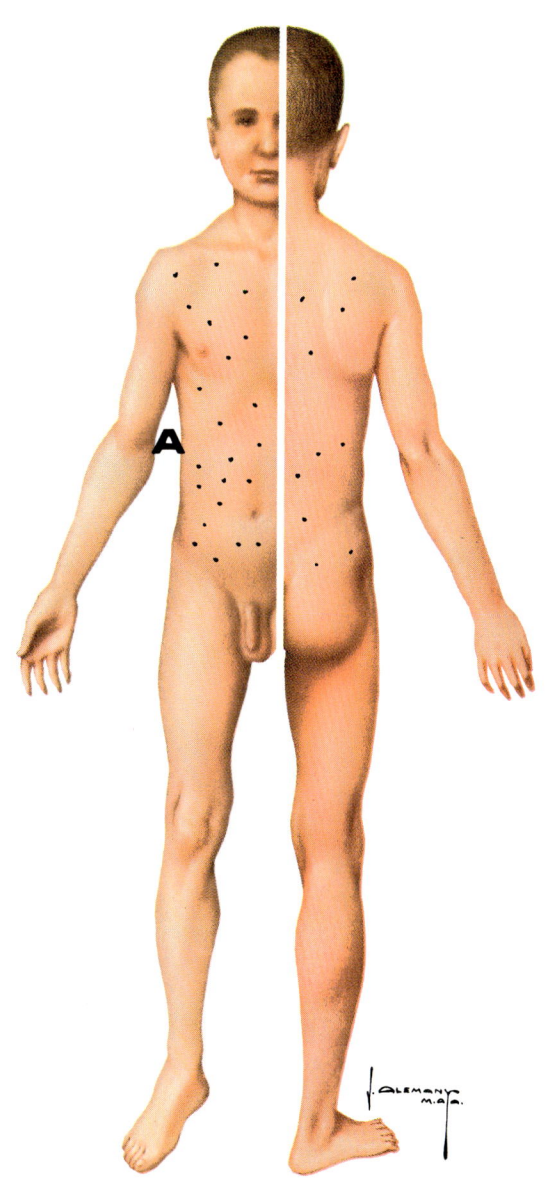

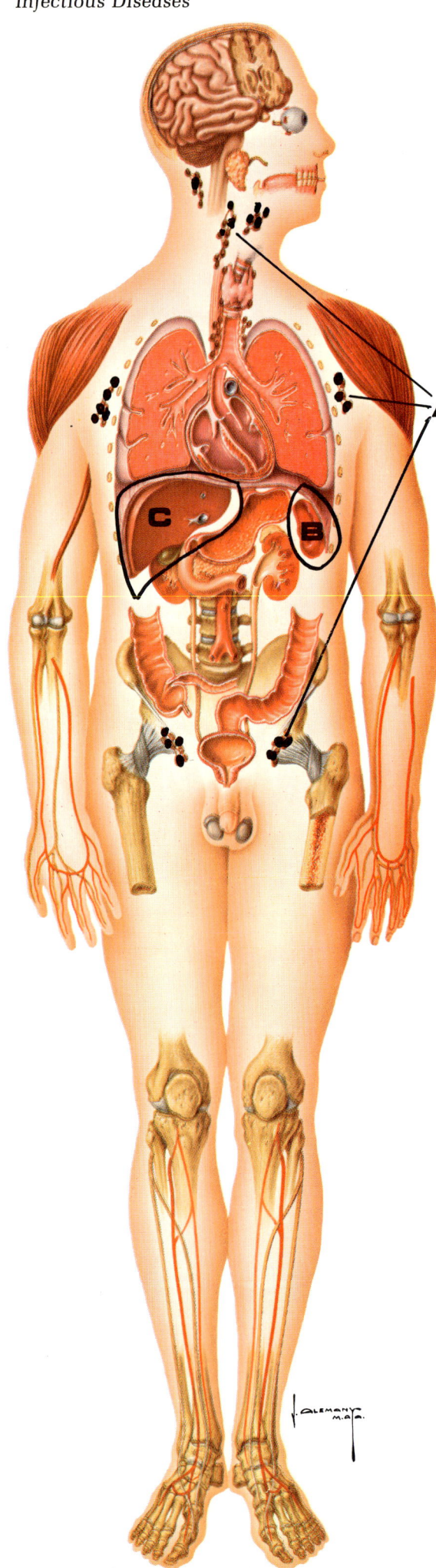

Brucellosis

A 36-year-old white farmer was referred for admission because of intermittent chills and fever of 6 weeks' duration. The temperature usually rose in the afternoon. In addition, he had had progressive weakness, loss of appetite, and generalized aches and pains. His wife complained that he was very "edgy."

Physical examination revealed a temperature of 101° F., generalized adenopathy (A) and a palpable spleen 3 cm. below the left subcostal margin (B).

Laboratory examination revealed a WBC of 5,300 cells/cu. mm., with a relative lymphocytosis, and a rising titer of brucellin agglutinins on 2 successive sera. Repeated blood cultures were negative.

Differential Diagnosis:
1. Infectious mononucleosis
2. Typhoid fever
3. Leukemia
4. Tuberculosis
5. Histoplasmosis
6. Collagen diseases
7. Sarcoidosis
8. Lymphoma
9. Malaria

Clinical Note. The symptoms listed in this case make it easy to understand why these patients are labeled psychoneurotic. Hepatomegaly (C) is not rare, but central and peripheral nerve, bone, vascular, and pulmonary lesions are infrequent. Blood cultures should be taken in all cases. As many as 50 per cent may be positive. The skin test is an unreliable method of diagnosis.

Pathology. The organs of the reticuloendothelial system are involved by lymphoid hyperplasia, focal necrosis, and nodular granulomas similar to tubercles but without caseation. The organisms exist intracellularly.

Gonorrhea

A 17-year-old Negro male complained of pain and swelling of 2 days' duration in his left knee. History revealed that 2 weeks prior to admission he had experienced burning on urination and a yellowish urethral discharge (A). He had gone to his local physician and had received an injection of penicillin. He was then asymptomatic until 4 days prior to admission, when he developed chills and fever, and pain in both wrists and the left ankle. This disappeared when he developed the symptoms in his left knee (B). He admitted to contact 3 weeks prior to admission.

Physical examination revealed a swollen, warm, and tender left knee with pain on the slightest flexion and extension. There was a whitish urethral discharge.

Laboratory study revealed negative cultures of joint fluid, but the gonococcal complement-fixation test was positive.

Treatment. Pain and swelling subsided gradually after a 2-week course of 600,000 units of procaine penicillin twice daily.

Differential Diagnosis:
1. Reiter's disease
2. Rheumatoid arthritis
3. Serum sickness
4. Gout
5. Rat-bite fever
6. Rheumatic fever
7. Brucellosis
8. Collagen disease

Clinical Note. This complication of gonorrhea is uncommon now, but a single injection of penicillin is not adequate to prevent it. Distinction from rheumatoid arthritis is difficult at times because of sterile joint fluid and the migratory nature of the arthritis. The complement-fixation test is very useful.

Pathology. There are hyperemia and polymorphonuclear exudate of the urethral mucosa. Extension of urethral inflammation to the prostate, epididymis, and seminal vesicles is not uncommon if untreated. Gonococcal endocarditis (C), another complication, is now very rare. Although there is increase of neutrophils and protein in the joint fluid, the only reaction in the synovium is hyperemia in the early stages.

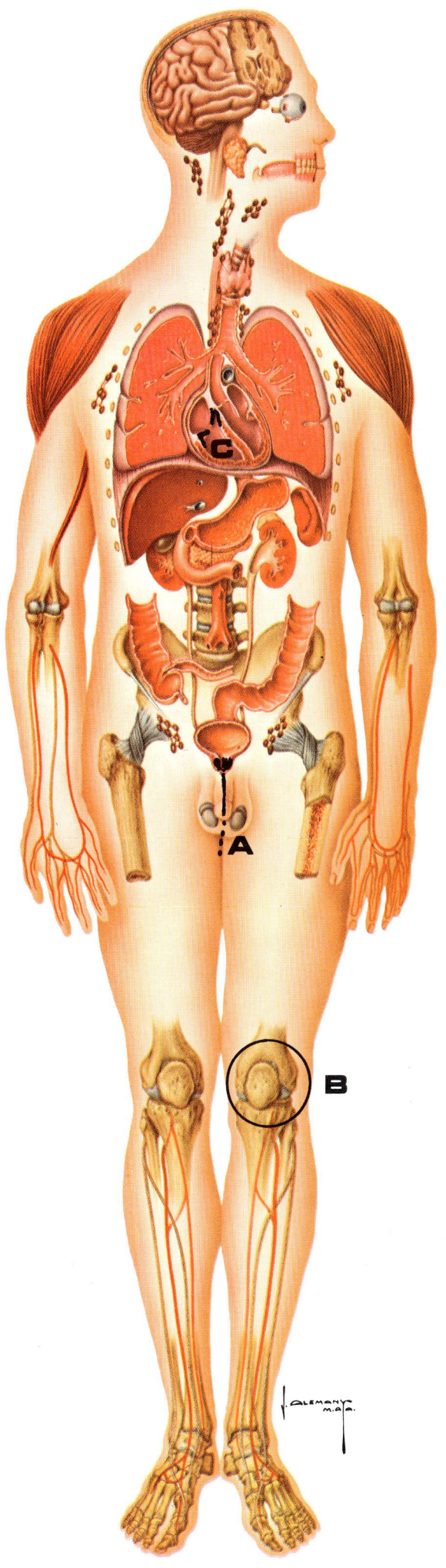

150 · Infectious Diseases

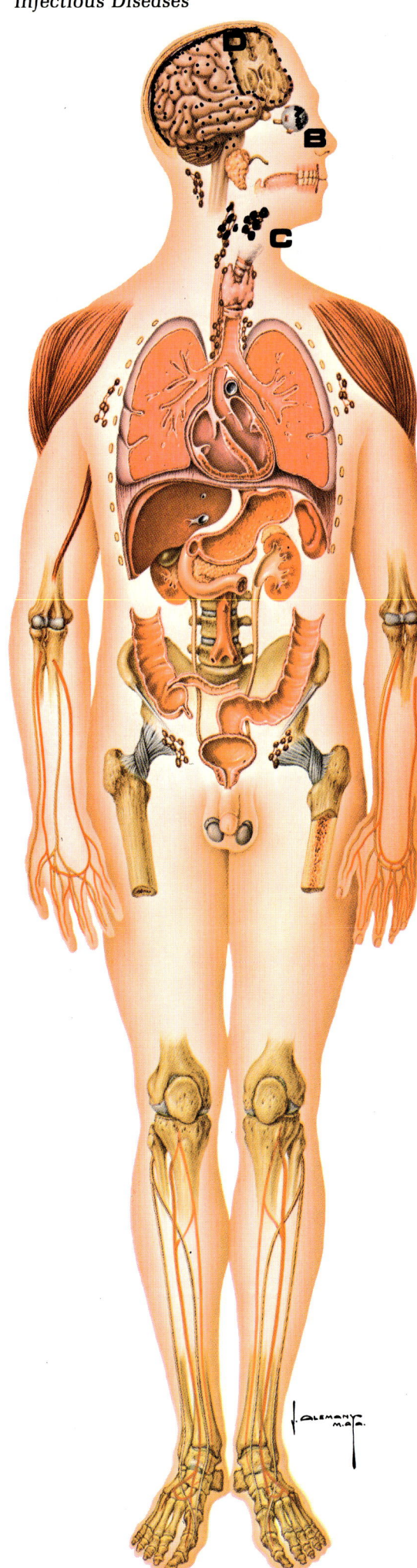

Listeriosis

A 32-year-old white male developed generalized headache, stiff neck, and fever. He had experienced a mild sore throat for 3 days prior to admission.

Physical examination revealed an injected throat and tonsils (A) and conjunctiva (B), marked bilateral cervical adenopathy (C), nuchal rigidity, and a positive Kernig's sign, indicating meningeal involvement (D).

Laboratory examination of the spinal fluid revealed 750 cells/cu. mm., most of which were neutrophils, a protein of 110 mg. and a sugar of 44 mg. per cent. Culture revealed a diphtheroid bacillus, but rabbit inoculation produced a characteristic keratoconjunctivitis.

Treatment with penicillin was effective.

Differential Diagnosis:
1. Infectious mononucleosis
2. Streptococcal pharyngitis
3. Miliary tuberculosis
4. Meningococcemia
5. Typhoid fever

6. Pneumococcal meningitis
7. Aseptic meningitis
8. Poliomyelitis
9. Leptospirosis
10. Brucellosis
11. Cryptococcosis
12. Viral encephalitis

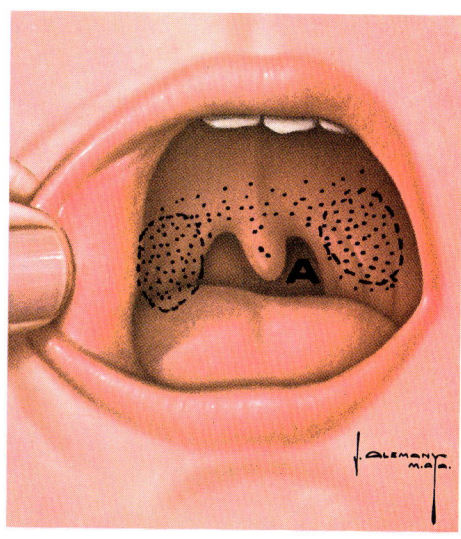

Clinical Note. This disease has a marked similarity to infectious mononucleosis. Both may involve the throat, lymph nodes, liver, spleen, and meninges. However, listeriosis most commonly presents as a meningitis, whereas infectious mononucleosis presents with a sore throat and cervical adenopathy. Infectious mononucleosis involves the liver and spleen more consistently. Conjunctivitis is peculiar to listeriosis. The isolation of the *Listeria* bacillus from the throat, blood, bone marrow, or urine and a negative heterophil antibody titer will make the distinction. Listeriosis has been accused of presenting as a mild influenza-like syndrome, a chronic urethritis, papular skin lesion, pneumonia and empyema. Any organ of the body may be involved.

Pathology. The bacillus provokes both acute suppurative and chronic granulomata, with focal necrosis in the involved tissues.

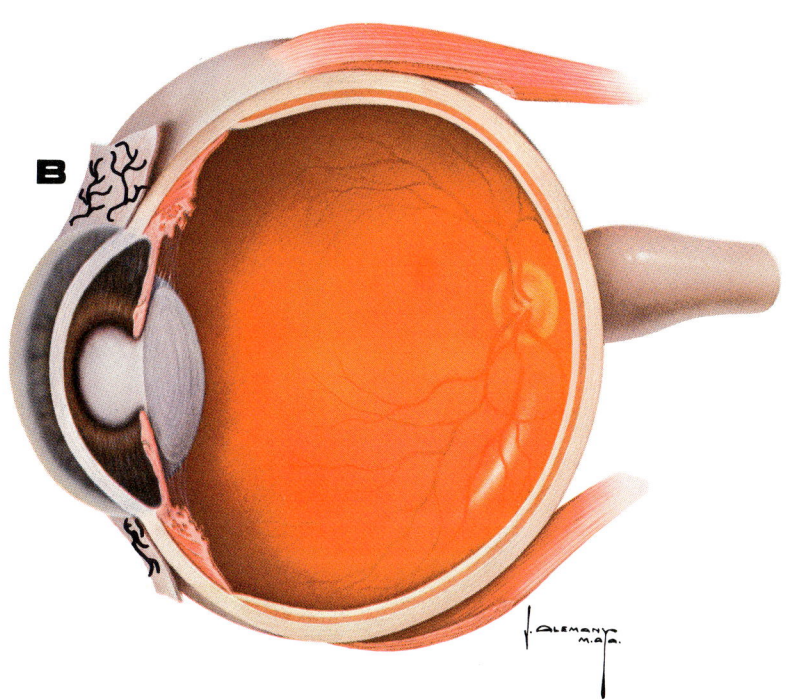

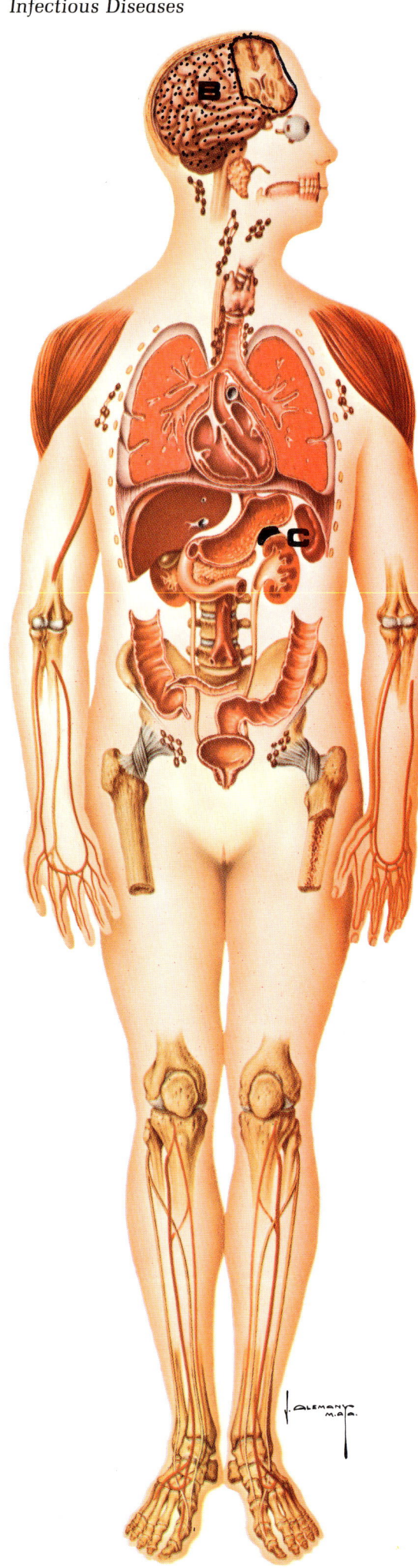

Meningococcemia

A 6-year-old white female was brought to the emergency room in a confused and irritable state. One hour prior to admission she had experienced a grand mal convulsion. In addition, the mother had noted that the child was feverish and had had a mild rash for 2 days prior to admission. There was no history of an upper respiratory infection.

Physical examination disclosed a spotty, generalized rash (A) which did not blanch on pressure; irritability and delirium, nuchal rigidity (B) with a positive Kernig's and Brudzinski's signs, and hyperactive reflexes throughout.

Laboratory examination revealed the cerebrospinal fluid was under a pressure of 350 mm. and contained 7,500 WBC/cu. mm., almost all of them neutrophils. A smear revealed gram-negative intracellular diplococci, and both blood and CSF culture grew out meningococci.

Treatment. She recovered on large doses of sulfasoxazole intravenously.

Differential Diagnosis:
1. Measles encephalitis
2. Typhoid fever

3. Epidemic typhus
4. Rocky Mountain spotted fever
5. Subacute bacterial endocarditis
6. Brucellosis
7. Bacterial meningitis of other causes
8. Subarachnoid hemorrhage
9. Toxic and infectious encephalopathies
10. Gonococcal meningitis

Clinical Note. A history of previous upper respiratory infection is present in 75 per cent of the cases. Unlike typhoid fever rash, this rash is purpuric, except in the early stage, and does not blanch on pressure. Meningitis cases constitute a small percentage of meningococcal infections, a point not commonly realized. More usual is the mild meningococcemia with fever and rash but no other clinically evident metastatic foci. The adrenal gland is a frequent site of metastatic involvement (Waterhouse-Friderichsen syndrome) (C).

Pathology. The skin involvement is characterized by damage to the capillary endothelium, with inflammation of the vessel wall, hemorrhage, and thrombosis. The meninges are coated with a purulent exudate of neutrophils, and there is intense hyperemia. The exudate extends to involve the ventricles. The adrenal glands are involved by hemorrhage, again due to capillary damage.

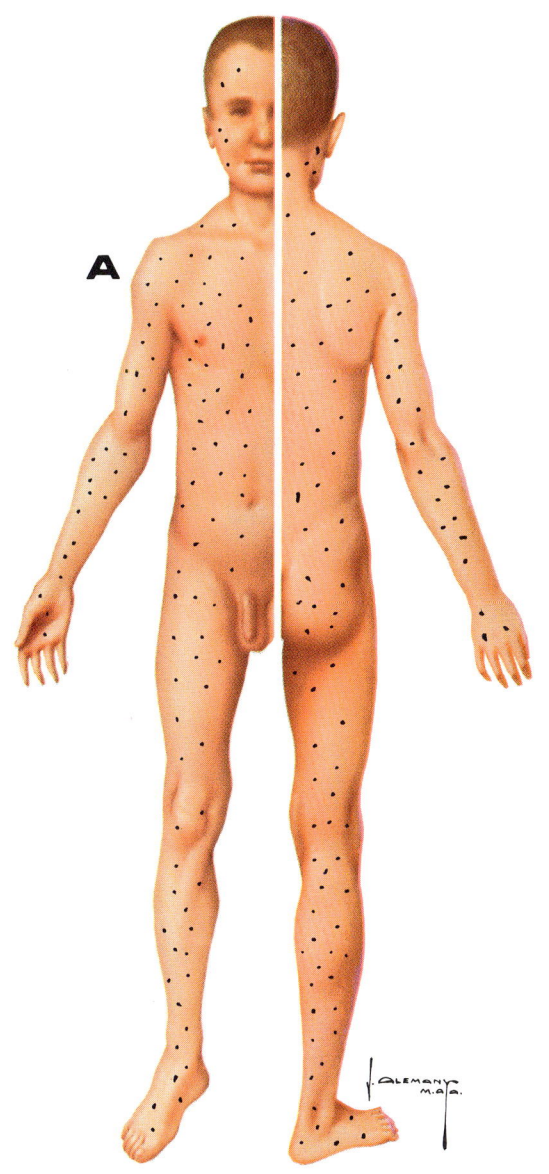

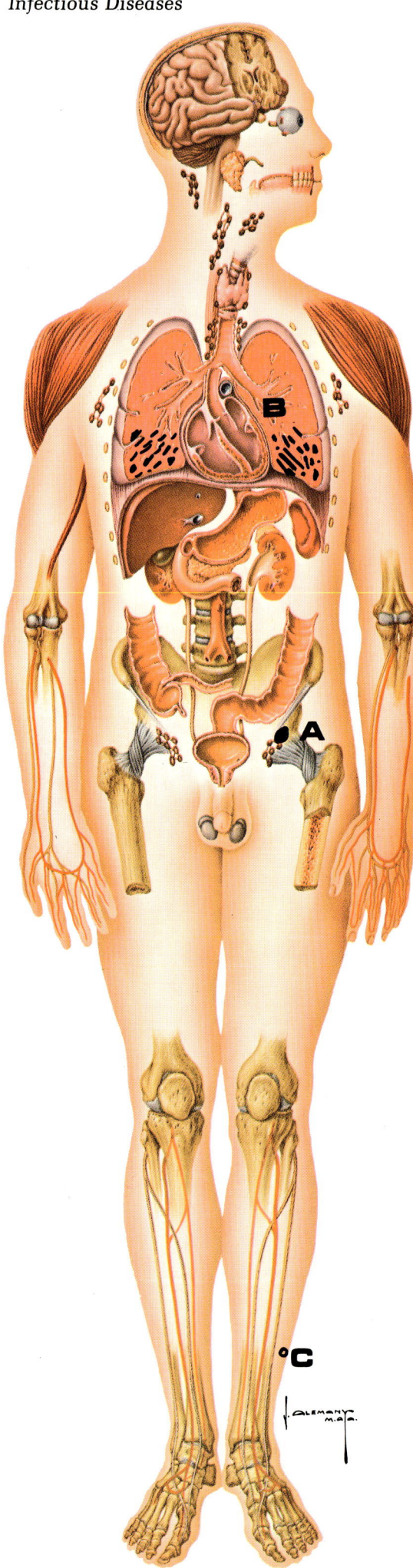

Plague

A 24-year-old Filipino, who had just arrived from the Far East, developed severe fever, generalized aches and pains, and a painful swelling in his left groin.

Physical examination revealed a swollen, tender left inguinal node (bubo) (A), and crepitant and sibilant rales over both lower lobes (B). Although no site of a fleabite was seen, it was presumed to be on the left lower leg (C).

Laboratory examination revealed a leukocytosis and gram-negative bacilli in aspirates from the left inguinal node, which grew out on blood agar and gave a positive test on guinea pig inoculation.

X-ray examination of the chest revealed scattered infiltrations in both lower lobes.

Treatment with chloramphenicol was ineffective.

Differential Diagnosis:
1. Tularemia
2. Lymphogranuloma venereum
3. Sporotrichosis
4. Other bacterial pneumonias
5. Malaria
6. Filariasis
7. Glanders
8. Staphylococcal cellulitis

Clinical Note. The combination of lymphatic and lung involvement is seen in tularemia; but in tularemia the skin becomes indurated and ulcerated at the site of entry of the organism. Although pulmonary involvement is usually secondary in tularemia, except in laboratory workers, plague pneumonia is often primary and spreads from person to person. Laboratory confirmation is easy, but not quick enough, and the clinician must start treatment on the basis of his clinical diagnosis. Bacteremia invariably follows the bubo, but clinical manifestations of renal, cerebral, or gastrointestinal involvement are rare.

Pathology. Microscopic changes in the bubo are an intense hemorrhagic inflammation with neutrophils, progressing to necrosis and a gelatinous edema of contiguous connective tissues and small vessel engorgement. The early lung lesions in the secondary type of pneumonia are perivascular foci of inflammatory cells and colonies of *Pasteurella pestis*. Lobar consolidation with a hemorrhagic exudate takes place so fast that the primary and secondary type become indistinguishable.

Miliary Tuberculosis

A 3-year-old Negro infant developed spiking afternoon fever and shortness of breath. On the day of admission the child became comatose. The mother had recently been discharged from a tuberculosis sanitorium.

Physical examination revealed a comatose child in acute distress with nuchal rigidity, indicating meningitis (A), hepatosplenomegaly (B), choroidal tubercles on ophthalmoscopic examination (C), and generalized lymphadenopathy (D).

Laboratory examination of gastric washings revealed tubercle bacilli on culture, also a normal white count and differential, and elevated spinal fluid lymphocytes and protein. Spinal fluid culture revealed acid-fast bacilli.

Chest x-ray revealed diffuse, finely discrete nodules in the lungs (E).

Differential Diagnosis:
1. Disseminated histoplasmosis
2. Leukemia
3. Sickle cell anemia
4. Multiple myeloma
5. Sarcoidosis
6. Syphilis
7. Cryptococcosis
8. Subacute bacterial endocarditis
9. Collagen diseases

Clinical Note. Hematogenous spread here is fulminating in contrast to syphilis. The liver and spleen are not always palpable, and the tuberculin test is often negative. Blood cultures are usually negative.

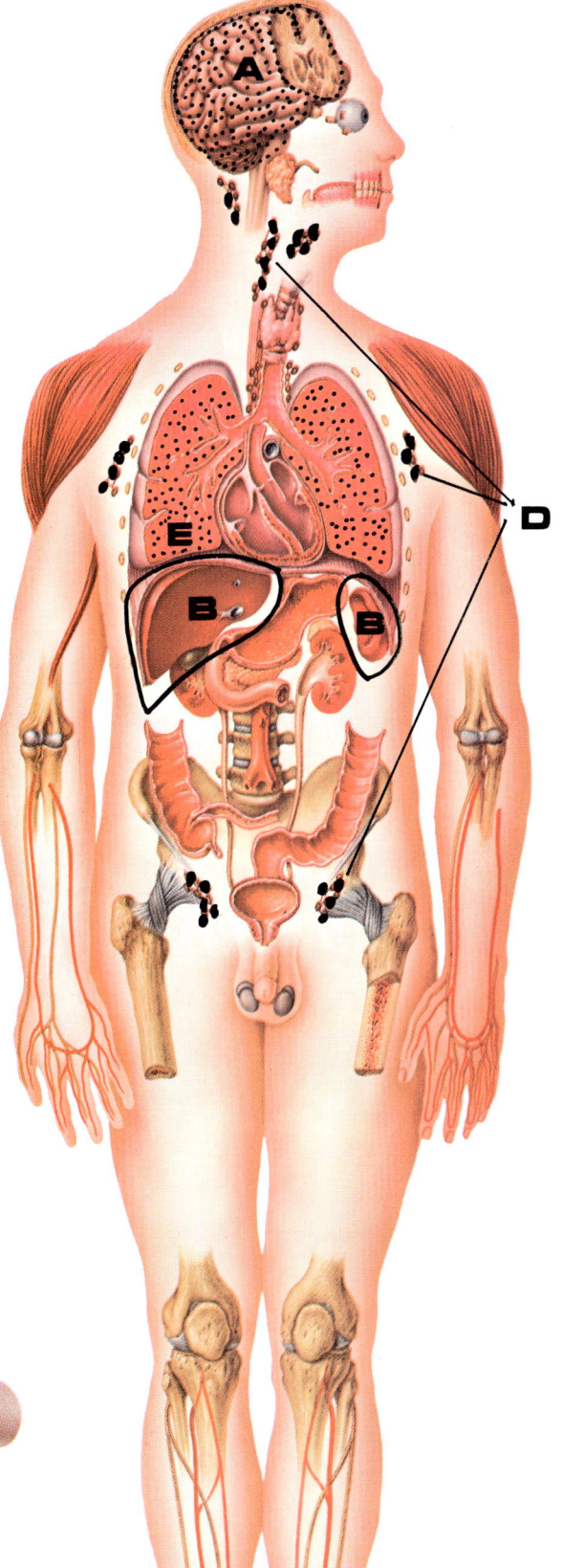

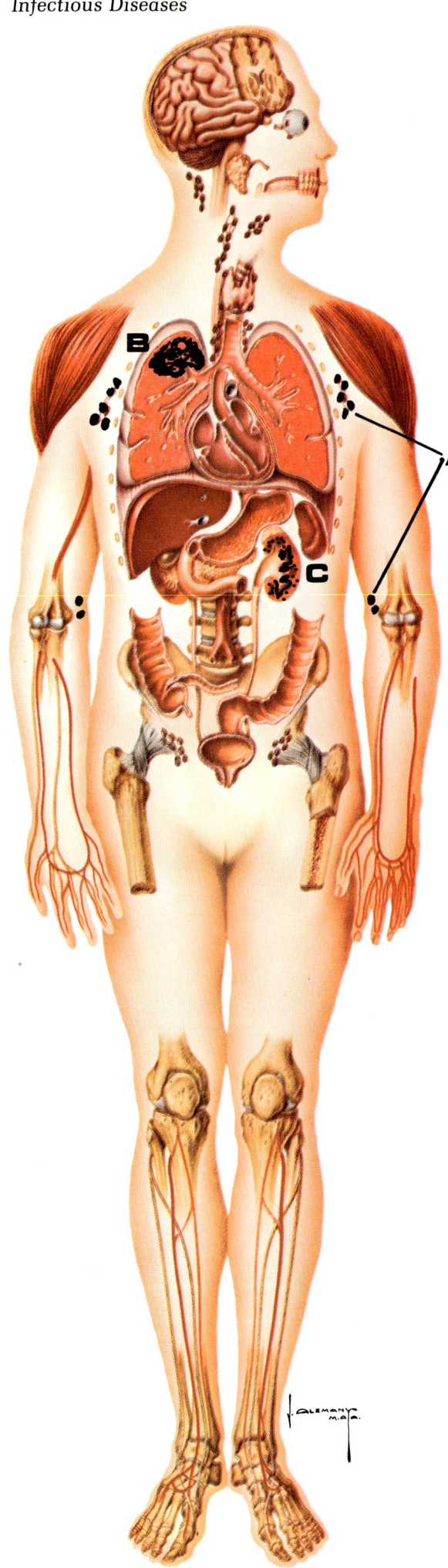

Pulmonary Tuberculosis

A 29-year-old white female complained of chronic cough and intermittent bloody sputum for 2 months prior to admission. She had lost 20 pounds of weight.

Physical examination revealed a few crepitant rales in the right upper lobe and bilateral axillary and epitrochlear adenopathy (A).

Laboratory examination revealed positive sputums and cultures for acid-fast bacilli and a positive tuberculin test.

Urinalysis revealed numerous red cells, and a culture revealed acid-fast bacilli.

X-ray examination of the chest revealed a right upper lobe infiltrate (B), and intravenous pyelography revealed calcification of the pyramids and calicectasis on the left (C).

Treatment with PAS and isoniazid was effective.

Differential Diagnosis:
1. Pulmonary infarction
2. Bronchogenic carcinoma
3. Bronchiectasis
4. Bronchial adenoma
5. Coccidioidomycosis
6. Histoplasmosis
7. Mitral stenosis with failure
8. *Klebsiella* pneumonia

Clinical Note. Hemoptysis should mean tuberculosis, neoplasm, or bronchiectasis until proved otherwise. Not every case of tuberculosis shows a positive sputum culture or smear, and therapy must be begun if the x-ray picture is typical. Gastric washings and bronchoscopy may yield positive results in these cases.

The author has been struck by the similarity of the stages of tuberculosis to those of syphilis although tuberculosis does not proceed systematically from primary to secondary to tertiary. The primary stage of tuberculosis is usually the lung, whereas syphilis usually involves the genitals. Both involve the regional lymph nodes. In contrast to syphilis, the primary stage of tuberculosis rarely clears spontaneously; rather it extends to the pleura, trachea, and sometimes the larynx locally. Both may disseminate through the blood, and this may be considered the secondary stage in both. However, hematogenous tuberculosis is much more violent than hematogenous syphilis and usually occurs in childhood. In the present case the spread through the blood to the kidney was asymptomatic. The localization in the kidney would be analogous to the tertiary stage of lues, in which spirochetes infiltrate the brain, liver, or aorta, etc. Tuberculosis may spread to the pericardium, peritoneum, musculoskeletal system, and gastrointestinal tract. Like lues, the "tertiary" stage of tuberculosis may be silent. Unlike syphilis, tuberculosis of the skin is uncommon. Both, however, invade the central nervous system, but clinical meningitis is more common in tuberculosis.

Pathology. Wherever tuberculosis occurs, the most common lesion is the granuloma. This consists of the giant cells of Langhans, surrounded by caseation necrosis and a border of epithelioid cells. This in turn is surrounded by lymphocytes and fibroblasts. The significant feature is the caseation necrosis, as all other granulomata (sarcoidosis, etc.) may have the other characteristics. The lesions are often calcified.

158 · Infectious Diseases

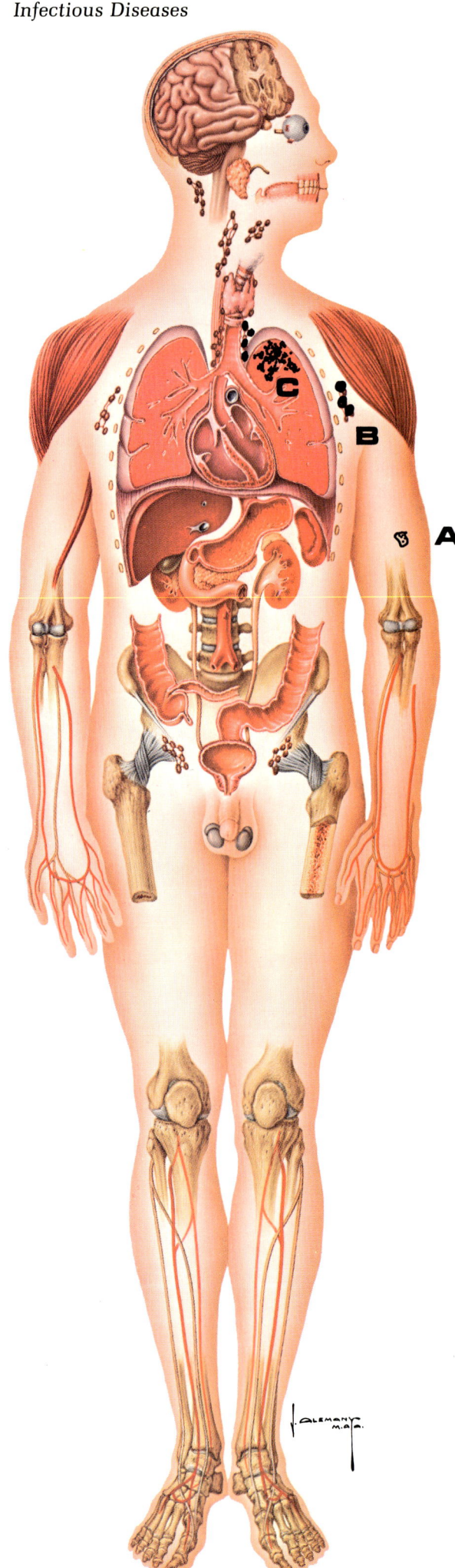

Tularemia

A 36-year-old hunter developed fever, headache, and generalized aches and pains. He had noted a small red papule on his left upper arm 5 days previously.

Physical examination revealed an indurated ulcer of his left arm (A), left axillary adenopathy (B), and a temperature of 103° F.

Laboratory examination revealed a sedimentation rate of 37 mm./hr., a 4+ CRP (C-reactive protein), but a normal white count. A culture of exudate from the ulcer was positive for *Pasteurella tularensis*. Both the Foshay skin test and the serum agglutination reaction were also positive.

X-ray examination of the chest revealed rounded infiltrations of the left upper lobe and left hilar adenopathy (C).

Treatment with streptomycin was effective.

Differential Diagnosis:
1. Rocky Mountain spotted fever
2. Sporotrichosis
3. Rat-bite fever
4. Syphilis
5. Infectious mononucleosis
6. Tuberculosis
7. Anthrax

Clinical Note. This patient probably was infected by a tick or deer fly; more often the hunter gets infected while cleaning the infected dead animal. Pneumonia occurs in at least 30 per cent of cases, and generalized adenopathy, hepatomegaly, and splenomegaly are common. But how many diseases with hepatomegaly present initially a cutaneous lesion? As in many fungal diseases, the portal of entry may be through the lungs (particularly in laboratory workers) or the intestinal tract (by ingestion of infected tissues). The eye may be attacked initially, and intense edema and chemosis develop with loss of vision. A rash is uncommon, which makes differentiation from Rocky Mountain spotted fever a lot easier.

Pathology. The granuloma of tularemia is a mass of necrotic neutrophils surrounded by a ring of epithelioid cells. There may be lymphoid hyperplasia in the vicinity of the lesion.

SPIROCHETES

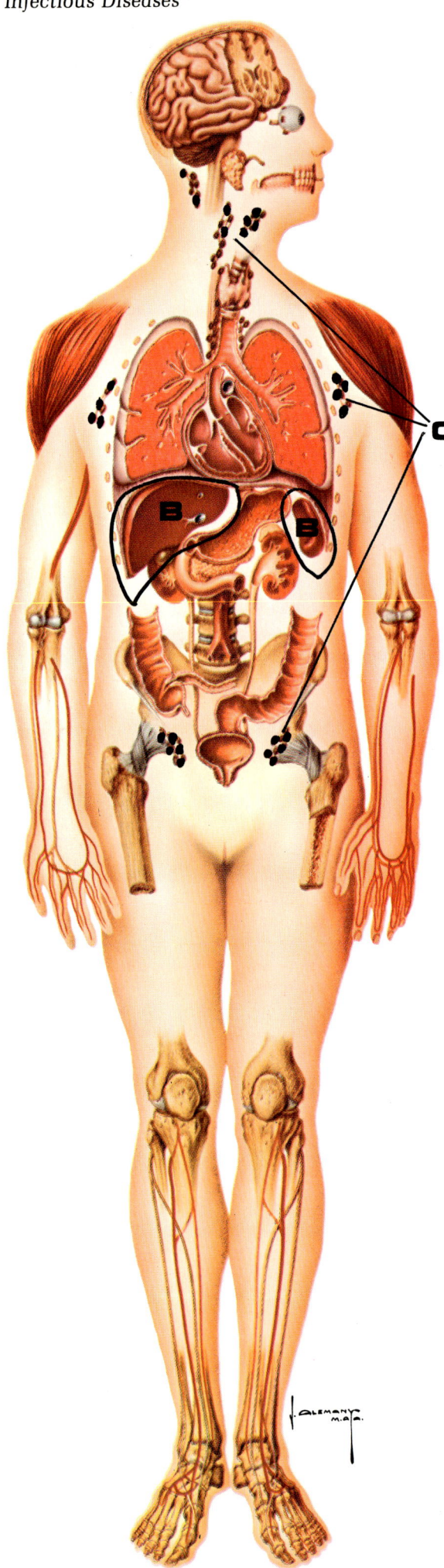

Relapsing Fever

A 28-year-old white female who had just returned from the West developed a high fever, intense headache, nausea and vomiting, and a hacking cough. Two days later she developed a rash on her trunk and extremities.

Physical examination revealed a temperature of 103° F., rose-colored spots of the trunk and extremities (A), hepatosplenomegaly (B), and mild generalized lymphadenopathy (C).

Laboratory examination revealed a leukocytosis, a weakly positive Wassermann, and spirochetes of *Borellia recurrentis* were demonstrated in the blood. Mice inoculation was also positive.

Treatment with chlortetracycline was effective.

Differential Diagnosis:
1. Typhoid fever
2. Rat-bite fever
3. Infectious mononucleosis
4. Leptospirosis

5. Leukemia
6. Thrombocytopenia purpura
7. Malaria
8. Typhus fever
9. Lupus erythematosus
10. Syphilis
11. Serum sickness

Clinical Note. As in malaria and rat-bite fever, the relapsing quality of the temperature and other symptoms in this disorder help to clarify the diagnosis. The period of remission may be as long as 10 days. The relapse is less severe, but may be accompanied by other systemic manifestations such as jaundice, conjunctivitis, iritis, uterine hemorrhages, pneumonia, neuritis, or arthritis. Unlike the result in other spirochetal diseases, the examination of the blood in this disorder is usually rewarding. These infections come from lice and soft ticks in this country.

Pathology. The spleen is enlarged and contains numerous small infarcts and spirochetes. There is fatty degeneration of the liver and congestion. Occasionally there is bile stasis.

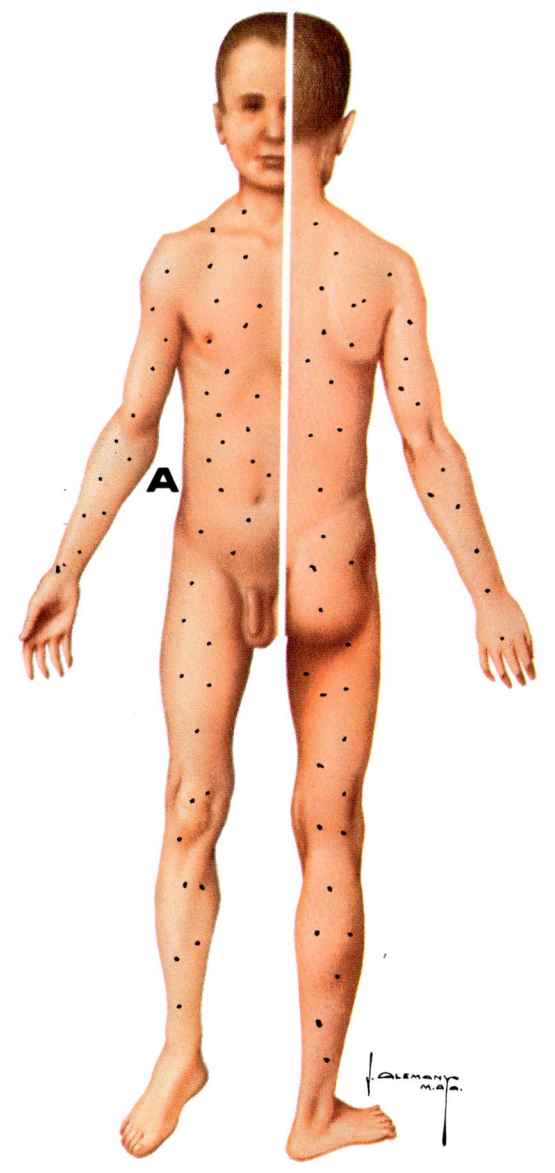

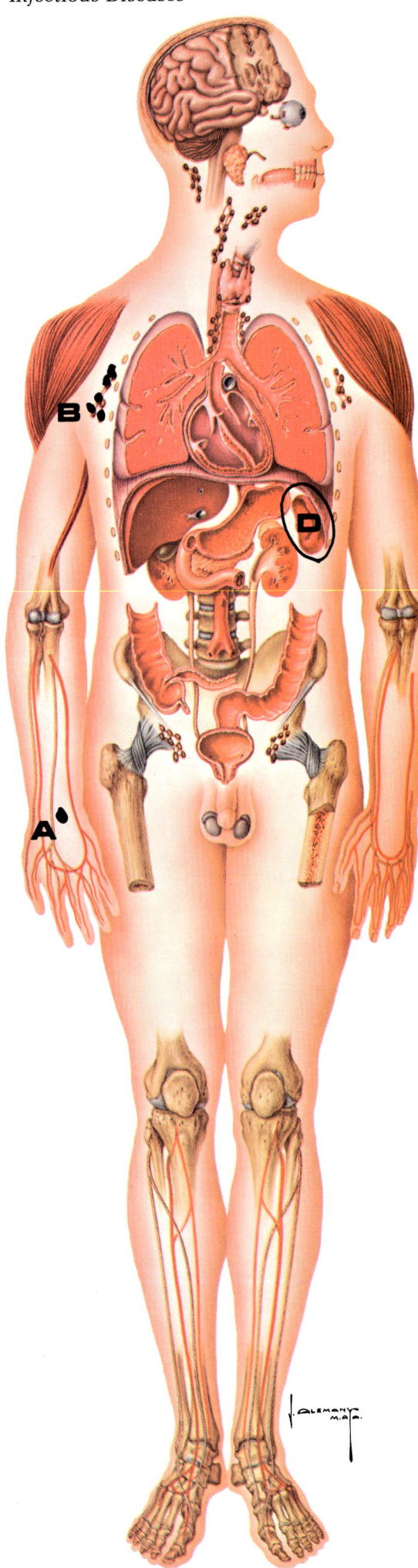

Spirillary Rat-Bite Fever

A 32-year-old white male garbage collector developed an acute painful and swollen nodule on his right wrist 5 days prior to admission. He had been bitten by a rat at the same site 2 weeks previously.

Physical examination revealed a temperature of 102° F., the swollen indurated nodule (A), right axillary adenopathy (B), and a generalized maculopapular rash (C). There was also splenomegaly (D).

Laboratory examination revealed leukocytosis, a weakly positive Wassermann, and a positive guinea pig inoculation test for *Spirillum minus*.

Treatment with penicillin was effective.

Differential Diagnosis:
1. Streptobacillary fever
2. Infectious mononucleosis
3. Agranulocytosis
4. Typhoid fever
5. Miliary tuberculosis

6. Histoplasmosis
7. Brucellosis
8. Hodgkin's disease
9. Rocky Mountain spotted fever
10. Lupus erythematosus
11. Letterer-Siwe disease
12. Serum sickness
13. Meningococcemia
14. Syphilis
15. Pretibial fever

Clinical Note. The history of a rat bite makes the diagnosis easy, but without that history, splenomegaly and rash can mean many things. Although *Spirillum minus* can produce arthralgias, frank arthritis is unusual, in contrast to symptoms in streptobacillary fever. The rash is almost always present, in contrast to the findings in other diseases caused by animal bites (tularemia, etc.). The spirochete cannot be cultured from the blood or detected on a blood smear, and so animal inoculation is crucial to the diagnosis.

Pathology. There are hyperemia and edema of the bite site with subsequent round cell infiltration and necrosis of the epithelium. A vegetative endocarditis has been reported.

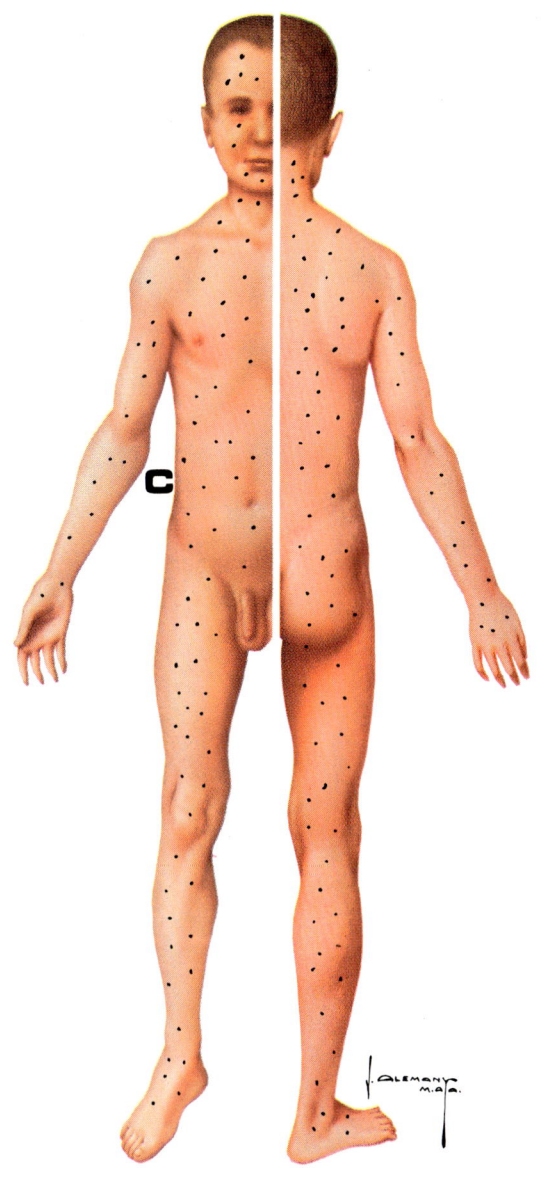

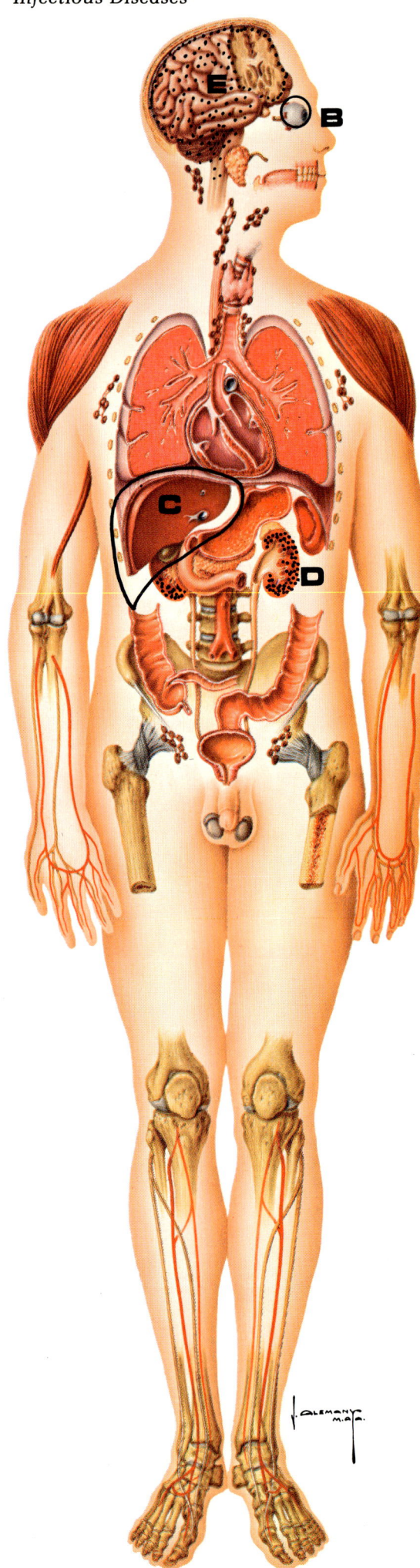

Weil's Disease

A 29-year-old Negro sewer worker complained of severe headache, muscular cramps, photophobia, and fever 6 days prior to admission. On the day of admission he developed yellow eyes and felt generally a lot sicker.

Physical examination revealed suffusion of the conjunctivae (A), icteric sclerae (B), and tender hepatomegaly (C). There was moderate nuchal rigidity.

Laboratory examination revealed a white count of 22,400 cells/cu. mm., predominantly neutrophils; a BUN of 42 mg. per cent; elevated serum bilirubin, transaminase, and alkaline phosphatase; and albuminuria and microscopic hematuria, indicating renal involvement (D). Spinal fluid examination revealed 250 cells per cu. mm., most of which were lymphocytes, confirming the meningeal involvement (E). Guinea pig inoculation was positive for *Leptospira icterohaemorrhagicae*. A rising titer of agglutinating antibodies for leptospirosis was also demonstrated.

Treatment with antibiotics was unsuccessful, but the patient nevertheless recovered.

Differential Diagnosis:
1. Viral hepatitis
2. Toxic hepatitis
3. Hemolytic anemias
4. Ascending cholangitis
5. Leukemia
6. Infectious mononucleosis
7. Porphyria
8. Carcinoma of the pancreas
9. Other causes of obstructive jaundice
10. Metastatic carcinoma
11. Yellow fever

Clinical Note. Infectious mononucleosis is the only other condition that may produce an aseptic meningitis with liver involvement to the extent of jaundice, but infectious mononucleosis does not cause renal involvement and a high BUN. On the other hand, malaria may manifest with a hepatorenal syndrome (black-water fever) and focal or diffuse cerebral involvement without meningitis. The suffusion of the conjunctivae and the muscular aches, particularly in the arms and calves, are the most distinctive findings. Only a few patients with leptospirosis, regardless of what the strain is, develop Weil's disease (Weil's "syndrome" might be a better name for it). The majority manifest merely headache, fever, conjunctival infection, and muscular aches, and are better in a week. Leptospirosis may manifest also as pretibial fever or merely as an aseptic meningitis. In pretibial fever the predominant findings are a rash and splenomegaly.

Pathology. The muscle tissue shows focal degeneration with very little cellular reaction. The liver shows bile stasis, some cytoplasmic degeneration, and hepatocellular regeneration. Attending necrosis and degeneration of the renal tubules is a diffuse interstitial nephritis.

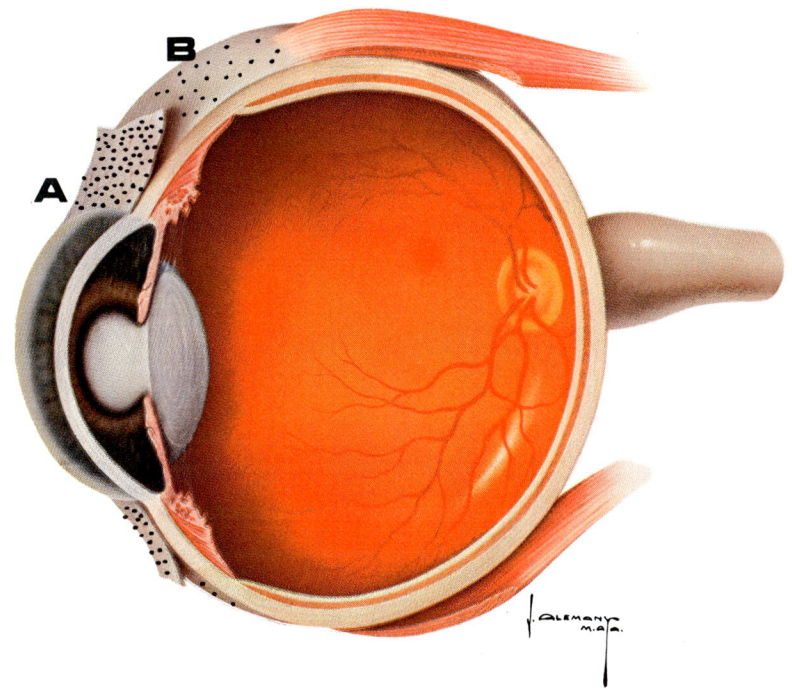

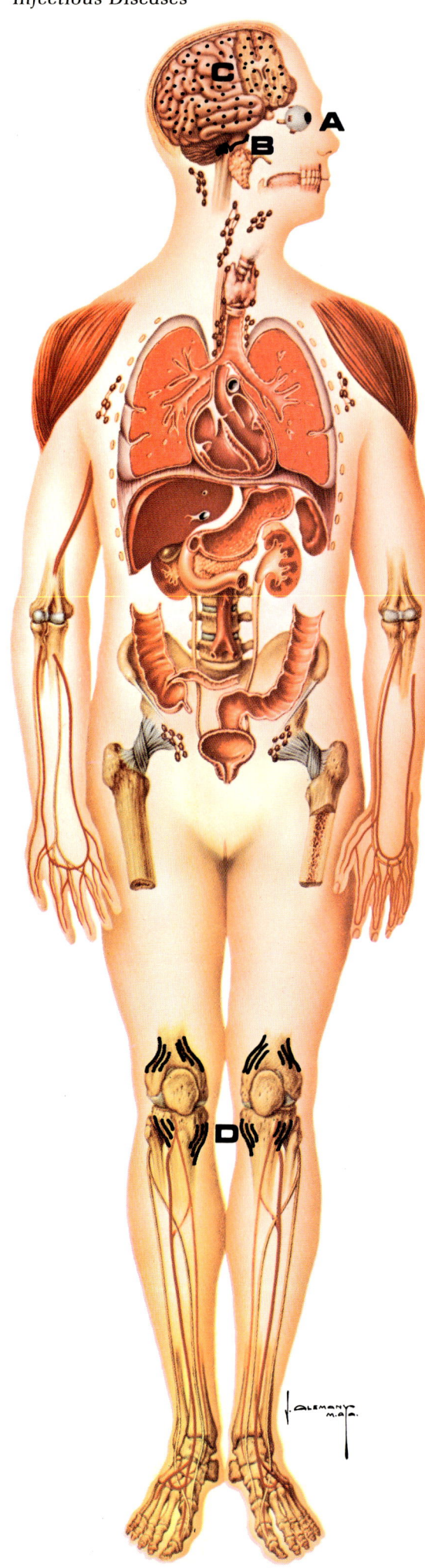

Congenital Syphilis

A 14-year-old white female complained of pain and redness of both eyes. Her performance in school had been poor in the previous 2 years. Her mother was known to have a positive Wassermann.

Physical examination revealed bilateral interstitial keratitis (A), bilateral nerve deafness (B), thickening, tenderness, and roughening of both tibia, and mental retardation, indicating cerebral involvement (C).

Laboratory examination revealed a positive Wassermann.

X-ray examination of the femurs and tibia showed periosteal thickening in layers (D).

Treatment with penicillin and steroids was beneficial.

Differential Diagnosis:
1. Sarcoidosis
2. Tuberculosis
3. Rubella in utero
4. Gargoylism
5. Arachnodactyly
6. Sjögren's syndrome
7. Leprosy
8. Galactosemia
9. Vitamin A deficiency
10. Fanconi syndrome

Clinical Note. Here there is eye, bone, and central nervous system involvement, as in gargoylism; but the eye involvement is acute in onset, and a blood Wassermann should clear up the confusion, if there is any. Unusual facial features may appear in both. (The saddle nose and Hutchinson's teeth of congenital syphilis are now rare.) Paroxysmal cold hemoglobinuria can also occur. In early congenital syphilis there may be hepatosplenomegaly with mild jaundice and a maculopapular rash.

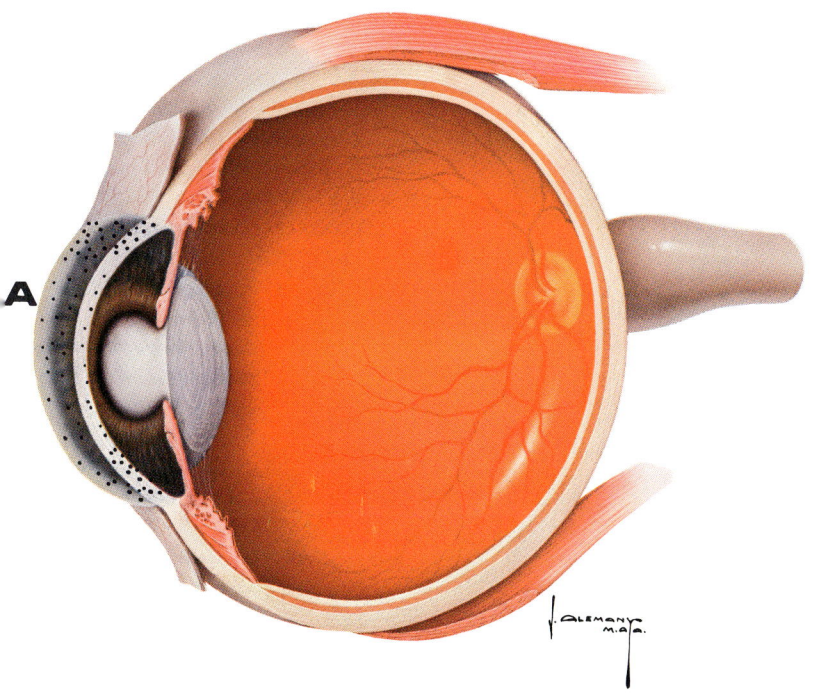

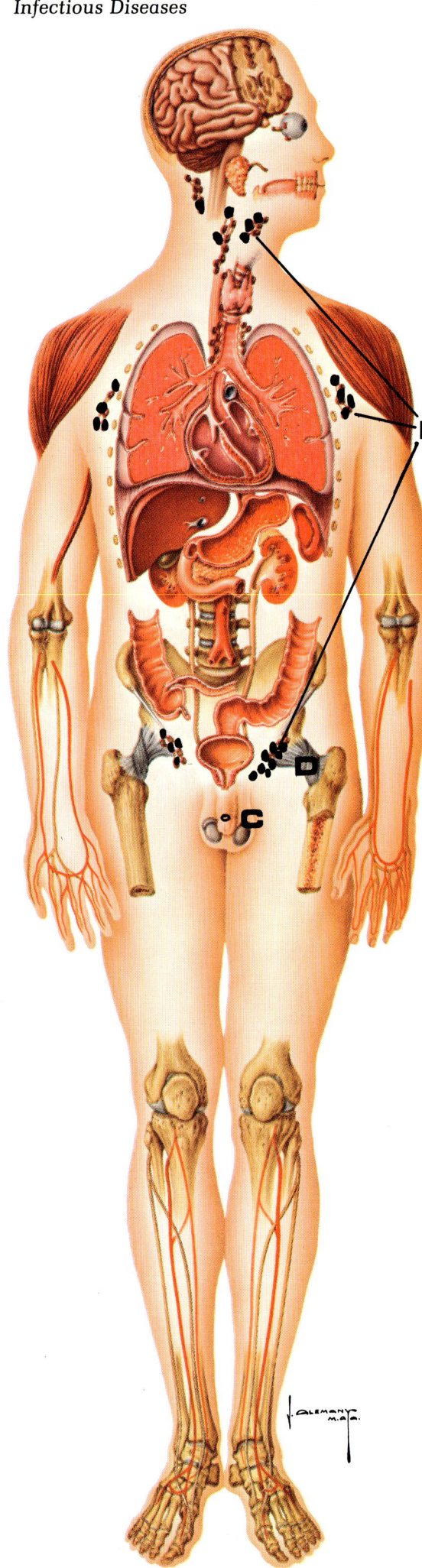

Syphilis, Case 1

A 24-year-old single male complained of a sore on his penis, which gradually cleared. Six weeks later he developed a generalized rash.

Physical examination revealed a generalized maculopapular rash, most prominent on the trunk and palms and soles (A), and generalized lymphadenopathy (B). Induration was noted under many of the papules. The primary lesion on the penis (C) and the prominent left inguinal adenopathy (D) are also demonstrated here.

Laboratory examination revealed a positive FTA-ABS and *Treponema pallidum* immobilization test (TPI).

Treatment with penicillin produced complete recovery.

Differential Diagnosis:
1. Chancroid
2. Lymphogranuloma inguinale
3. Lymphogranuloma venereum
4. Gonorrhea
5. Tularemia
6. Hodgkin's disease
7. Serum sickness
8. Reiter's disease
9. Pellagra
10. Yaws
11. Actinomycosis
12. Measles
13. Filariasis
14. Infectious mononucleosis
15. Rocky Mountain spotted fever

Clinical Note. The prevalence of this disease in unmarried young adults, prostitutes, and homosexuals is helpful in diagnosis. Not all patients develop clinical signs of secondary lues and thus may present with the tertiary stage. Lymphadenopathy is very common in the second stage, particularly posterior cervical. The skin lesions vary in size, but induration is common. Condylomata lata (E) (papillomatous lesions of the anogenital area) appear in this stage. Primary lesions may appear anywhere on the body. A large number of diseases are associated with biologic false positive Wassermann reactions. Now that more specific serologic tests are available, no one should be labeled with a diagnosis of secondary or tertiary lues without confirmation by one of these tests (TPI, FTA-ABS, etc.). Systemic symptoms are rare and help to distinguish primary and secondary lues from other infectious diseases.

Pathology. The primary lesion of the genitalia is at first a papule, which then breaks down into an ulcer with surrounding induration. Microscopically, there is a mononuclear infiltration at the ulcer base, surrounded by a vascular and fibroblastic reaction. Endothelial and fibroblastic proliferation of the adjacent small blood vessels produces an obliterative endarteritis. The mucocutaneous lesions of secondary syphilis have the same appearance histologically of primary syphilis except that the mononuclear cell reaction is not as intense.

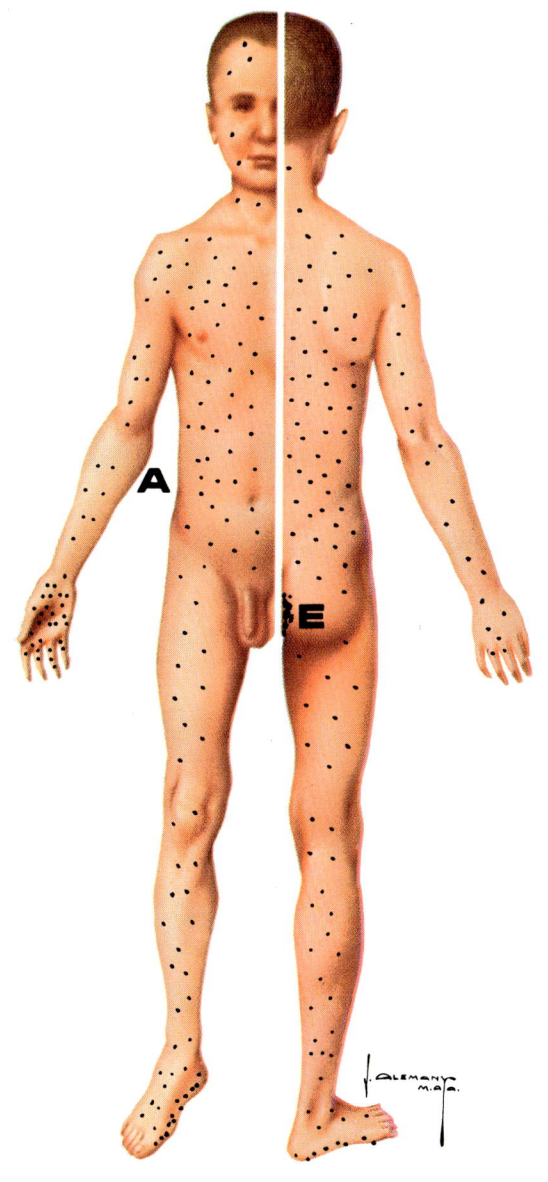

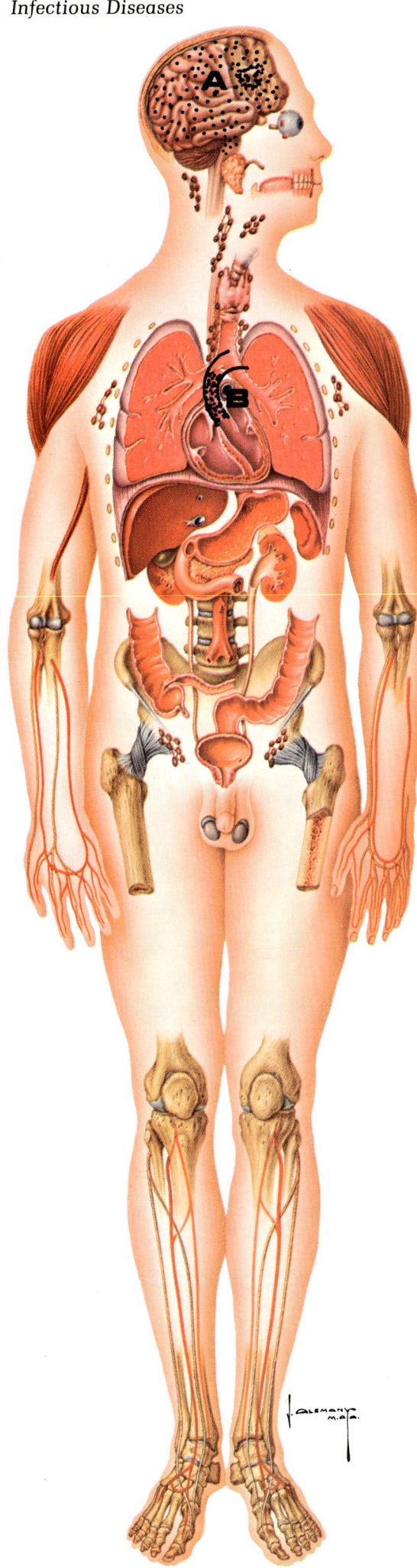

Syphilis, Case 2

A 54-year-old Negro male was brought to the psychiatric clinic because his family complained he had become very hostile and aggressive lately and heard voices that weren't there.

Physical examination revealed bilateral Argyll Robertson pupils, fine tremors of the face and tongue, slurred speech, and bilateral Babinski signs, all indications of involvement of the central nervous system (A). In addition, there was a grade III aortic diastolic murmur, indicating involvement of the aortic valves (B).

Laboratory examination revealed a positive TPI and a positive FTA-ABS test on the spinal fluid. The spinal fluid also revealed a first zone colloidal gold reaction, an elevated protein, and 135 cells/cu. mm., mostly lymphocytes.

Treatment with penicillin was beneficial.

Differential Diagnosis:
1. Wernicke's encephalopathy
2. Alcoholic intoxication
3. Brominism
4. Lead encephalopathy
5. Wilson's disease
6. Space-occupying lesion of the cerebral cortex
7. Cerebral arteriosclerosis
8. Alzheimer's disease
9. Leptospirosis
10. Collagen diseases
11. Tuberculosis
12. Beriberi
13. Subacute bacterial endocarditis
14. Sickle cell anemia
15. Trypanosomiasis

Clinical Note. The tip-off in this case was the heart murmur of aortic insufficiency. It is not frequently appreciated that neurologic and cardiovascular involvement often occur together. Other neurologic syndromes such as tabes dorsalis, meningitis, cerebral thrombosis, and gummas occur in tertiary lues. Gummas may also appear in the skeleton and liver. Almost any organ of the body can be affected by tertiary lues.

Pathology. The brain is atrophied, the meninges and ependyma thickened, and microscopically the nerve cell population is reduced and replaced by glial tissue. There is perivascular cuffing of mononuclear cells. The microglia are rod-shaped and contain increased amounts of iron. The proximal aorta is dilated, and microscopically the vasa vasorum are thickened (obliterative endarteritis), and the elastic and smooth muscle of the media are destroyed and replaced by fibrous scarring.

MYCOSES

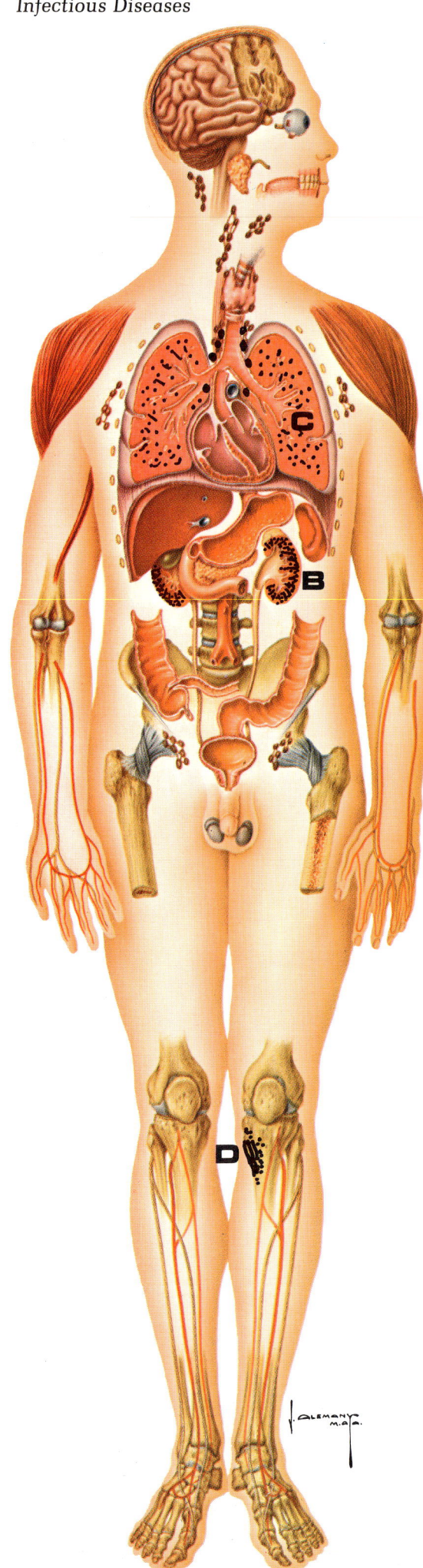

North American Blastomycosis

A 28-year-old Negro male complained of persistent rash of the face and hands for several months. He complained also of an occasional dry cough and fever.

Physical examination revealed multiple granulomatous ulcerating lesions of the face, hands, and top of the feet (A).

Laboratory examination of material from the skin lesions revealed budding yeast cells on direct examination and characteristic colonies of *Blastomyces dermatitidis* on culture. A skin test for blastomycosis was positive. Pyuria and proteinuria indicated renal involvement (B).

X-ray examination of the chest revealed mottled, irregular densities scattered throughout with hilar adenopathy (C). X-ray of the tibia revealed a few circumscribed lytic areas with periosteal reaction (D).

Treatment with amphotericin B was effective.

Differential Diagnosis:
1. Tuberculosis
2. Sarcoidosis
3. Syphilis
4. Basal cell carcinoma
5. Metastatic carcinoma or sarcoma
6. Lupus erythematosus
7. Acne vulgaris
8. Leprosy
9. Weber-Christian disease

Clinical Note. In this case we have a combination of pulmonary and skin lesions clinically, which is the most common presentation of this disease. Tuberculosis and bronchogenic carcinoma with skin metastasis may present in this way, also, as may sarcoidosis and lupus erythematosus less frequently. The urinary tract and bone are the next most frequent tissues to be involved. Do not be fooled by negative cultures or skin tests! Dermatologists are reminded to take chest x-rays routinely.

Pathology. Although there is more tissue reaction than in cryptococcosis, cavitation and calcification in the lungs are still rare. The main reaction is suppurative and epithelioid granulomata, whether in the skin or other tissue.

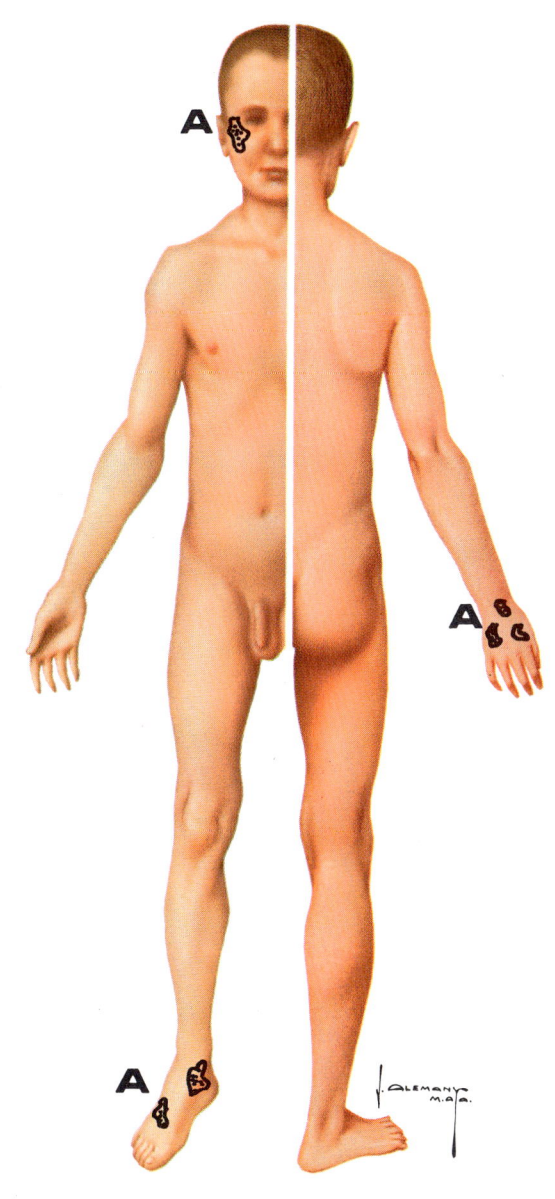

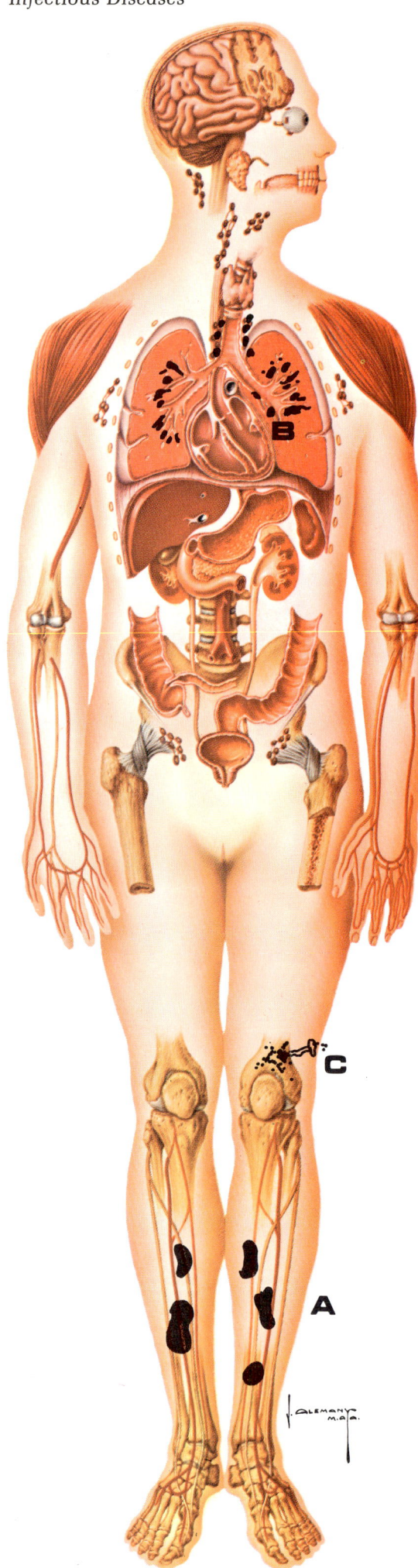

Coccidioidomycosis

A 28-year-old white female developed fever, backache, headache, and a dry cough 3 days prior to admission. On the day of admission she developed a rash of both legs.

Physical examination revealed a few sibilant rales over the right lower lobe and large, tender hard macules over both shins (A).

Laboratory examination revealed eosinophilia, and a sputum culture was positive for *Coccidioides immitis*. The coccidioidin skin test and complement-fixation tests were also positive.

X-ray examination of the chest revealed patchy peribronchial infiltration and bilateral hilar adenopathy (B).

Treatment with amphotericin B was effective.

Differential Diagnosis:
1. Tuberculosis
2. Histoplasmosis
3. Loeffler's syndrome
4. Actinomycosis
5. Blastomycosis
6. Sarcoidosis
7. Typhoid fever
8. Primary atypical pneumonia

Clinical Note. In addition to lung and skin manifestations, there may be bone involvement (C) in the disseminated form, which is fortunately rare. The skin may be involved with ulcers, abscesses, or fistulous tracts all the way from skin to bone, as in actinomycosis. The majority of cases, as in histoplasmosis, present with a mild flu-like syndrome having respiratory involvement that disappears spontaneously or is completely asymptomatic. Like tuberculosis, coccidioidomycosis may have cardiac, meningeal, and other visceral organ involvement; but such cases are exceedingly rare.

Pathology. The primary reaction is suppurative, but chronic granulomas with both caseation necrosis and giant cells may occur, leading in some cases to cavitation in the lungs.

Cryptococcosis

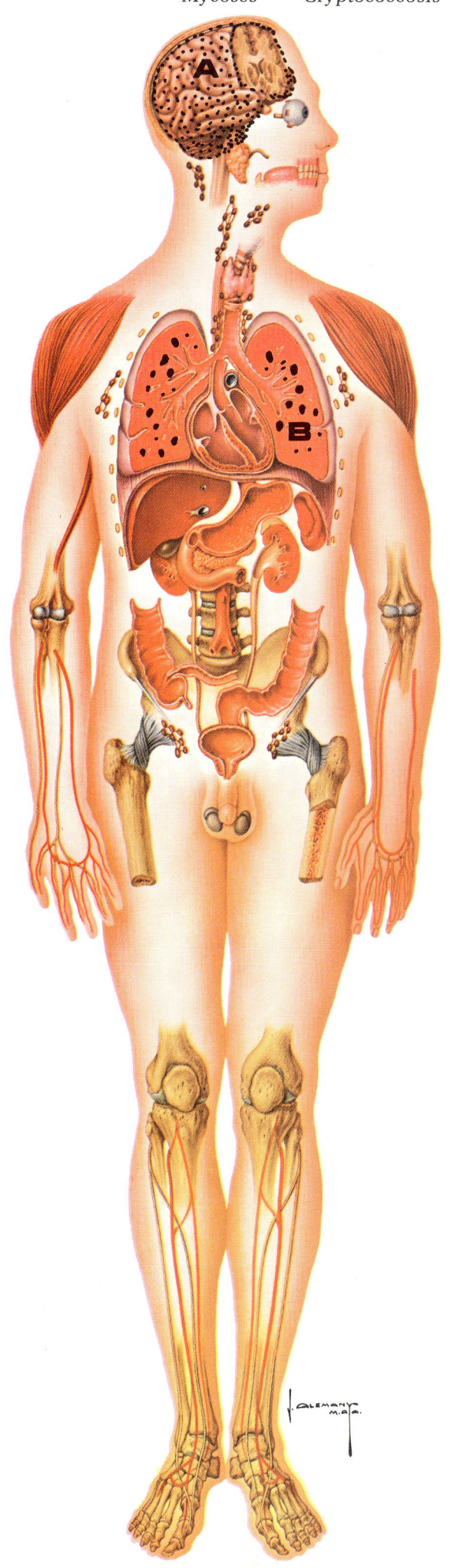

A 47-year-old white male farmer complained of severe constant generalized headache and stiff neck for 2 weeks prior to admission. He also had a nonproductive cough and occasional chills.

Physical examination revealed a temperature of 101° F. and definite nuchal rigidity as signs of meningeal involvement (A), and poor visual acuity bilaterally; but the chest was clear.

Laboratory examination revealed increased lymphocytes and protein and, on an India ink preparation, spherical fungal cells in the spinal fluid, which grew typical colonies of *Cryptococcus neoformans* on Sabouraud's medium.

X-ray examination of the chest revealed nodular infiltrates of both lungs (B) of various sizes.

Treatment with amphotericin B was effective.

Differential Diagnosis:
1. Tuberculosis
2. Sarcoidosis
3. Subarachnoid hemorrhage
4. Leptospirosis
5. Viral meningitis
6. Cervical spondylosis
7. Nocardiosis
8. Histoplasmosis
9. Coccidioidomycosis
10. Lymphoma
11. Pneumococcal pneumonia
12. Syphilitic meningitis

Clinical Note. Here we have lung (B) and meningeal involvement; but in some cases there may be renal, bone, and skin involvement. This combination, which along with fever and an insidious onset may be found in tuberculosis and nocardiosis, is rarely found with the other mycoses. It emphasizes the importance of a chest x-ray in cases of meningitis. Since spinal fluid culture may be difficult, urine is frequently cultured as well. This disease should be suspected in cases of lymphoma, leukemia, and diabetes.

Pathology. The lung shows very little cellular reaction, and thus suppuration, necrosis, and caseation with cavitation are rare, and hilar adenopathy is late. The meningeal reaction is at the base of the brain and may lead to compression of the cranial nerves and hydrocephalus, simulating a tumor.

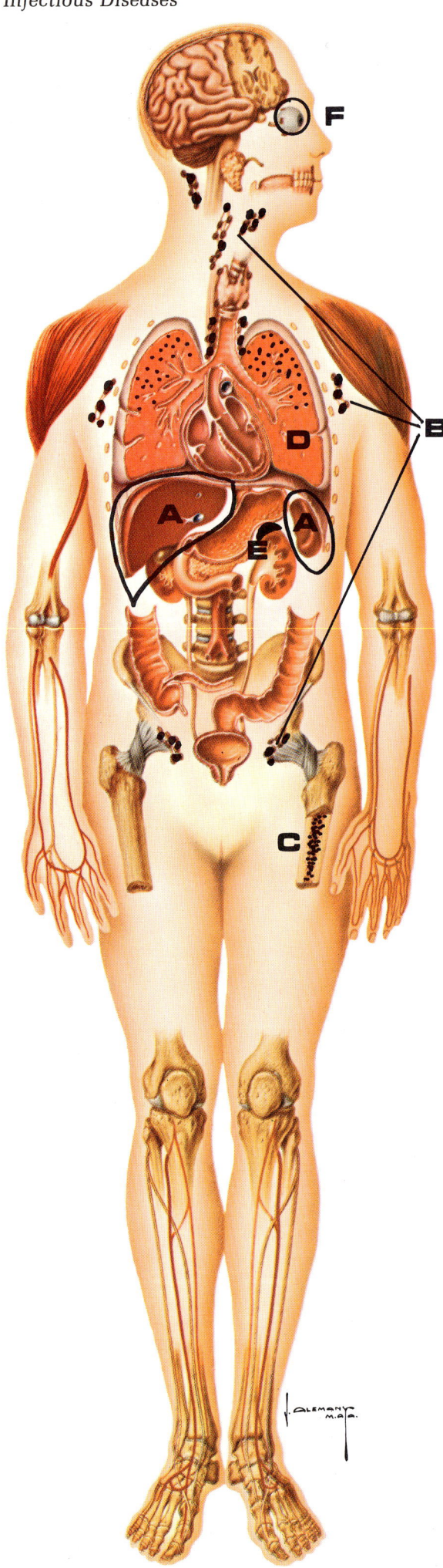

Disseminated Histoplasmosis

An 18-year-old white female complained of increasing fatigue and weight loss with spiking fever almost daily for 1 month. She had cleaned out her mother's chicken coop a couple of months before.

Physical examination revealed a fever of 102° F., hepatosplenomegaly (A) without jaundice, generalized lymphadenopathy (B), and a few scattered sibilant rales over the chest.

Laboratory examination revealed a normocytic anemia, leukopenia, and positive skin test and complement-fixation test for histoplasmosis. A bone marrow examination revealed the yeast form of *Histoplasma capsulatum* (C), explaining the anemia and leukopenia.

X-ray examination of the chest revealed a few small infiltrates in both upper lung fields and bilateral hilar adenopathy (D).

Treatment with amphotericin B was unsuccessful, and she died in adrenal insufficiency, indicating infiltration of the adrenal glands (E).

Differential Diagnosis:
1. Tuberculosis
2. Sarcoidosis
3. Gaucher's disease
4. Lupus erythematosus
5. Hodgkin's disease
6. Leukemia
7. Typhoid fever
8. Brucellosis
9. Infectious mononucleosis
10. Schistosomiasis
11. Cooley's anemia
12. Malaria
13. Amyloidosis

Clinical Note. Contrary to popular belief, the disseminated form of histoplasmosis is unusual. Most cases of the disease show asymptomatic pulmonic involvement or manifest with fever, cough, and mild pulmonary infiltration. A chronic cavitary form indistinguishable from pulmonary tuberculosis also occurs. Typical multiple miliary calcifications found on x-ray examination are usually a sign of old healed histoplasmosis infection. Similar calcifications may occur in the liver and spleen.

What other systemic diseases present with lung, liver, spleen, lymph node, and hematologic involvement? Miliary or hematogenous tuberculosis may mimic this disease exactly, and infiltration of the adrenal glands is common in both. Involvement of the skin is more common in miliary tuberculosis; but lesions of the mucosa of the mouth, larynx, and gastrointestinal tract can occur in histoplasmosis just as they do in tuberculosis. Both diseases cause granulomatous uveitis (F). Sarcoidosis may cause similar involvement, but more frequently it affects the nervous system, skin, and bones.

Pathology. After following the above discussion, it should not surprise the reader that the yeast forms provoke a tissue reaction similar to that of tuberculosis with epithelioid cells, caseation necrosis, giant cells, and proliferation of lymphocytes.

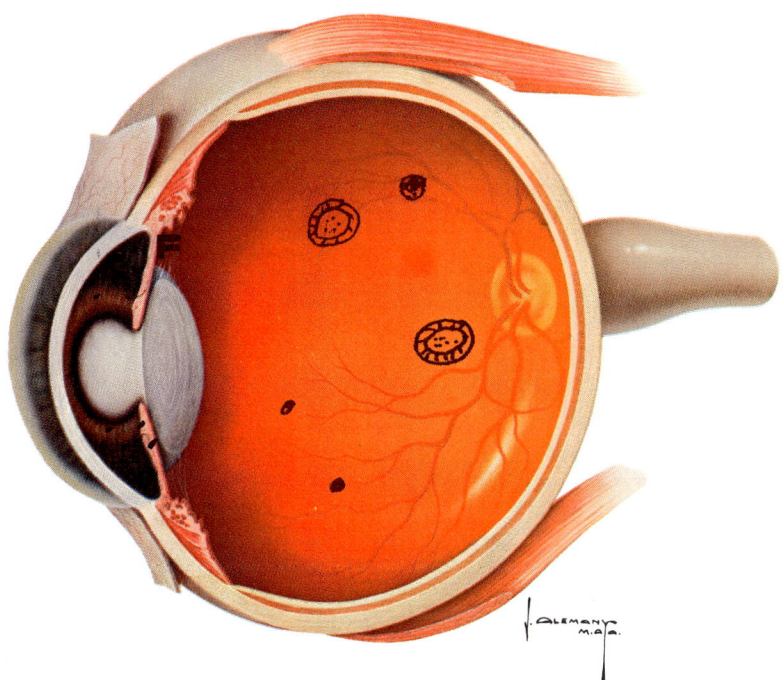

178 · Infectious Diseases

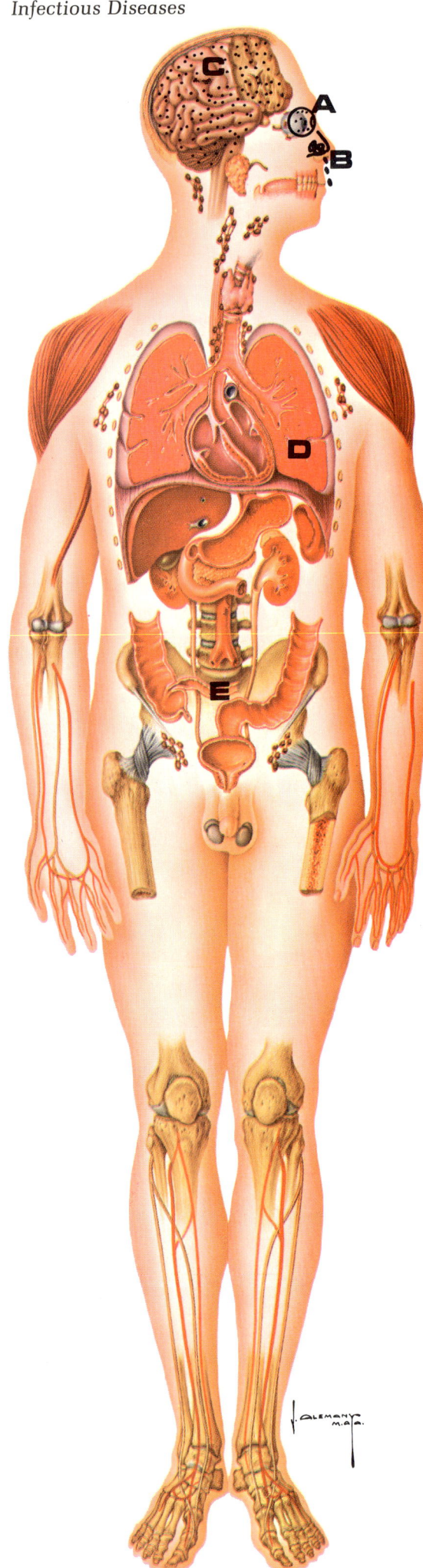

Mucormycosis

A 43-year-old white male diabetic developed a purulent nasal discharge which failed to respond to antibiotics. Two days prior to admission he developed right periorbital swelling and double vision.

Physical examination revealed right periorbital edema, chemosis, exophthalmos (A), oculomotor palsy, and gangrenous ulceration of the nasal mucosa (B).

Laboratory examination revealed the characteristic mycelia on culture of the nasal discharge.

X-ray examination of the sinuses revealed an opacified right maxillary antrum.

Treatment with amphotericin B was unsuccessful, and the patient died of meningoencephalitis (C).

Differential Diagnosis:
1. Wegener's granulomatosis
2. Actinomycosis
3. Tuberculosis
4. Acute bacterial sinusitis
5. Hyperthyroidism
6. Nasopharyngeal carcinoma
7. Retro-orbital neoplasm
8. Rhinosporidiosis
9. Glanders

Clinical Note. Instead of stubbornly persisting in treating cases of resistant sinusitis with antibiotics, especially with underlying diabetes, leukemia, or lymphoma, one should get a culture on Sabouraud's medium or a mucosal biopsy. In one third of the cases this disease spreads to involve the brain, heart, and kidneys. It has a great affinity for arteries, producing a purulent arteritis and thrombosis in the internal carotid artery, the pulmonary artery, or the coronary artery. Although it customarily invades the body through the nose or sinuses, it may make its initial insult in the lung (D) or intestinal tract (E), just as actinomycosis does.

What other systemic disease affects the nasal passages, the lung, and the arteries in a similar way? Wegener's granulomatosis, of course.

Pathology. There may be acute inflammation and suppuration of the tissue and blood vessels in the orbit, lungs, central nervous system, heart, skin, kidney, and gastrointestinal tract.

Nocardiosis

A 48-year-old white male was brought for examination because his wife had noted he had episodes during which he would smack his lips and not respond to questions. He had had intermittent low-grade fever, night sweats, and cough productive of purulent and occasionally blood-streaked sputum for 2 months previously.

Physical examination revealed dullness, loss of palpable fremitus, diminished breath sounds over the right lower lobe, and a temperature of 101° F.

Laboratory examination revealed *Nocardia asteroides* in the sputum culture; aside from a protein of 65 mg. per 100 ml., the spinal fluid was normal. However, an EEG revealed a right temporal lobe focus.

X-ray examination of the chest revealed a dense nodular infiltrate of the right lower lobe and right pleural effusion (A); angiography revealed a space-occupying lesion of the right temporal lobe.

Treatment. This lesion proved to be an abscess (B) on craniotomy. The patient was also treated with long-term sulfonamides.

Differential Diagnosis:
1. Tuberculosis
2. Cryptococcosis
3. Sarcoidosis
4. Carcinoma of the lung with metastasis
5. *Klebsiella* pneumonia
6. Typhoid fever
7. Histoplasmosis
8. Chromoblastomycosis

Clinical Note. Although clinical evidence of pulmonary disease is present in 75 per cent of these cases, only 25 per cent manifest pleural involvement. The brain is the most common organ of dissemination, but the liver, kidney, spleen, and subcutaneous tissues may also be involved. This disease, like other fungal infections, is often seen in diabetics and patients with lymphoma or leukemia.

Pathology. The organism does not regularly produce sulfur granules, and the granulomatous reaction rarely contains giant cells or caseation necrosis. Cavitation and miliary lesions are uncommon. The pulmonary lesions may extend to the pleura and ribs, but fistulous tracts to the skin occur less frequently than in actinomycosis.

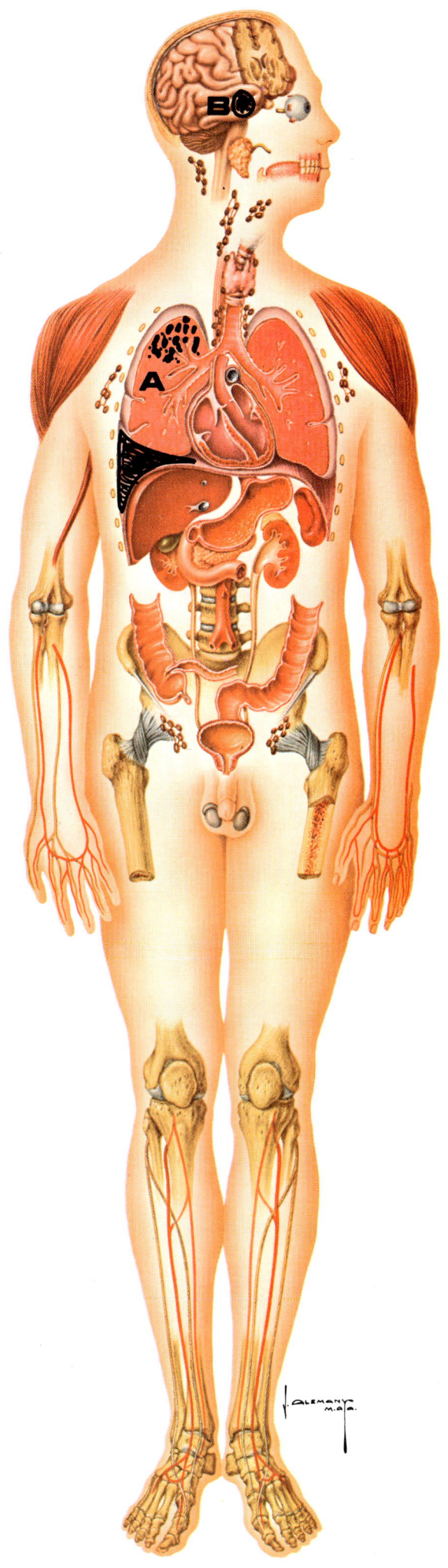

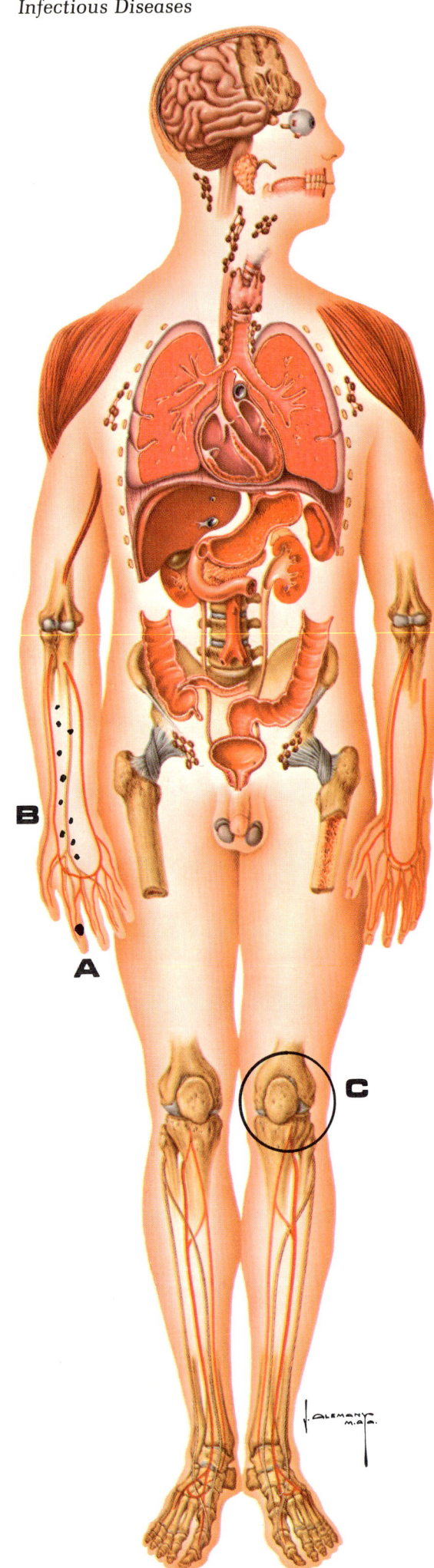

Sporotrichosis

A 28-year-old white male laborer complained of a painful swelling on his right index finger. He had lacerated his finger two weeks previously; but though it had healed sufficiently to go back to work, on the day of admission he developed a swollen left knee joint.

Physical examination revealed a tender reddish nodule of the right index finger (A) with a chain of small subcutaneous nodes running up his right wrist and forearm (B). The left knee joint was swollen and tender (C).

Laboratory examination revealed *Sporotrichum schenckii* in a culture from the aspirate of the nodule on the finger and the synovial fluid.

Treatment with potassium iodide was effective.

Differential Diagnosis:
1. Tularemia
2. Staphylococcal cellulitis
3. Tuberculosis
4. Cat-scratch disease
5. Syphilis
6. South American blastomycosis
7. Actinomycosis
8. Maduromycosis
9. Rat-bite fever
10. Gonorrhea
11. Glanders

Clinical Note. Here we have skin, lymphatic, and joint involvement, a combination seen in gonorrhea and rat-bite fever; but in gonorrhea the portal of entry is consistently the genitalia. Tularemia presents with a cutaneous ulcer; instead of producing multiple lesions along the lymph vessels, however, it causes regional and subsequently generalized lymphadenopathy. If allowed to continue untreated, the subcutaneous lesions of sporotrichosis may extend to bone, just as in actinomycosis. The fungus may spread hematogenously to bone, eye, lungs, gastrointestinal tract, and central nervous system. Like actinomycosis and other fungi, it may enter the body via the lung or gastrointestinal tract.

Pathology. Reactions to the fungus are varied, including acute suppuration and granulomata with epithelioid and giant cells.

PARASITES

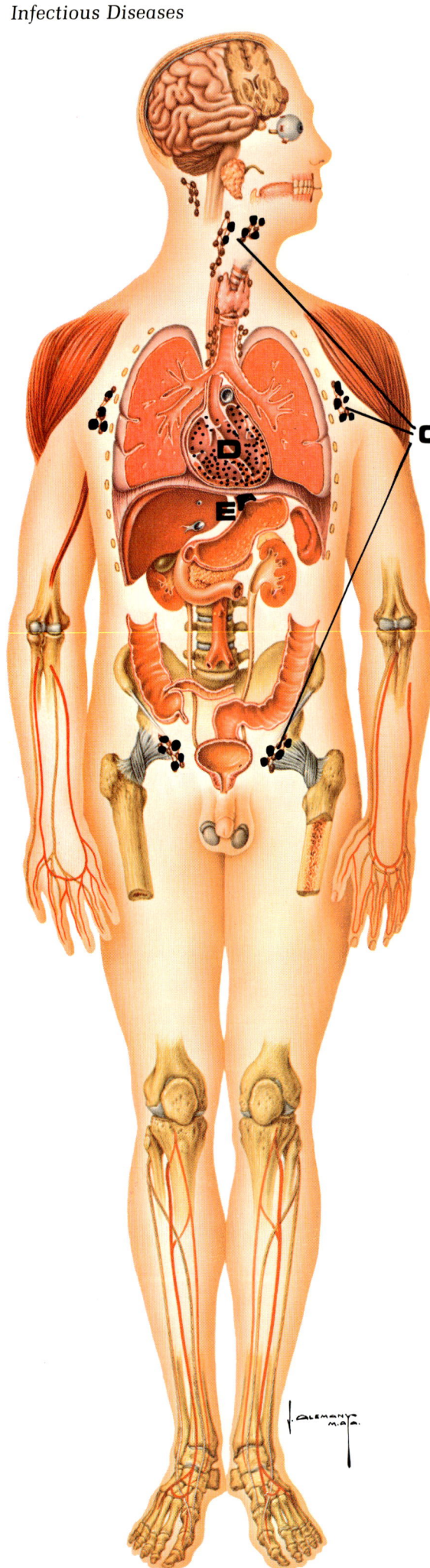

Chagas' Disease

A 13-year-old Brazilian male developed a swollen right eye (from the bite of a reduviid bug) and fever.

Physical examination revealed right periorbital edema and injected lids (Chagas-Romaña sign) (A), a temperature of 101° F., a macular rash of the proximal extremities and trunk (B), and generalized lymphadenopathy (C).

Laboratory examination revealed trypanosomes on the blood smears. An electrocardiogram revealed frequent ventricular extrasystoles, indicating myocarditis (D).

Treatment with primaquine was ineffective.

Differential Diagnosis:
1. Trichinosis
2. Rheumatic fever
3. Idiopathic myocarditis
4. Cavernous sinus thrombosis
5. Orbital cellulitis
6. Orbital tumor
7. Myxedema
8. Acute glomerulonephritis
9. Amyloidosis
10. Beriberi
11. Tuberculosis
12. Syphilis

Clinical Note. Here is a disease remarkably similar to rheumatic fever except that the initial lesion in rheumatic fever occurs in the throat (a streptococcal pharyngitis). Both produce a variety of skin lesions and in their acute stages may cause myocarditis and central nervous system involvement (Syndenham's chorea and Chagas' meningoencephalitis). Both have chronic stages with cardiac involvement; but in Chagas' disease the myocardium is the principal site of disease, whereas in rheumatic fever progressive endocarditis is the principal lesion. Chagas' disease may involve also the lower portion of the esophagus (E), producing achalasia, and the colon. The initial lesion of Chagas' disease may be in the skin, and rarely there is an initial onset with polyserositis and edema. When laboratory examination of the blood is negative, cultures, animal inoculation and a complement-fixation test should be performed before the disease is definitely ruled out.

Pathology. The myocardium shows an interstitial inflammation with mononuclear cells, *Trypanosoma cruzi* organisms, and destruction of muscle fibers. The endocardium and pericardium may also be involved.

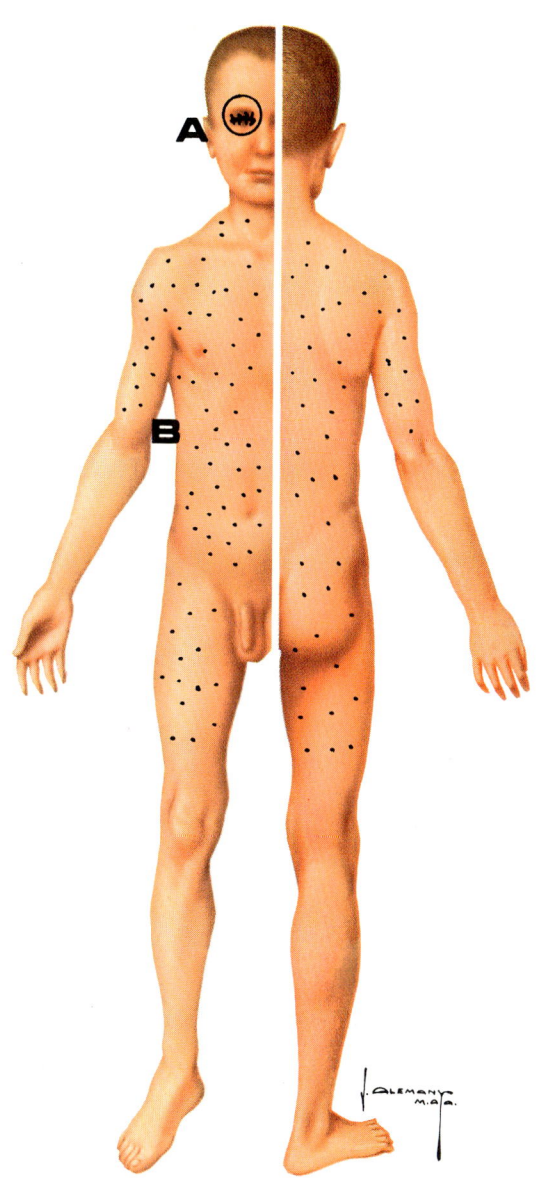

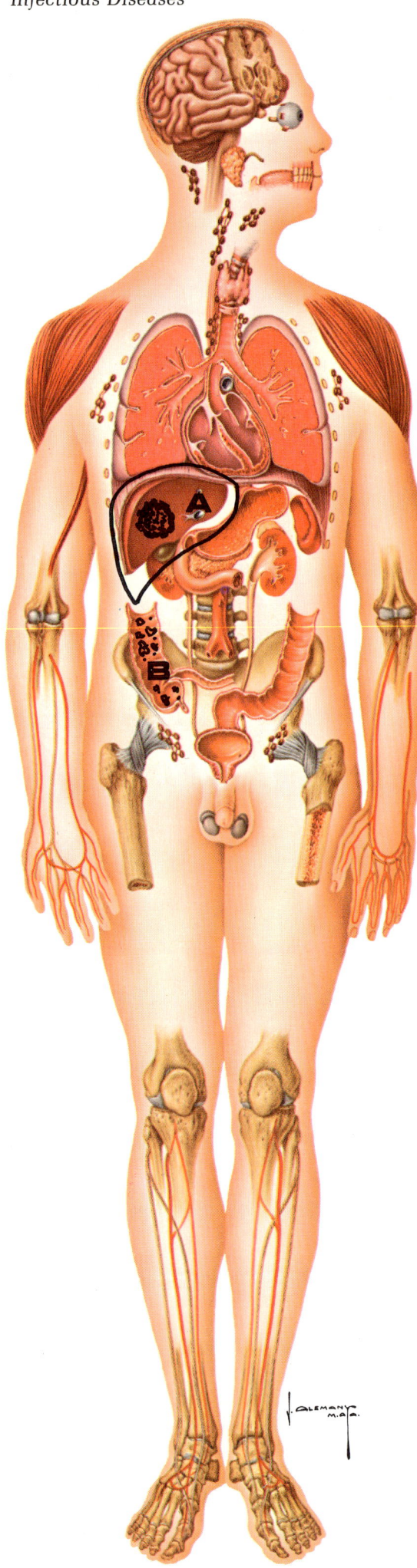

Amebiasis

A 34-year-old Negro male complained of recurrent fever and chills for the past 3 months. For several months he had also had intermittent diarrhea with blood and mucus at times.

Physical examination revealed tenderness in the right upper quadrant and a large tender liver (A) due to an abscess.

Laboratory examination revealed a moderate leukocytosis, numerous amoebic trophozoites in a fresh warm cathartic stool, and a positive complement-fixation reaction to *Entamoeba histolytica*.

X-ray examination of the chest revealed elevation and fixation of the right leaf of the diaphragm, and a barium enema revealed a narrow, irregular cecum caused by amebic ulcerations (B).

Treatment with chloroquine was effective.

Differential Diagnosis:
1. Ulcerative colitis
2. *Salmonella* infections
3. Mucous colitis
4. Carcinoid syndrome
5. Carcinoma of the large bowel
6. Zollinger-Ellison syndrome
7. Celiac disease
8. Regional enteritis
9. Other intestinal parasites
10. Hyperthyroidism
11. Viral hepatitis

Clinical Note. A spiking temperature is often the only symptom of this disease. There may be tenderness in the right upper quadrant. As many as one third of the patients do not have diarrhea at all. Both the sigmoidoscopic examination and the barium enema are negative in the majority of cases. In most cases only a warm stool obtained by inducing diarrhea will be diagnostic. The complement-fixation test has been abandoned in most laboratories. Involvement of the cecum and ascending colon is typical of this disorder, in contrast to ulcerative colitis. The spread to the liver is similar to that found in carcinoid syndrome and carcinomas of the large bowel. An acute and chronic hepatitis has been described. The lung may be involved by direct extension.

Pathology. Although the ulcers usually involve the right side of the large bowel, they may extend throughout the bowel. The lesion begins in the mucosa in contrast to the sequence in ulcerative colitis. Hemorrhage, perforation, and stricture are uncommon. The amebic abscess of the liver develops from coalescence of necrotic areas.

Cysticercosis

A 32-year-old Mexican farmer sustained a grand mal seizure.

Physical examination revealed left-sided hemiparesis, indicating involvement of the right cerebral hemisphere (A).

Laboratory examination revealed eosinophilia, and the eggs of *Taenia solium* were found in the stool. Spinal fluid examination revealed 110 white cells per cu. mm. with a high percentage of eosinophils. A biopsy of subcutaneous tissue was positive for cysticerci.

Treatment with quinacrine hydrochloride was helpful.

Differential Diagnosis:
1. Trichinosis
2. Schistosomiasis
3. Brain tumor
4. Cerebral abscess
5. Idiopathic epilepsy
6. Hypoglycemia, of various causes
7. Hypocalcemia, of various causes
8. Collagen disease
9. Cerebral infarction
10. Tuberculosis
11. Syphilis
12. Cryptococcosis

Clinical Note. Cysticercosis in man is almost always due to *T. solium*, but a few cases due to *T. saginata* have been reported. The infection involves most the subcutaneous tissues (B) and muscle (C) (like Trichinosis), but its presence in these areas is infrequently recognized clinically. The brain, eyes, lungs, and peritoneum may also be involved. The live parasite causes little tissue reaction, but when it dies, there are reaction and encapsulation, and eventually calcification. Surgical removal is often necessary in cases with cerebral involvement. Only 25 per cent of these cases can be diagnosed by examining the stool for eggs. Biopsy is the only way to be sure about the rest. Intestinal infection by the adult worm is often unnoticed.

Pathology. As mentioned, when the larva dies, there is mononuclear cell reaction with fibrosis, encapsulation, and finally calcification. Man usually gets the infection by eating infected pork. The adult worms develop in the intestines (D) and produce eggs which pass with the stools. If the person is not careful to wash after bowel movements, the eggs are passed from anus to mouth and ingested. The eggs hatch into cysticerci in the upper bowel, where they invade the bloodstream and lymphatics.

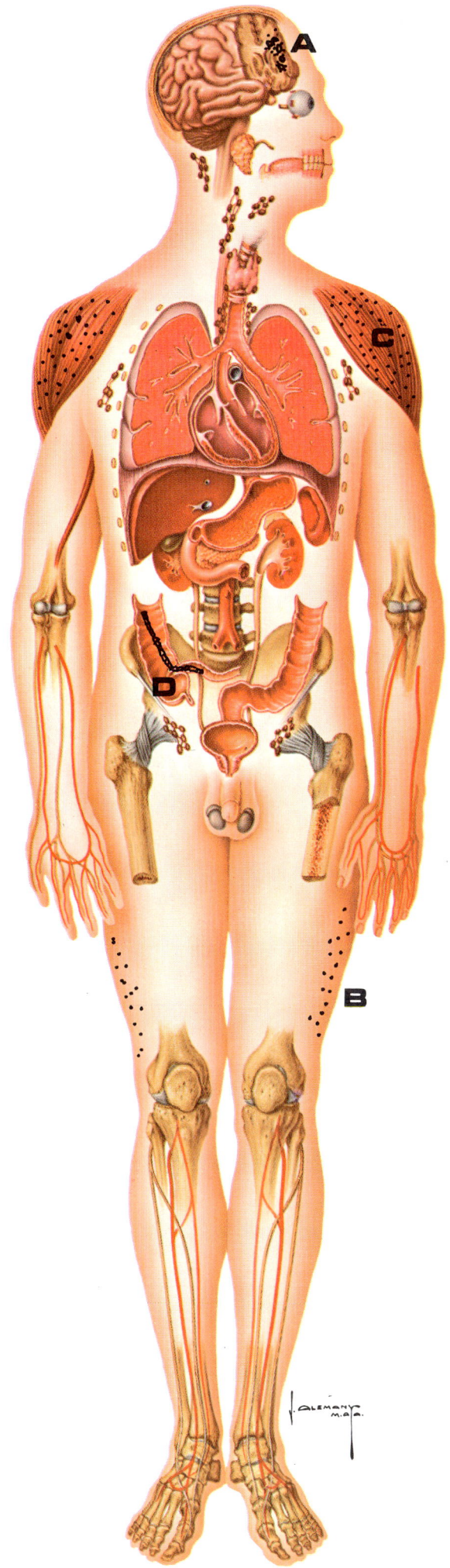

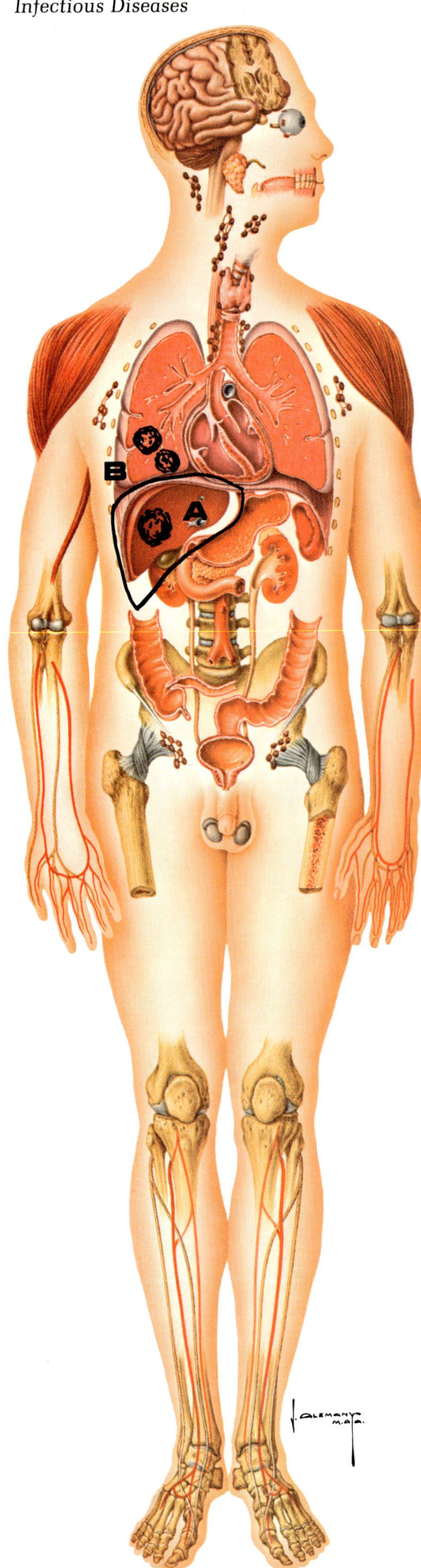

Echinococcosis

A 36-year-old Australian farmer complained of a persistent chronic cough and occasional hemoptysis.

Physical examination revealed a few crepitant and sonorous rales of the right lung and hepatomegaly without jaundice (A); otherwise the man was in surprisingly good health.

Laboratory examination revealed a slight eosinophilia, a positive Casoni skin test for echinococcosis, and a positive complement-fixation test for echinococcosis.

X-ray examination of the chest revealed 2 round radiopaque densities, 4 cm. in diameter, in the right lower lobe (B).

Surgical removal of the pulmonary cysts was effective.

Differential Diagnosis:
1. Tuberculosis
2. Coccidioidomycosis
3. Paragonimiasis
4. Bronchogenic carcinoma
5. Pulmonary embolism
6. Actinomycosis
7. Amebiasis
8. Kala-azar
9. Schistosomiasis
10. Histoplasmosis
11. Q-fever
12. Infectious mononucleosis
13. Silicosis
14. Hodgkin's disease

Clinical Note. Although the liver is the most common site of invasion, the lungs, bone, kidney, and, rarely, the brain may be involved. These patients may harbor the cysts for years with very few symptoms unless they rupture, when toxic manifestations commonly occur. The cysts may be visualized in the liver on x-ray if they become calcified. Liver function tests are usually unaltered. Puncture for diagnostic purposes is contraindicated because it may induce manifestations such as anaphylactic shock. Surgical removal is not always effective, and cysts in bone are best left alone. Man probably gets the infection by handling infected soil or dogs whose fur is contaminated.

Pathology. The cysts induce a lymphocytic and histiocytic reaction, often with giant cells and eosinophils. Later there is peripheral fibrosis. The cyst itself is made up of two layers: the germinative layer and the laminated layer. As described above, the last forms a third layer of reaction and fibrous tissue.

Filariasis (Bancroftian)

A 24-year-old soldier complained of a large red swelling on the inner aspect of his left thigh and of fever, chills, and nausea. He had had several previous attacks of swelling, usually in the same place but occasionally in the scrotum and elsewhere.

Physical examination revealed a raised, indurated, red hot swelling, 12 cm. in diameter, of the left thigh (A) and generalized lymphadenopathy (B), particularly of the inguinal lymph nodes (C).

Laboratory examination of blood smears taken at night revealed several microfilariae, and there was a prominent eosinophilia.

Treatment with diethylcarbamazine was effective.

Differential Diagnosis:
1. Erysipelas
2. Urticaria
3. Lymphogranuloma venereum
4. Syphilis
5. Lymphedema
6. Phlebitis
7. Osteomyelitis
8. Diabetes mellitus
9. Scleroderma
10. Lupus erythematosus
11. Erythema induratum
12. Weber-Christian disease
13. Eczema, focal

Clinical Note. Most medical students get the misconception that the major manifestation of filariasis is elephantiasis. In fact, only a small percentage of cases develop an enlarged leg or scrotum (D). Even the breast or arm may be involved. It may take a year before microfilariae appear in the blood; hence a skin test and a complement-fixation test may have to be used to get a diagnosis. Lymph node biopsy is also of value. Man contracts the infection from the bite of an infected mosquito.

Pathology. The adult worms reside in the lymphatic tissues, where they invoke acute edema and obliterative endolymphangitis, with eosinophilia initially. Later there is granulomatous development with giant cells and mononuclear cell reaction. There may be an intense fibroblastic hyperplasia with obstructive thrombosis or fibrosis of the lymphatics.

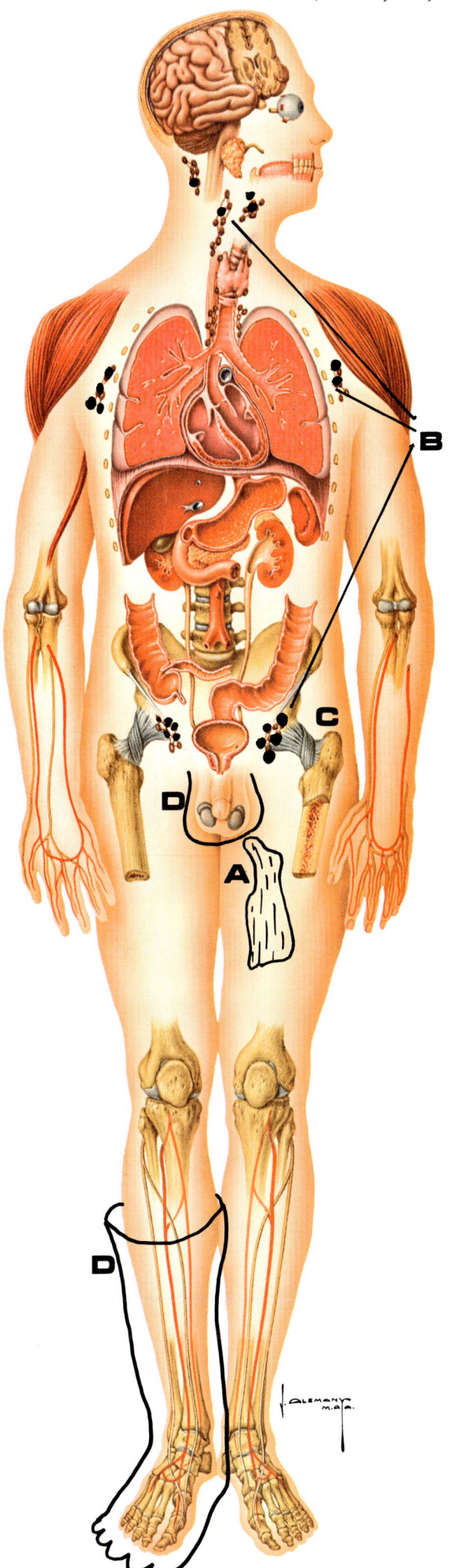

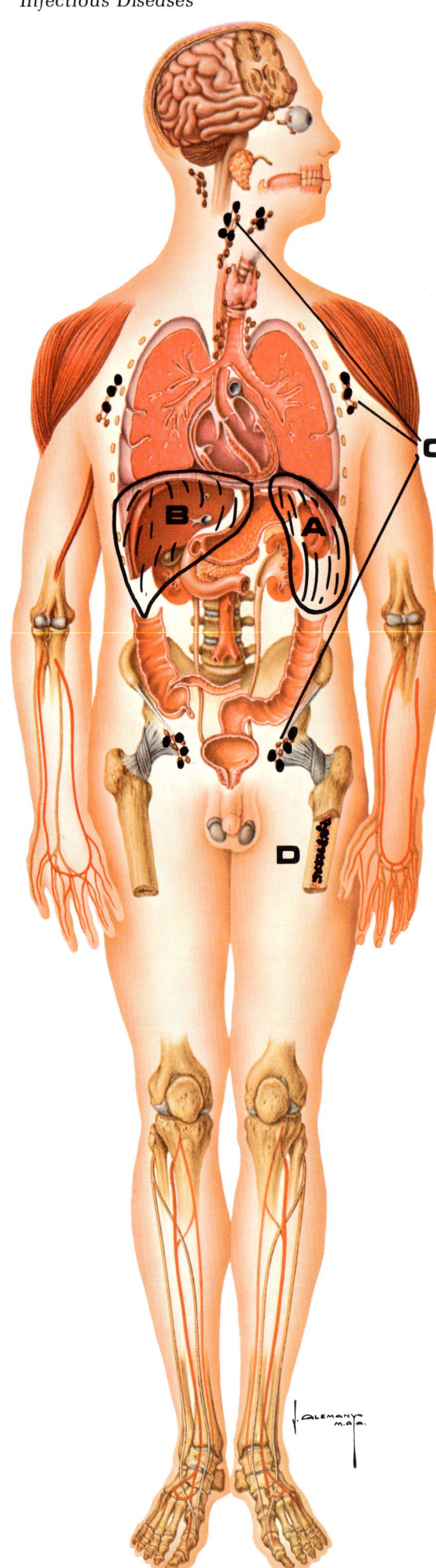

Kala-Azar

A 38-year-old Chinese was found to have on routine physical a large left upper quadrant mass. Careful questioning revealed that he had experienced intermittent fever, dizziness, anorexia, and some weight loss for at least a year.

Physical examination revealed a massive nontender spleen (A), hepatomegaly (B) without jaundice, and generalized lymphadenopathy (C).

Laboratory examination revealed anemia, leukopenia, and thrombocytopenia. Typical *Leishmania* forms were found in the blood smears.

Treatment with ethylstibamine was ineffective.

Differential Diagnosis:
1. Malaria
2. Schistosomiasis
3. Relapsing fever
4. Leptospirosis
5. Hodgkin's disease
6. Cirrhosis of the liver
7. Hemolytic anemias
8. Typhoid fever
9. Myeloid metaplasia
10. Gaucher's disease
11. Tuberculosis
12. Histoplasmosis
13. Brucellosis
14. Bacterial endocarditis

Clinical Note. Here is a protozoan that, like malaria, assaults the reticuloendothelial system in contrast to trypanosomiasis, which affects the heart and central nervous system. The discovery of the disease on a routine physical emphasizes that symptoms are vague and not usually incapacitating. Of course, the Chinese are used to living with parasites. Jaundice is rare, as would be expected since the main lesion is in the reticuloendothelial system. The pancytopenia is due not only to splenic enlargement but also to bone marrow invasion (D) and replacement by the organisms. In untreated cases skin lesions may develop, as in "oriental sore." The bite of the *Phlebotomus* sandfly usually goes unnoticed in contrast to the bite lesions in trypanosomiasis. When the organisms cannot be found on blood smears, animal inoculation or tissue aspiration and biopsy may supply the diagnosis. The spleen, liver, lymph nodes, or bone marrow may be good sources of the organisms.

Pathology. There is hyperplasia of the reticuloendothelial cells of the spleen and liver, where the *Leishmania* multiply intracellularly. There is replacement of the bone marrow by heavily parasitized reticuloendothelial cells.

Malaria

A 27-year-old soldier who had just returned from Vietnam 1 month prior to admission developed headache, backache, cough, and a low-grade temperature 1 week prior to admission. A diagnosis of viral influenza was made by his local doctor, and he was treated with symptomatic therapy. On the day of admission he developed a high temperature, chills, and severe headache and became slightly confused. A profuse sweat developed later.

Physical examination revealed a temperature of 104° F. and splenomegaly (A) without lymphadenopathy.

Laboratory examination revealed a leukopenia and thrombocytopenia, and *Plasmodium vivax* organisms were found on thick blood smears.

Treatment with chloroquine brought about a remission and assisted in the diagnosis.

Differential Diagnosis:
1. Kala-azar
2. Hemolytic anemias
3. Oroya fever
4. Hodgkin's disease
5. Infectious mononucleosis
6. Pernicious anemia
7. Reticuloendotheliosis
8. Lupus erythematosus
9. Leukemia
10. Typhoid fever
11. Histoplasmosis
12. Tuberculosis
13. Sarcoidosis
14. Other blood dyscrasias
15. Serum sickness

Clinical Note. Soldiers may not develop symptoms for some time after discharge because they are on malaria prophylaxis while in the service. When the patient presents with only splenomegaly, the list of differential diagnoses is long. However, the temperature curve is almost diagnostic although other diseases (rat-bite fever, etc.) may produce a relapsing temperature. Anyone with fever of unknown origin should be questioned about travel outside of the country, especially in this day of jet airline service. The liver (B) is usually involved in vivax malaria, but there is rarely jaundice. The fact that lymphadenopathy is uncommon in the early stages helps to rule out infectious mononucleosis. The stupor and confusion are not always due to the temperature. Falciparum malaria may cause focal and diffuse cerebral involvement (C) because of plugging of the small cerebral vessels. It is also the usual cause of black-water fever (hemoglobinuria) produced by extensive intravascular hemolysis. Now and then repeated smears must be done to establish the diagnosis. A therapeutic diagnostic test is sometimes useful.

Pathology. The spleen is slate-gray in color, and on cut-surface a brownish pulp exudes. This is made up mostly of parasitized erythrocytes. The liver is enlarged and dark, and the Kupffer cells are engorged with disintegrating parasites.

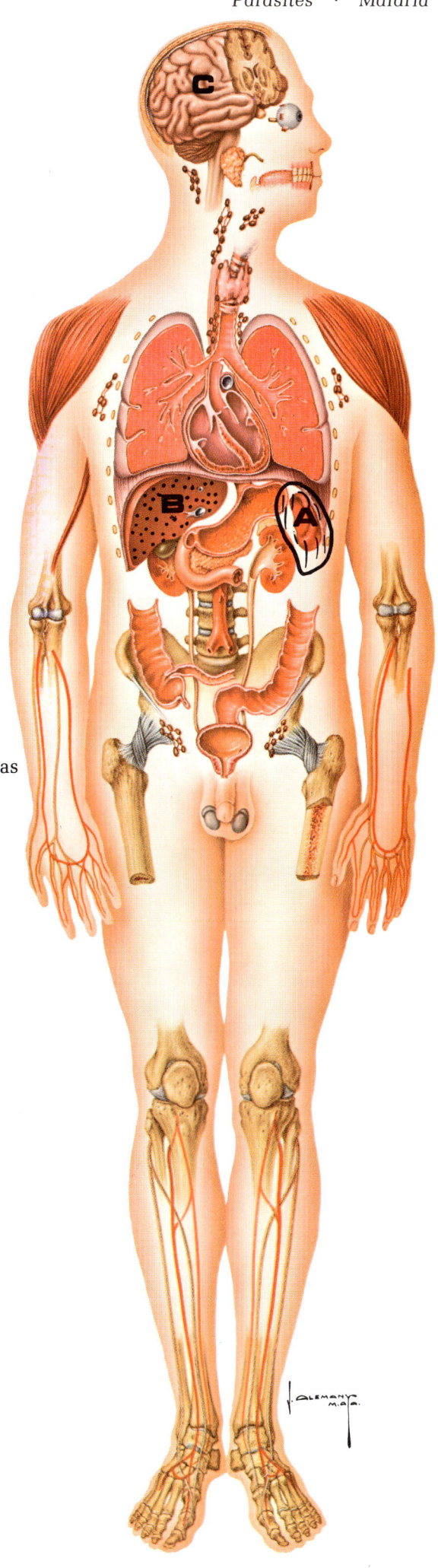

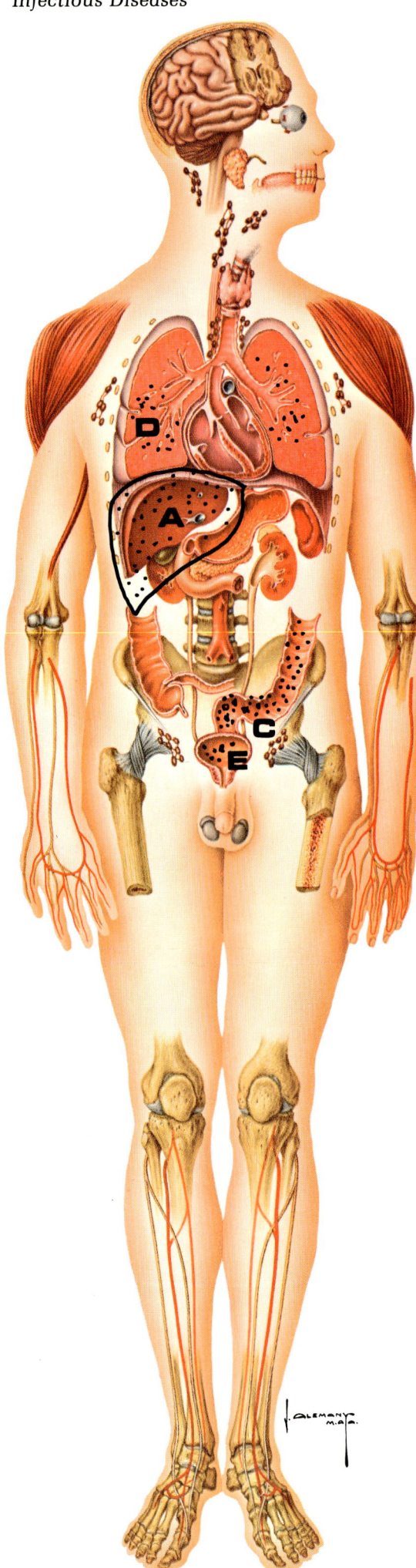

Schistosomiasis (S. Mansoni)

A 24-year-old West Indian developed severe itching and a macular rash of the legs after swimming in a nearby pond. Five weeks later he developed fever, sweats, and abdominal pain.

Physical examination revealed a temperature of 102° F., hepatomegaly (A), and generalized abdominal tenderness. There was a generalized urticaria (B). *Sigmoidoscopy* later revealed many small ulcerations (C).

Laboratory examination revealed an elevated thymol turbidity, a 4+ cephalin flocculation, and a high serum gamma globulin. There was eosinophilia, and *Schistosoma mansoni* eggs were found in the stools.

Treatment with stibophen was effective.

Differential Diagnosis:
1. Trichinosis
2. Viral hepatitis
3. Infectious mononucleosis
4. Ulcerative colitis
5. Whipple's disease
6. Carcinoid syndrome
7. Leptospirosis
8. Yellow fever
9. Malaria

10. Brucellosis
11. Amebiasis
12. Lupus erythematosus
13. Cirrhosis of the liver
14. Gaucher's disease
15. Serum sickness
16. Pernicious anemia
17. Hemochromatosis
18. Amyloidosis
19. Porphyria

Clinical Note. Although the involvement of the skin and liver are the principal lesions in the acute stage, as the disease progresses, the lungs may be involved by embolic eggs (D), and the intestines may become abscessed more and more and may rupture or fibrose. The spleen may be enlarged secondary to the progressive periportal cirrhosis of the liver. There may even be esophageal varices, occasionally convulsions, and hemiplegia and paraplegia may develop from cerebral involvement by the eggs. In S. haematobium infections particularly, there is painless hematuria due to bladder involvement (E).

Pathology. The eggs may be found in the liver, lungs, entire bowels, pancreas, spleen, urogenital organs, and brain. The eggs are the nucleus of pseudotubercles with foreign body giant cells surrounded by a ring of epithelioid cells and a second ring of lymphocytes and eosinophils. Outside this circle there may be fibroblastic proliferation in various stages.

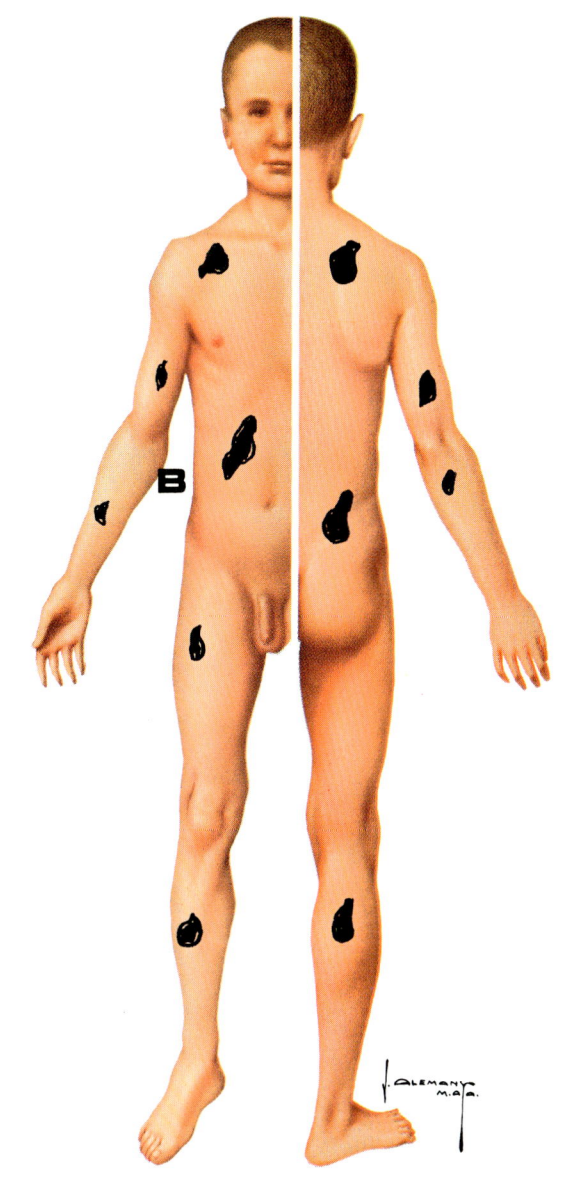

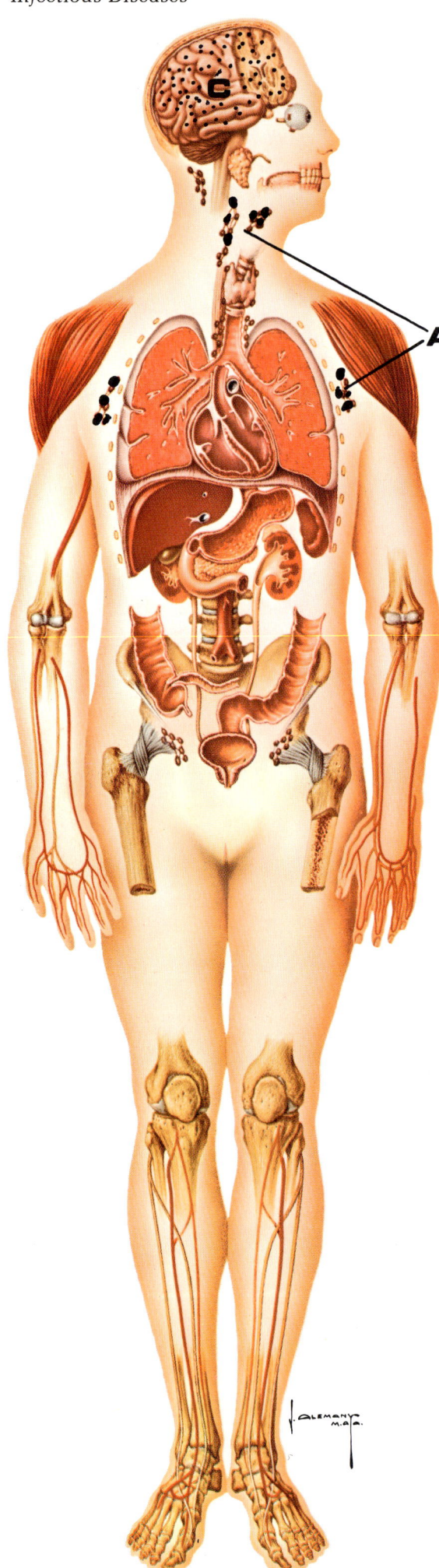

Toxoplasmosis

A 29-year-old white female developed swelling in her neck and moderate fever 14 days prior to admission. On the day of admission she noted blurring of the vision in her right eye.

Physical examination revealed cervical and axillary adenopathy (A), chorioretinitis in the right fundus (B), and tender muscles.

Laboratory examination revealed a Sabin-Feldman dye test positive to 1:1000. Later the toxoplasma complement-fixation test became positive.

Treatment with pyrimethamine and sulfamethazine was unsuccessful.

Differential Diagnosis:
1. Infectious mononucleosis
2. Listeriosis
3. Brucellosis
4. Syphilis
5. Tuberculosis
6. Sarcoidosis
7. Histoplasmosis
8. Tuberosclerosis
9. Sturge-Weber syndrome
10. Trichinosis
11. German measles

Clinical Note. There is tremendous similarity to infectious mononucleosis. The muscles may be involved by the encysted parasites, as in trichinosis. In the adult disseminated form there may be spread to the lungs, heart, brain, and liver. The congenital form is probably more common, and principally involved are the brain (C), producing mental retardation, convulsions, and cerebral calcifications, and the eye, affected with a more severe chorioretinitis.

Pathology. There is reticulum cell hyperplasia in the lymph nodes, perimacular coagulation necrosis of the retina and choroid with adjacent mononuclear cell infiltrates, and periventricular necrosis with a granulomatous reaction. Occasionally there may be a large spherical mass in the brain filled with parasites.

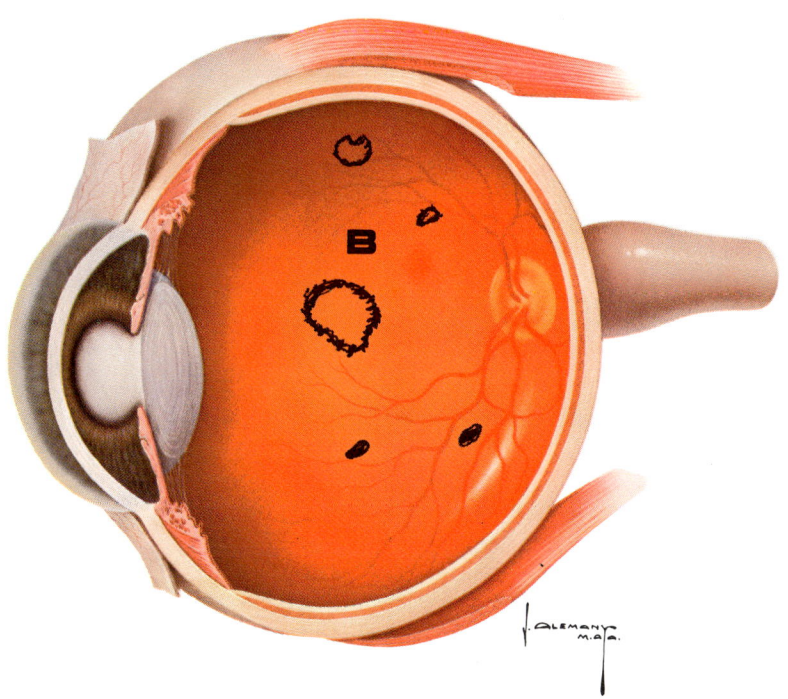

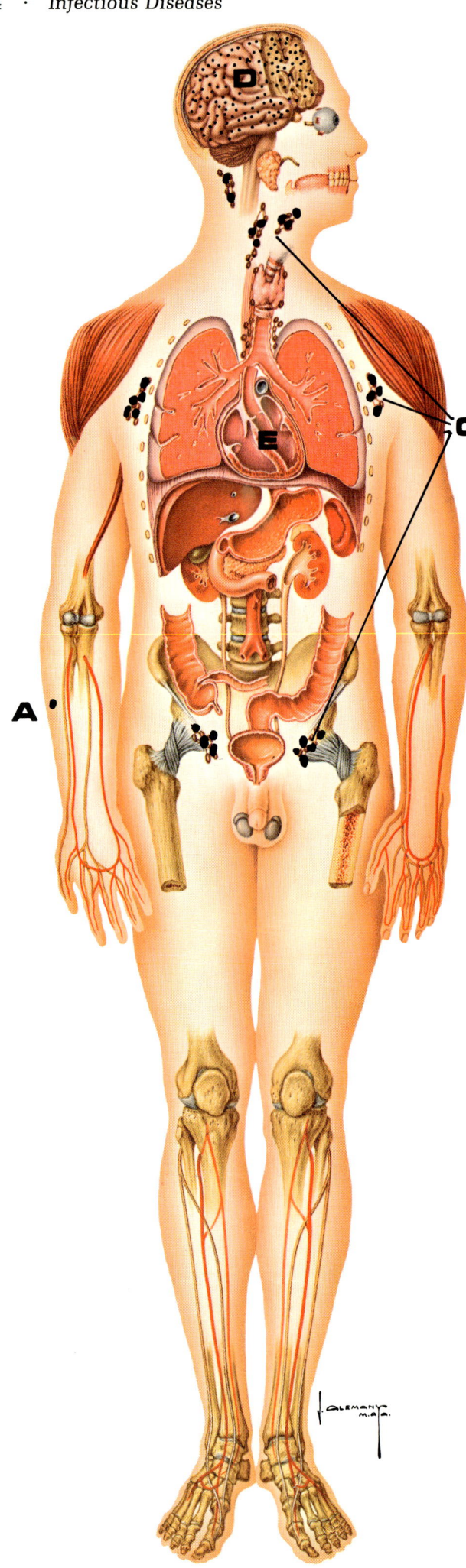

African Trypanosomiasis

A 25-year-old Negro male complained of fever, persistent headache, and a generalized rash. Three weeks previously he had noted a red swelling on his right forearm (A) (the bite of a *Glossina* fly).

Physical examination revealed a generalized erythematous maculopapular rash (B) and generalized lymphadenopathy (C); nuchal rigidity and tremors of his hands gave evidence of meningeal and nervous system involvement (D).

Laboratory examination revealed trypanosomes in the blood and cerebrospinal fluid and a spinal fluid cell count of 550 cells/cu. mm., most of which were lymphocytes.

Treatment with suramin sodium and tryparsamide was effective.

Differential Diagnosis:
1. Syphilis
2. Schistosomiasis
3. Malaria
4. Cysticercosis
5. Leptospirosis
6. Cryptococcosis
7. Tuberculosis
8. Viral meningitis
9. Poliomyelitis
10. Measles
11. Infectious mononucleosis
12. Yellow fever
13. Brucellosis

Clinical Note. The invasion of the skin and lymph nodes (at first local and then generalized) and then of the blood and central nervous system is typical. Splenomegaly is common but never as great as in leishmaniasis. A pancarditis (E) has been described. The lymph nodes are tender at first. Involvement of the central nervous system may lead to cerebellar ataxia or a pyramidal tract syndrome. Severe mental disturbances are common and simulate general paresis. The disease is usually fatal without treatment. When the organisms cannot be found in the blood, they are often found on lymph node aspiration or guinea pig inoculation.

Pathology. The meninges may be thickened and adherent, and the brain is edematous. There is perivascular cuffing of plasma cells on microscopic examination. Russell bodies (probably degenerated plasma cells) are seen in these areas throughout the brain. The myocardium may be be infiltrated with mononuclear cells and some adjacent scar formation.

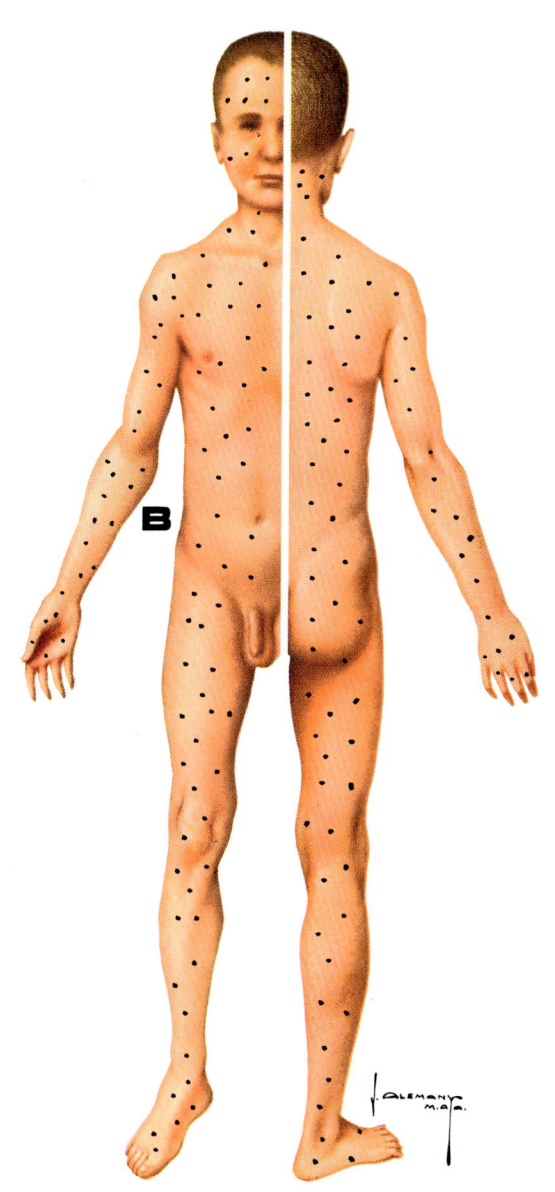

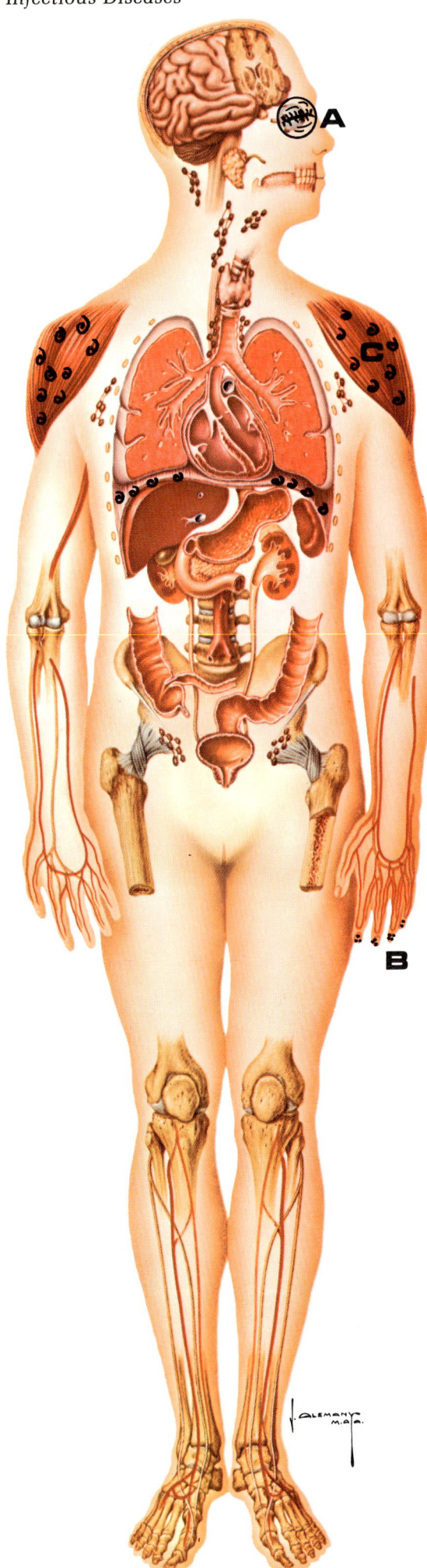

Trichinosis

A 28-year-old white female developed acute nausea and vomiting and diarrhea 1 week prior to admission; the condition was diagnosed as viral gastroenteritis. Careful questioning revealed that she had had sausage for lunch 2 days prior to this. The day before admission she developed swelling of her face, fever, and muscular pain and weakness.

Physical examination revealed periorbital edema (A), splinter hemorrhages (B) of the nails, and tender deltoid muscles.

Laboratory examination revealed eosinophilia, and biopsy of the deltoid muscle (C) was positive for *Trichinella* larvae.

Treatment with corticosteroids was helpful.

Differential Diagnosis:
1. Dermatomyositis
2. Periarteritis nodosa
3. Cysticercosis
4. Viral influenza
5. Serum sickness
6. Acute glomerulonephritis
7. Poliomyelitis
8. Subacute bacterial endocarditis
9. Sickle cell crisis
10. Porphyria

Clinical Note. Most of these cases, like those of poliomyelitis, go undiagnosed because too few of the larvae get to the muscles. Trichinosis is easily mistaken for dermatomyositis. There may be transient skin rashes in addition to the periorbital edema. The intradermal skin test is not too useful in diagnosis because it isn't positive for 2 weeks, and chronic cases of trichinosis are infrequently seen clinically since the symptoms clear after encystment of the larvae. Central nervous system involvement causing delirium and even hemiplegia is infrequent but reminds one of cysticercosis. This disease is felt to be one of the worst public health problems of our time.

Pathology. The larvae are most frequently found in the diaphragmatic, deltoid, intercostal, and cervical muscles. A ring of basophilic material forms around the larvae, the muscles undergo hydropic or hyaline degeneration, and there are edema and infiltration of all types of white cells in the connective tissues, with eventual encapsulation of the larva.

Chapter 8

Metabolic Diseases

This is another group of diseases which are for the most part hereditary. With the exception of gout and diabetes mellitus, they are rare. Genetic counseling may eradicate many of these disorders. They are usually due to a deficiency of a body enzyme or hormone, some of which may be deficient only in utero. Since there are hundreds of enzymes in the body metabolism, there must be hundreds more as yet unclassified or undescribed metabolic disorders.

The diagnosis of a few of these can be made clinically (Kayser-Fleischer ring in Wilson's disease, etc.), but once again the laboratory is absolutely essential to the diagnosis in most cases.

198 · *Metabolic Diseases*

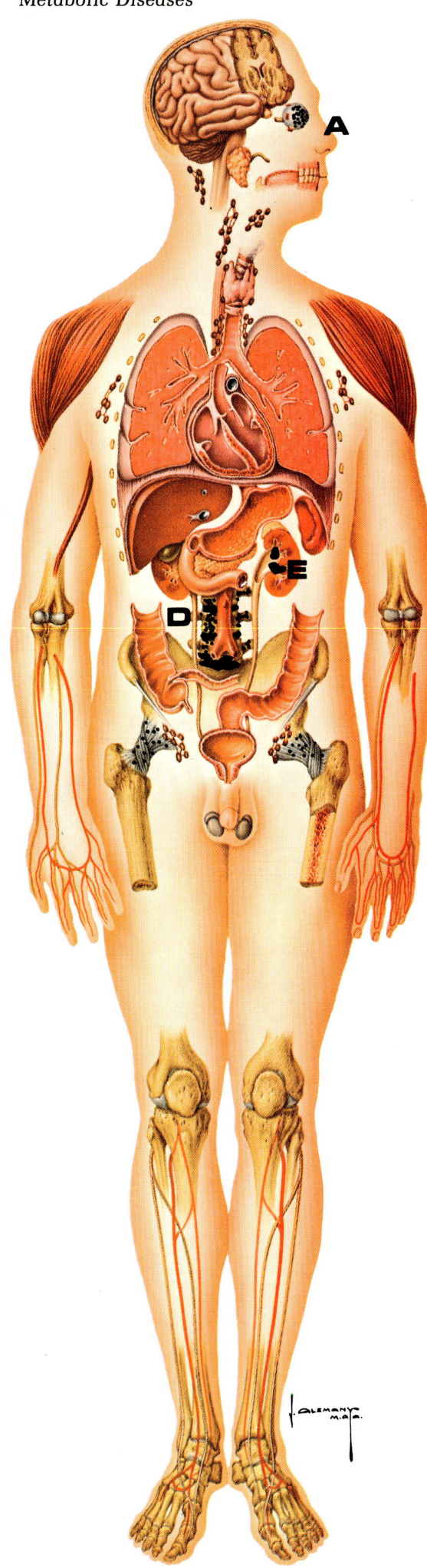

Alkaptonuria and Ochronosis

A 36-year-old white male had had dark-staining urine since childhood. Now he complained of frequent pain in his right hip. His father had been troubled with a similar condition all his life.

Physical examination revealed light brown pigmentation of both sclera (A), bluish discoloration of the external ears (B), and brownish pigmentation of the skin (C).

Laboratory examination revealed that the urine turned dark on adding alkali, and it reduced Benedict's solution. Homogentisic acid was isolated from the urine.

X-ray examination revealed degenerative osteoarthritic changes in both hip joints and calcification of the intervertebral disks (D).

Differential Diagnosis:
1. Rheumatoid arthritis and spondylitis
2. Cystinosis
3. Osteoarthritis
4. Osteogenesis imperfecta
5. Metastatic carcinoma
6. Multiple myeloma

Clinical Note. This condition is due to a lack of homogentisic acid oxidase, which normally destroys the homogentisic acid. It is often diagnosed in infancy by the dark urine on the diapers. The intense calcification of the intervertebral disks, as seen in this case, is pathognomonic of the disease. This is a benign disease and does not shorten life appreciably.

Pathology. Deposits of the excess homogentisic acid on the cartilages, tendons, joints, skin, and other connective tissues account for the clinical findings. That which is excreted in the urine may occasionally form stones (E).

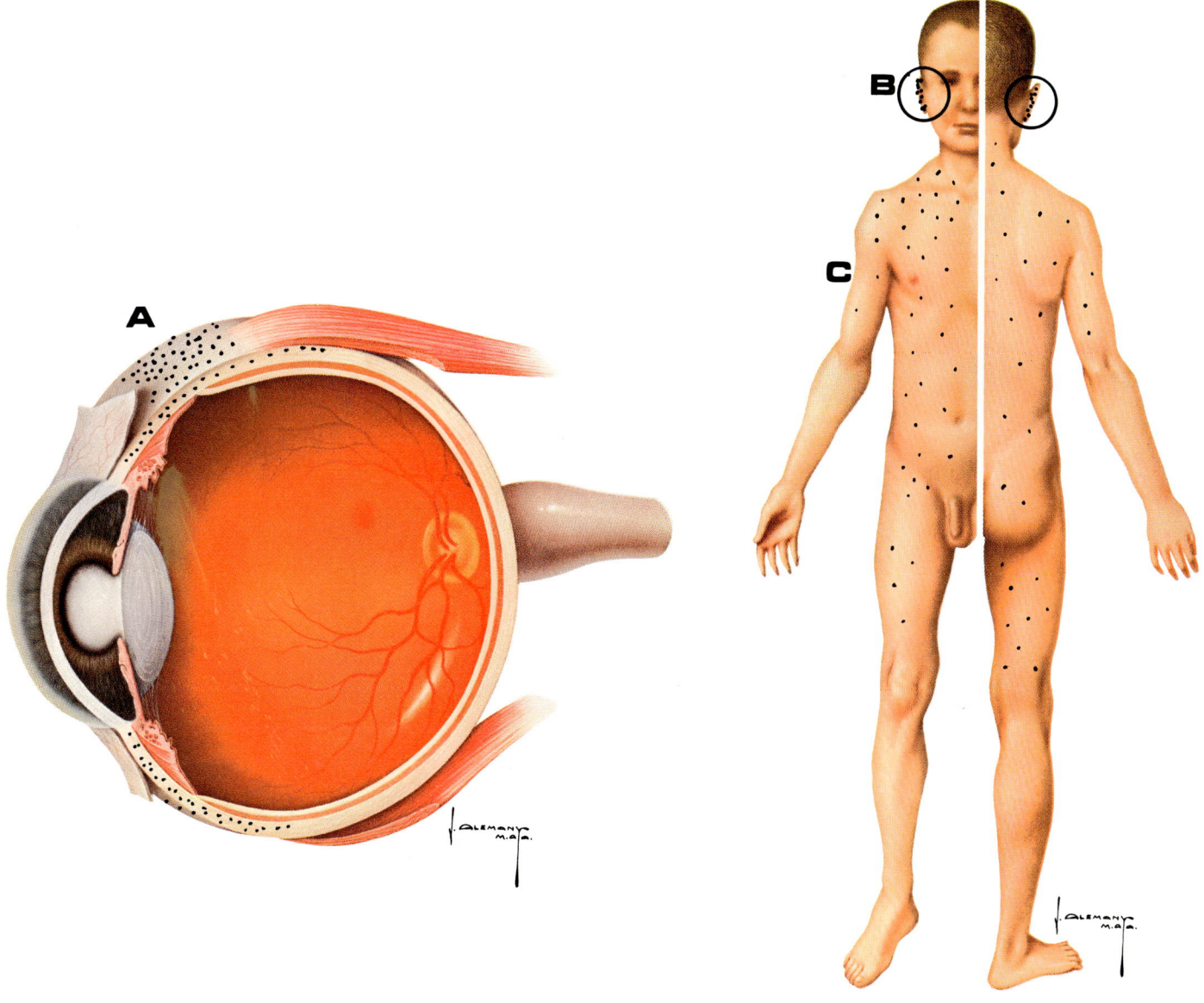

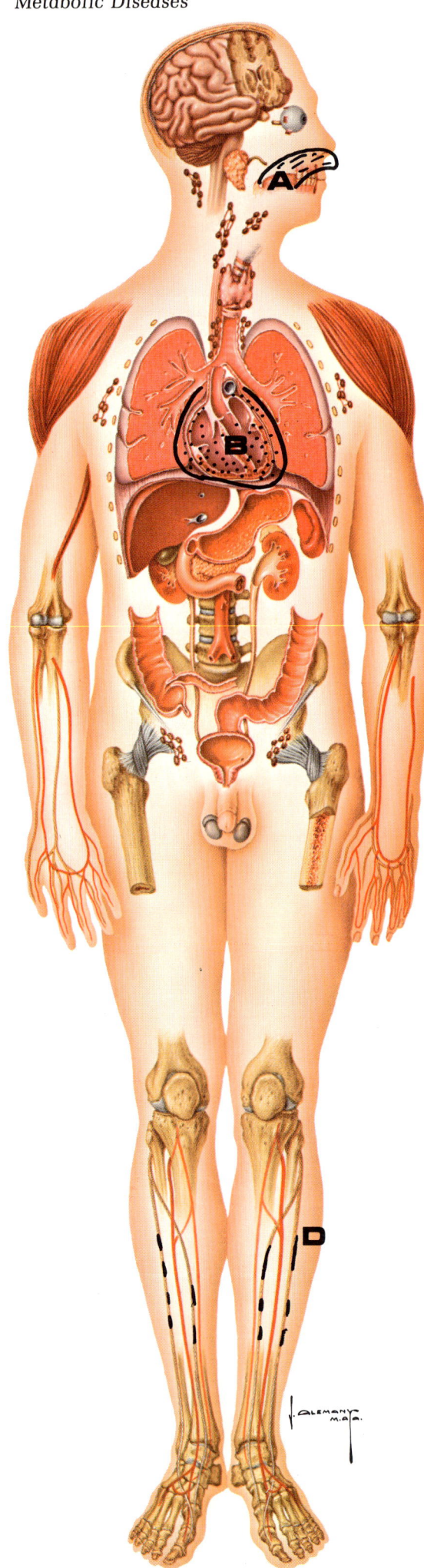

Primary Systemic Amyloidosis

A 52-year-old white male complained of increasing shortness of breath, swelling of the legs, and palpitations. He had noted that his speech became thick at times in the previous 2 weeks.

Physical examination revealed macroglossia (A), bilateral crepitant rales over the lungs, cardiomegaly (B), 2+ pitting edema of both legs, and waxy nodules of the skin about the neck, eyelids, and upper and lower extremities (C).

Laboratory examination revealed an equivocal Congo red test. Gingival and lingual biopsy revealed the amyloid deposits.

Differential Diagnosis:
1. Secondary amyloidosis
2. Congestive heart failure due to atherosclerotic heart disease
3. Glycogen storage disease
4. Hemochromatosis
5. Rheumatic heart disease
6. Subacute bacterial endocarditis
7. Beriberi
8. Myxedema
9. Constrictive pericarditis

Clinical Note. There is a sharp contrast in the involvement here as compared with that of secondary amyloidosis, and yet both may involve the liver, spleen, and kidneys. These two types of amyloidosis are analogous to glycogen storage disease of the von Gierke's type, which involves the liver, and to generalized glycogenosis, which involves the heart. There is a tendency of clinicians to regard every case of congestive heart failure without obvious valvular involvement as due to atherosclerotic heart disease. This is the reason that this condition is so frequently overlooked. Since no treatment is available, this is not critical. However, beriberi and hypothyroidism are two causes of heart failure that can be treated and therefore should be remembered.

Pathology. The amyloid deposits have a predilection for cardiac, skeletal, and smooth muscle, particularly the smooth muscle of the medium-sized and small blood vessels throughout the body. Neuropathies (D) are common in the familial form of this disease. The distribution of the amyloid deposits in multiple myeloma is similar to that in primary systemic amyloidosis.

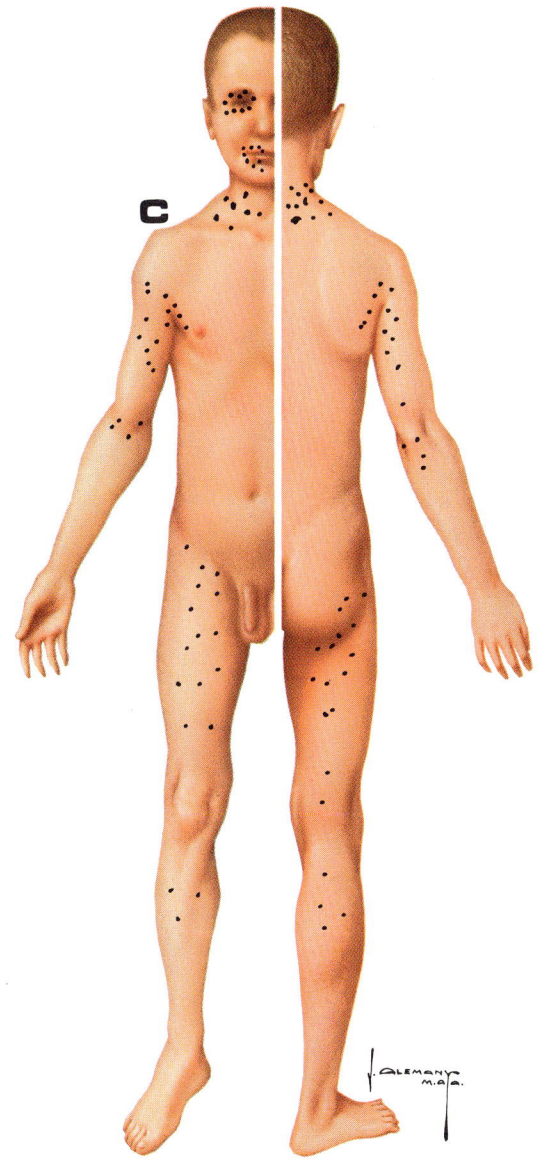

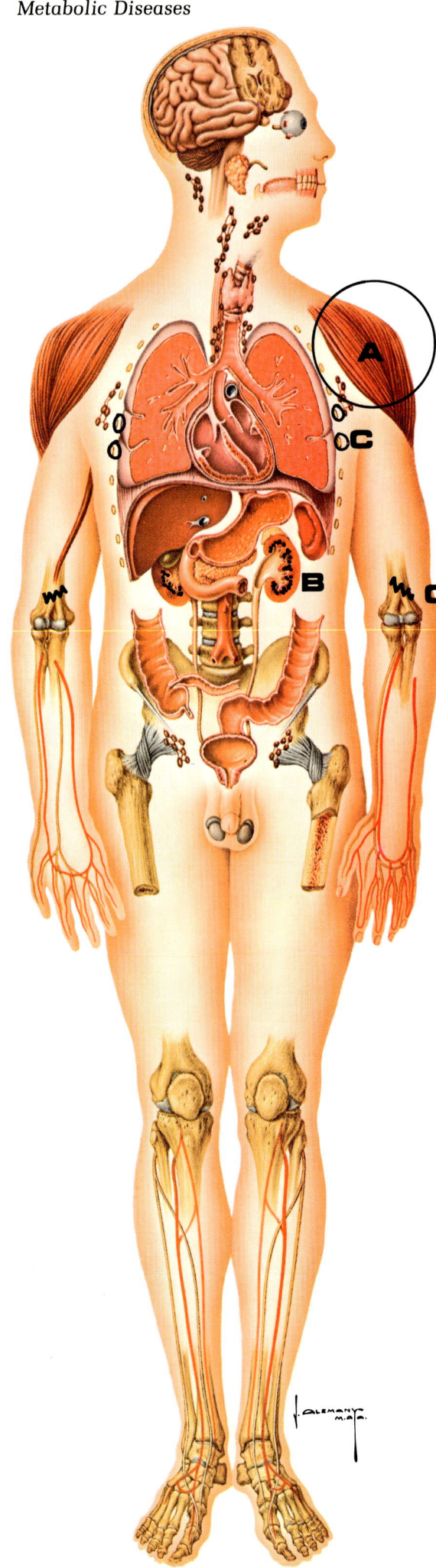

Renal Tubular Acidosis

A 16-year-old white male complained of periodic muscular weakness (A) and fatigue over the past year. He had been hospitalized for treatment of a renal calculus 6 months previously.

Physical examination revealed generalized hyporeflexia and a waddling gait, but was otherwise unremarkable.

Laboratory examination revealed a reduced serum potassium, bicarbonate, and phosphate, a normal serum calcium, and a high alkaline phosphatase. The urine was persistently alkaline, and there was hypercalcuria.

X-ray examination revealed nephrocalcinosis (B), osteomalacia, and symmetrical fractures of the ribs and humeri (C).

Treatment with alkalinizing mixtures of citrates, calcium, and potassium salts, and with vitamin D was very successful.

Differential Diagnosis:
1. Familial periodic paralysis
2. Lignac-Fanconi syndrome
3. Hyperparathyroidism
4. Acetazolamide toxicity
5. Chronic renal failure
6. Infectious mononucleosis

Clinical Note. The differential diagnosis of fatigue in young adults can be fascinating if conditions like this are always considered. The presence of nephrocalcinosis distinguishes this condition from the Lignac-Fanconi syndrome. The normal serum calcium helps to differentiate it from hyperparathyroidism, but this distinction is sometimes difficult.

Pathology. Except for the nephrocalcinosis and osteomalacia, with the pathologic fractures mentioned above, there are no distinct pathologic changes. The tubular defect is physiologic rather than anatomic and based on an inability to excrete hydrogen ion.

Secondary Amyloidosis

A 56-year-old white male had had recurrent pulmonary tuberculosis for several years. In the past 3 months he had noted increased swelling of legs and eyelids and, to a lesser extent, the rest of his body.

Physical examination revealed periorbital edema, hepatosplenomegaly (A), and ascites with 4+ pitting edema of both lower extremities (B).

Laboratory examination revealed marked albuminuria and waxy and granular casts in the urine, indicating renal involvement (C). There was a positive Congo red test. Rectal and liver biopsies were both positive for amyloid deposits.

Treatment was limited to cure of the underlying disorder.

Differential Diagnosis:
1. Glycogen storage disease
2. Laennec's cirrhosis
3. Nephrotic stage of glomerulonephritis
4. Kimmelstiel-Wilson's disease
5. Lupus erythematosus
6. Lipoid nephrosis, idiopathic
7. Bilateral renal vein thrombosis

Clinical Note. When the nephrotic syndrome is manifested in the course of a chronic infection of any system, particularly bone, amyloidosis should be suspected. The finding of associated hepatosplenomegaly makes the diagnosis very likely. Contrast the location of the deposits in this disorder with those in primary amyloidosis (page 200). Jaundice is as rare in this disorder as it is in other diseases in which foreign or native material deposits in the liver, such as Wilson's disease, glycogen storage disease, and hemochromatosis.

Pathology. The deposits occur primarily in the liver, spleen, kidney, and adrenal glands (D), principally about the walls of capillaries and arterioles. The deposits lead to compression and atrophy of the parenchymal cells in these organs. Yet clinical adrenal insufficiency is rarely due to the amyloidosis in these glands, but tuberculous involvement of these glands may cause it. The lymph nodes, pancreas, prostate, thyroid gland, and gastrointestinal tract may also be involved.

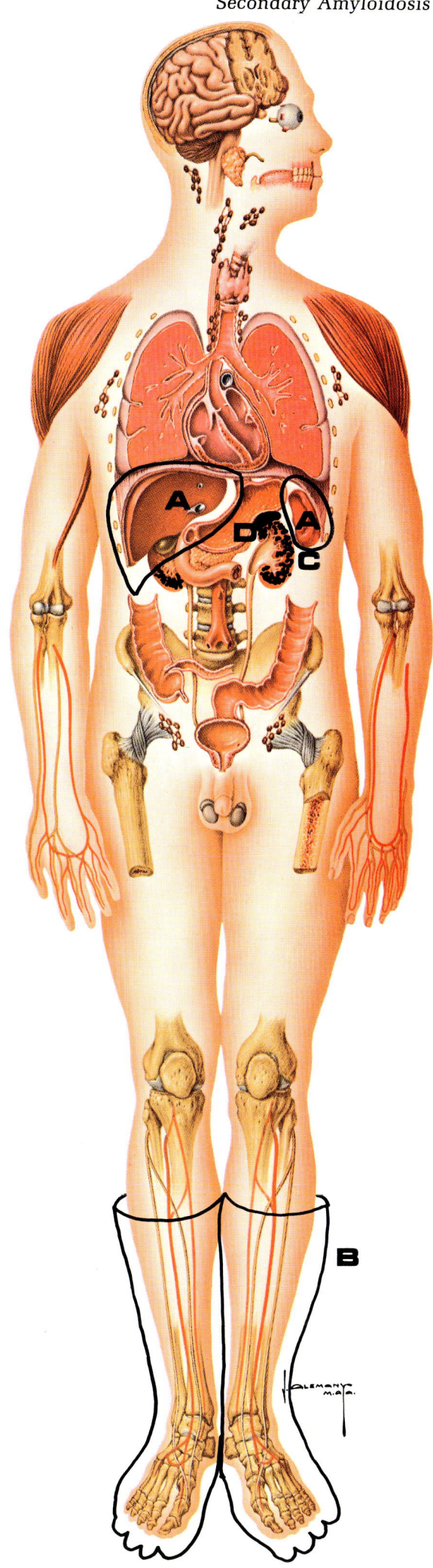

204 · *Metabolic Dieases*

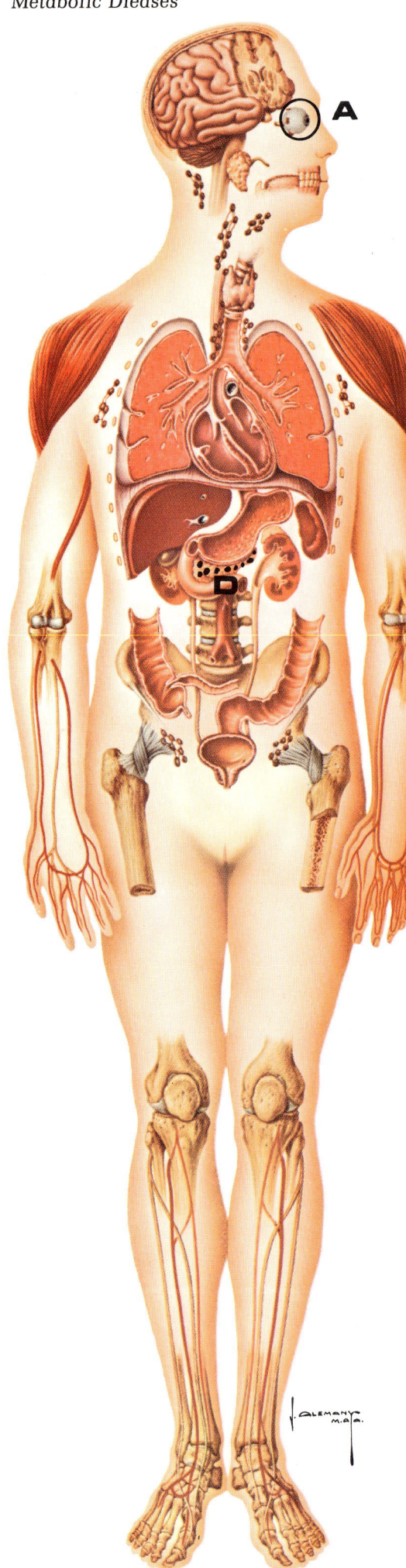

Diabetes Mellitus, Case 1

A 56-year-old white female complained of increasing blurred vision and bifrontal headaches. Her grandmother had died of diabetes mellitus.

Physical examination revealed elevated pressure on tonometry in both eyes, indicating glaucoma (A), and perimacular berry hemorrhages and microaneurysms (B).

Laboratory studies revealed a FBS of 175 mg. per cent and 3+ sugar in her urine.

Treatment with pilocarpine and acetazolamide was effective in controlling the glaucoma.

Differential Diagnosis:
1. Sturge-Weber syndrome
2. Iritis
3. Scleritis
4. Conjunctivitis

Clinical Note. All cases of glaucoma should have a fasting blood sugar. The diabetic retinopathy in this case *made* the diagnosis certain, but it is not always present. Cataracts also may be present (C).

Pathology. Hyalinization and fibrosis were found in many of the islet cells (D).

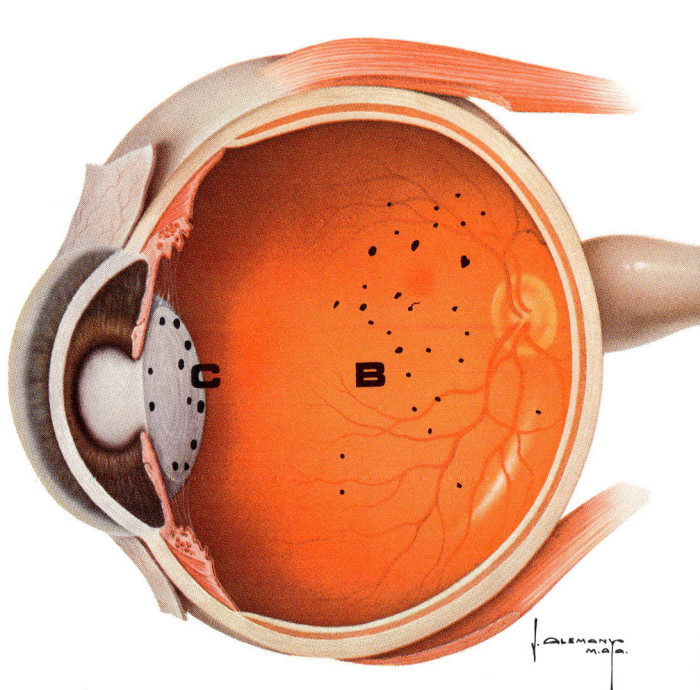

Diabetes Mellitus, Case 2

A 45-year-old white male complained of profound thirst and excessive appetite, frequency of urination, weight loss, and weakness for several months.

Physical examination revealed hemorrhages and microaneurysms in both fundi (A), bilateral atrophy of the interossei muscles, indicating ulnar neuropathy (B), diminished dorsalis pedis and tibialis pulses bilaterally, indicating peripheral arteriosclerosis (C).

Laboratory examination revealed a blood sugar of 450 mg. per cent, a CO_2 of 17 mEq./L., and acetone in the blood and urine.

Differential Diagnosis:
1. Hyperthyroidism
2. Hyperparathyroidism
3. Diabetes insipidus
4. Chronic nephritis
5. Addison's disease
6. Chronic congestive heart failure
7. Celiac disease

Clinical Note. The polydypsia, polyphagia, polyuria, and weight loss are quite typical of this disease, but also characterize hyperthyroidism. Polyneuropathy likewise is common, but it may be a mononeuritis, too, particularly oculomotor or femoral. The acidosis was not severe enough in this case to cause coma, but this undoubtedly would have developed with further procrastination. Premature peripheral arteriosclerosis and atherosclerosis are common.

Pathology. There is hydropic degeneration of the islet cells in various areas of the pancreas, but other areas are normal (D). The neuropathy may be due to one of three things: metabolic degeneration, ischemia due to arteriolarsclerosis of the vasa nervorum, or rupture of the vasa nervorum.

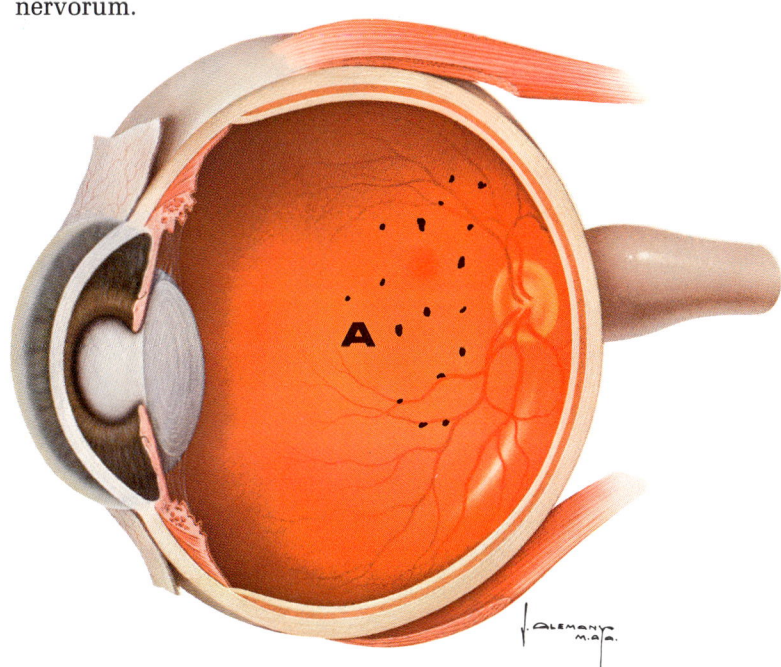
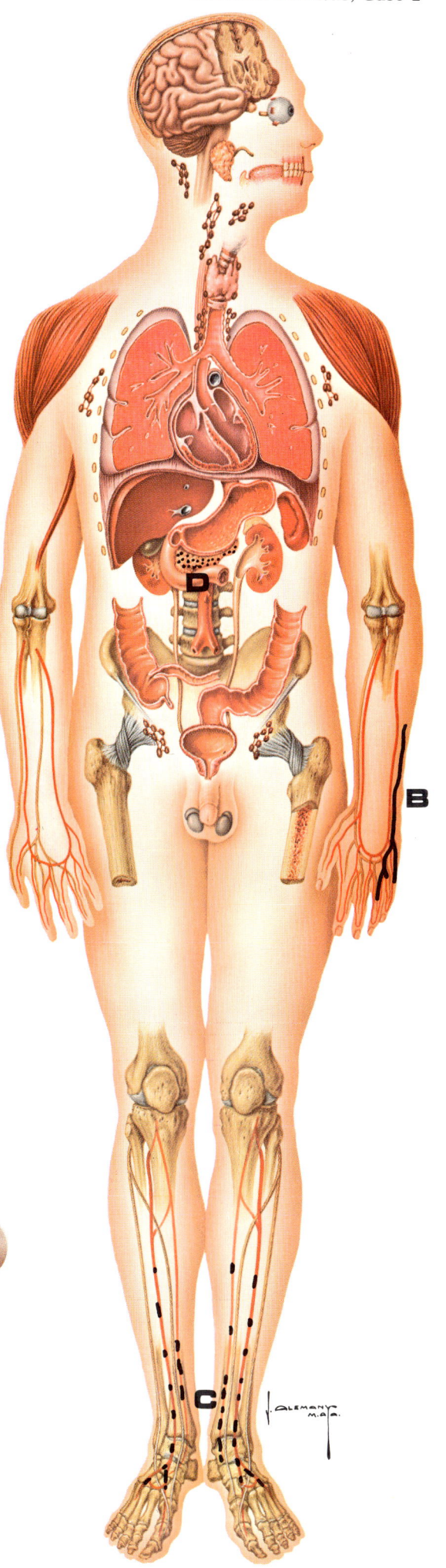

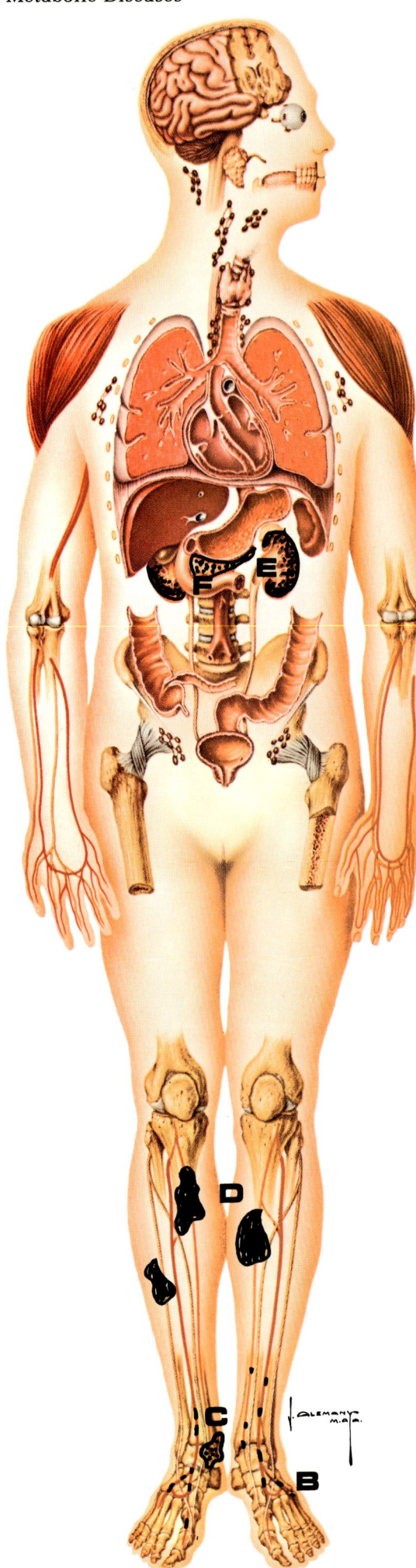

Diabetes Mellitus, Case 3

A 62-year-old white female complained of a painful draining ulcer of her right leg. She was known to have had diabetes mellitus of a severe nature for some time.

Physical examination revealed bilateral diabetic retinopathy (A), diminished dorsalis pedis and tibialis pulses bilaterally (B), a necrotic ulcer, 6 cm. in diameter, over her right medial malleolus (C), and sharply defined, reddish-brown plaques over the anterior tibiae bilaterally (D).

Laboratory examination revealed a blood sugar of 205 mg., a BUN of 38 mg. per cent, a cholesterol of 410 mg. per cent, and an albumin of 3.2 gm. per cent. Urinalysis revealed numerous red cells, red cell and granular casts, and 4+ albuminuria.

Differential Diagnosis:
1. Arteriosclerosis obliterans
2. Varicose ulcers
3. Buerger's disease
4. Sickle cell anemia
5. Yaws
6. Syphilis
7. Fungal diseases
8. Tularemia

Clinical Note. This disease is the great mimicker of local disease. It may present as glaucoma to the ophthalmologist, as a chronic abscess or leg ulcer to the surgeon, as a neuropathy to the neurologist, as nephrosis to the nephrologist, and as an acute myocardial infarction to the cardiologist. There may be many other ways in which it can present. It certainly would be highly desirable to make a fasting blood sugar a routine test on all hospital admissions. This case is of interest because it presents with skin lesions of the lower legs, called *necrobiosis lipoidica*, and also with evidence of renal disease (E), probably Kimmelstiel-Wilson's disease. It is not unusual for sugar to be absent from the urine in this disease despite a high blood sugar because the renal threshold has been elevated by diseased glomeruli.

Pathology. The pancreas, as in case 1, shows changes (F). The arteriosclerotic lesions of the arteries are similar to those in arteriosclerosis obliterans without diabetes. The ulcers may be due to arteriosclerosis or microangiopathy, as in this case, in which only part of the foot is involved. Microscopic examination of the kidney reveals nodular hyaline infiltrates in the walls of the glomerular capillaries with, at times, complete occlusion of the lumen.

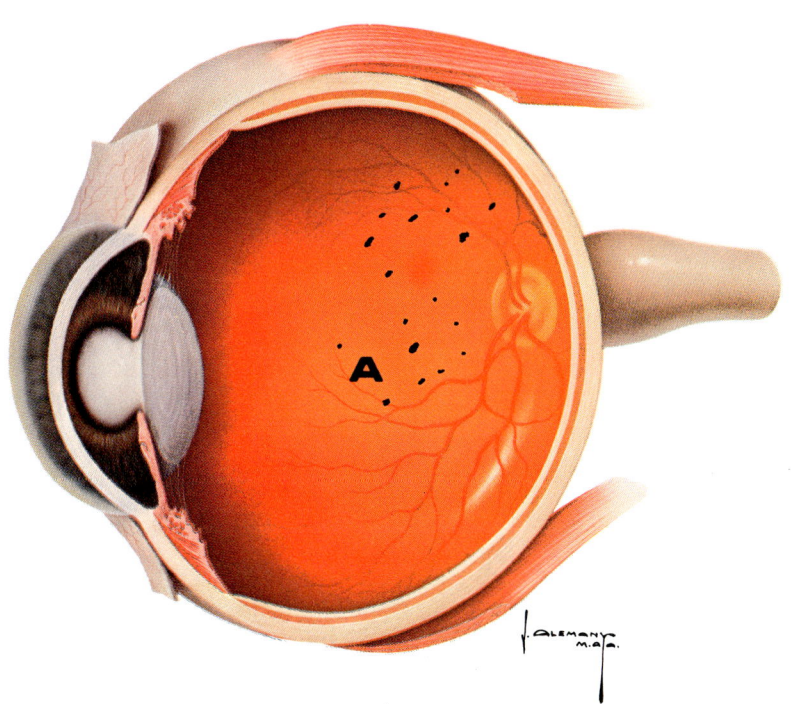

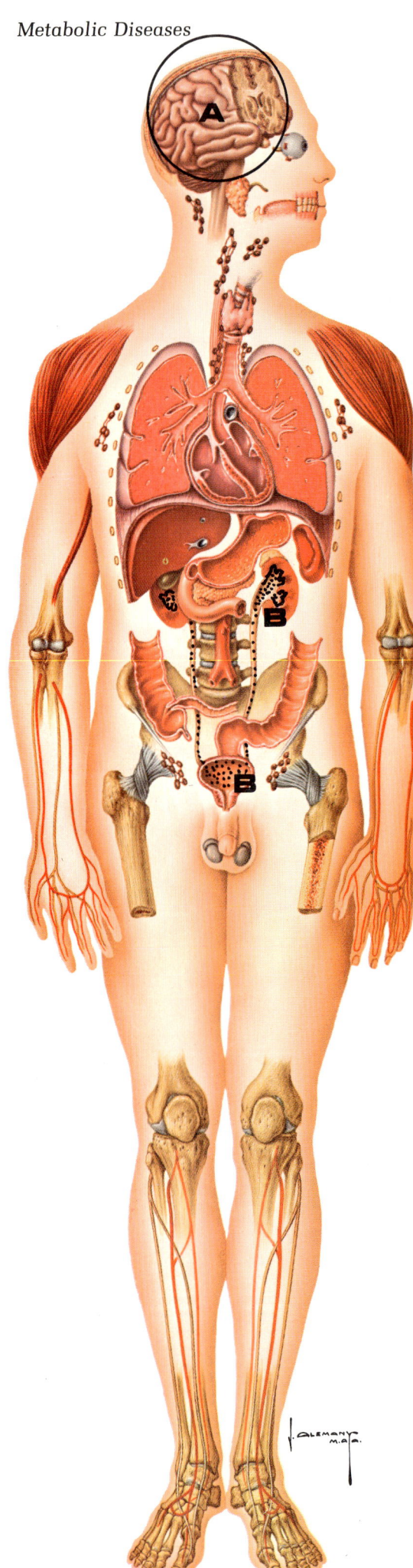

Diabetes Mellitus, Case 4

A 37-year-old white male was admitted to the hospital in a comatose state.

Physical examination revealed the coma (A), dilated fixed pupils, dry tongue, and mushy eyeballs, sweet odor to his breath, tachypnea, and diminished reflexes on all 4 extremities.

Laboratory examination revealed a blood sugar of 650 mg. per cent, ketonemia, a CO_2 of 8 mEq/L., and glycosuria and pyuria. A urine culture revealed a heavy growth of *Escherichia coli*, confirming the presence of a urinary tract infection (B).

Treatment of the acidosis and infection brought about recovery.

Differential Diagnosis:
1. Cerebrovascular disease
2. Septicemia
3. Insulin shock
4. Uremia
5. Pulmonary emphysema
6. Brain tumor
7. Epilepsy
8. Hypoparathyroidism
9. Hypopituitarism
10. Addisonian crisis
11. Meningoencephalitis
12. Alcoholism
13. Stokes-Adams syncope
14. Cerebral concussion

Clinical Note. Undoubtedly a severe pyelonephritis (B) had precipitated diabetic coma in this case. Infections from any source may do the same. Urinary tract infections are particularly common in the diabetic. Coma in the diabetic is not always due to acidosis or too much insulin. Diabetics with Kimmelstiel-Wilson's disease may go into uremic coma, and cerebrovascular accidents are more common in the diabetic. Severe renal papillary necrosis may produce sudden uremia and coma. No lesions of the pancreas are demonstrated here to emphasize that occasionally the pancreas may be normal.

Pathology. Microscopic examination of the kidneys reveals focal interstitial infiltration of leukocytes and lymphocytes with tubular destruction and abscess formation. When there is papillary necrosis, the papillae stand out as grayish-yellow infarcted areas and masses of bacteria; some plasma cells are prominent microscopically.

Glycogen Storage Disease (Von Gierke's Disease, etc.)

An 11-month-old white male was admitted to the neurology service because of frequent early-morning convulsions. The child had been a feeding problem for some time and was underweight and underdeveloped.

Physical examination revealed marked hepatomegaly (A) without jaundice or lymphadenopathy.

Laboratory examination revealed a blood sugar of 48 mg. per cent, acetonuria, and hyperlipemia. There was no significant increase of the blood sugar after glucagon and epinephrine. A liver biopsy revealed engorged liver cells, which stained positive for glycogen.

Treatment with frequent feeding, steroids, and glucagon was helpful.

Differential Diagnosis:
1. Idiopathic epilepsy
2. Space-occupying lesion of brain
3. Adrenal insufficiency
4. Hypopituitarism
5. Islet cell adenoma
6. Galactosemia
7. Hepatitis
8. Amyloidosis
9. Gaucher's disease
10. Cytomegalic inclusion disease

Clinical Note. Although this case illustrates the most common type of glycogen storage disease, it may present with primarily musculoskeletal involvement (B) (McArdle's disease) or cardiac muscle involvement (C), as in generalized glycogenosis. Less commonly, the brain and kidneys are involved. The absence of jaundice, cataracts, and mental retardation in most cases distinguishes this condition from galactosemia. Enzymatic assay of the liver and other tissues helps to distinguish whether the defect is due to lack of glucose-6-phosphatase (von Gierke's disease), lack of liver phosphorylase (Her's disease), lack of debrancher enzyme (limit dextrinosis), lack of muscle phosphorylase (McArdle's disease), or lack of brancher enzyme (amylopectinosis).

Pathology. There is increased intracellular glycogen in hepatic, renal, muscle, and brain cells with little cellular reaction to this non-foreign infiltrator.

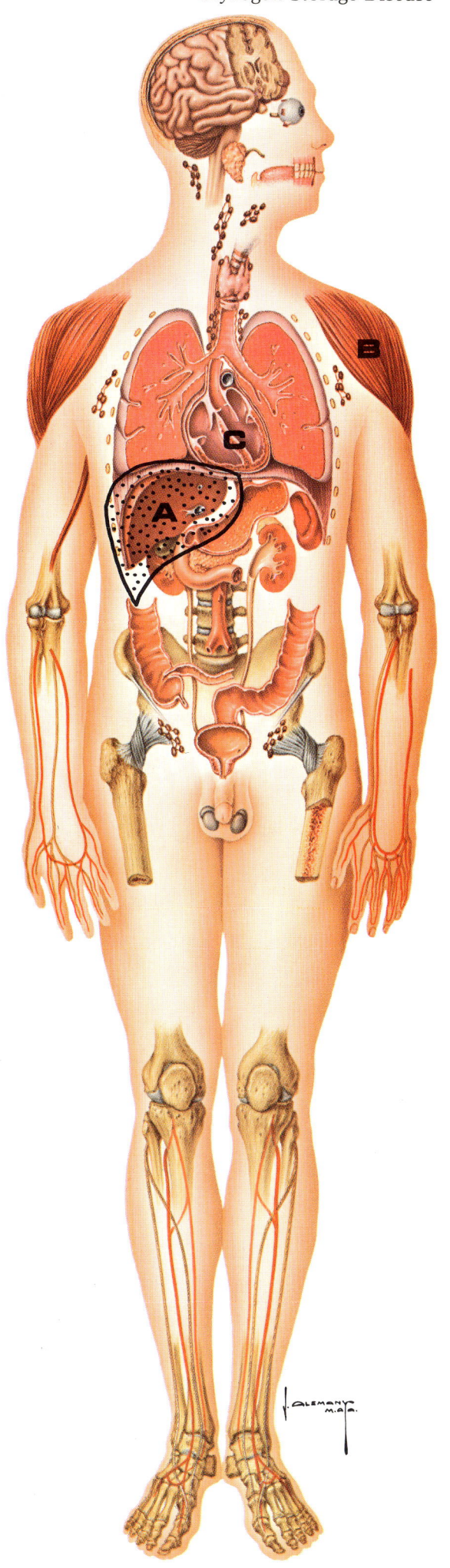

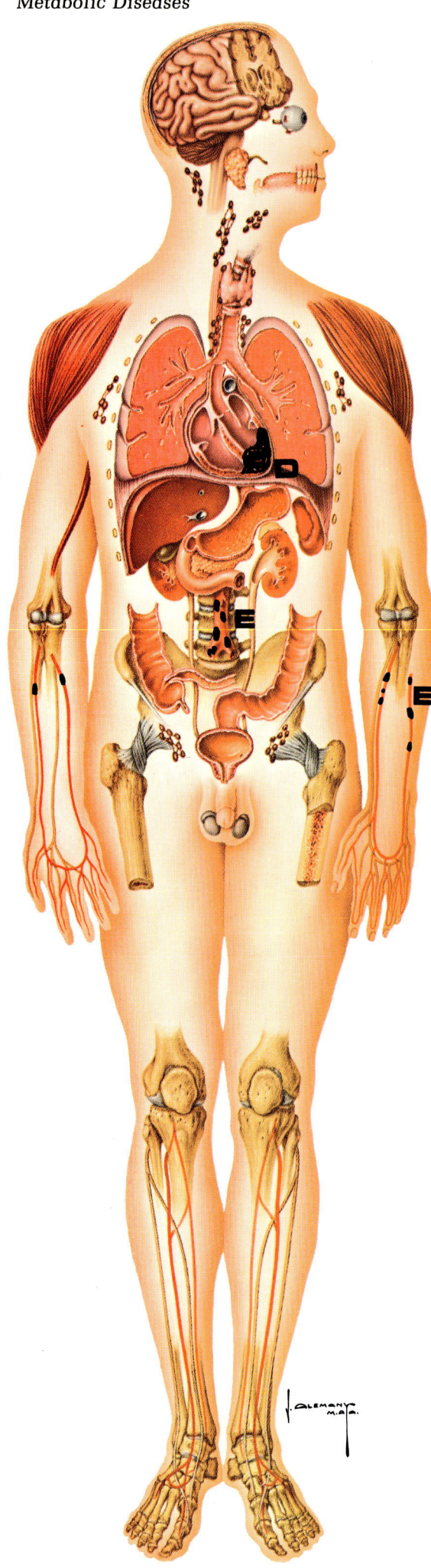

Essential Hypercholesterolemia

A 32-year-old white male complained of severe left precordial pain radiating down his left arm. His father had died of a myocardial infarction at an early age.

Physical examination revealed a pale, sweaty white male in acute distress, with xanthelasmas (A) bilaterally, arcus senilis (B), and tendon xanthomas of the hands and patellae (C).

Laboratory examination revealed a high transaminase and lactic dehydrogenase. An EKG revealed an acute myocardial infarction (D).

Treatment with a low cholesterol diet, Atromid-S and anticoagulants for the acute infarction was effective.

Differential Diagnosis:
1. Hypothyroidism
2. Pneumothorax
3. Essential hypertriglyceridemia
4. Pulmonary infarct
5. Diabetes mellitus
6. Pericarditis, idiopathic
7. Acute esophagitis

Clinical Note. Most of these cases are discovered accidentally when a routine annual physical discloses a high serum cholesterol, and investigation in the family reveals others with a high serum cholesterol and the skin manifestations listed above. About 60 per cent eventually manifest coronary artery disease.

Pathology. Microscopic examination of the involved tissues reveals the characteristic lipid-laden foam cells. There is premature atherosclerosis throughout the large arteries of the body (E).

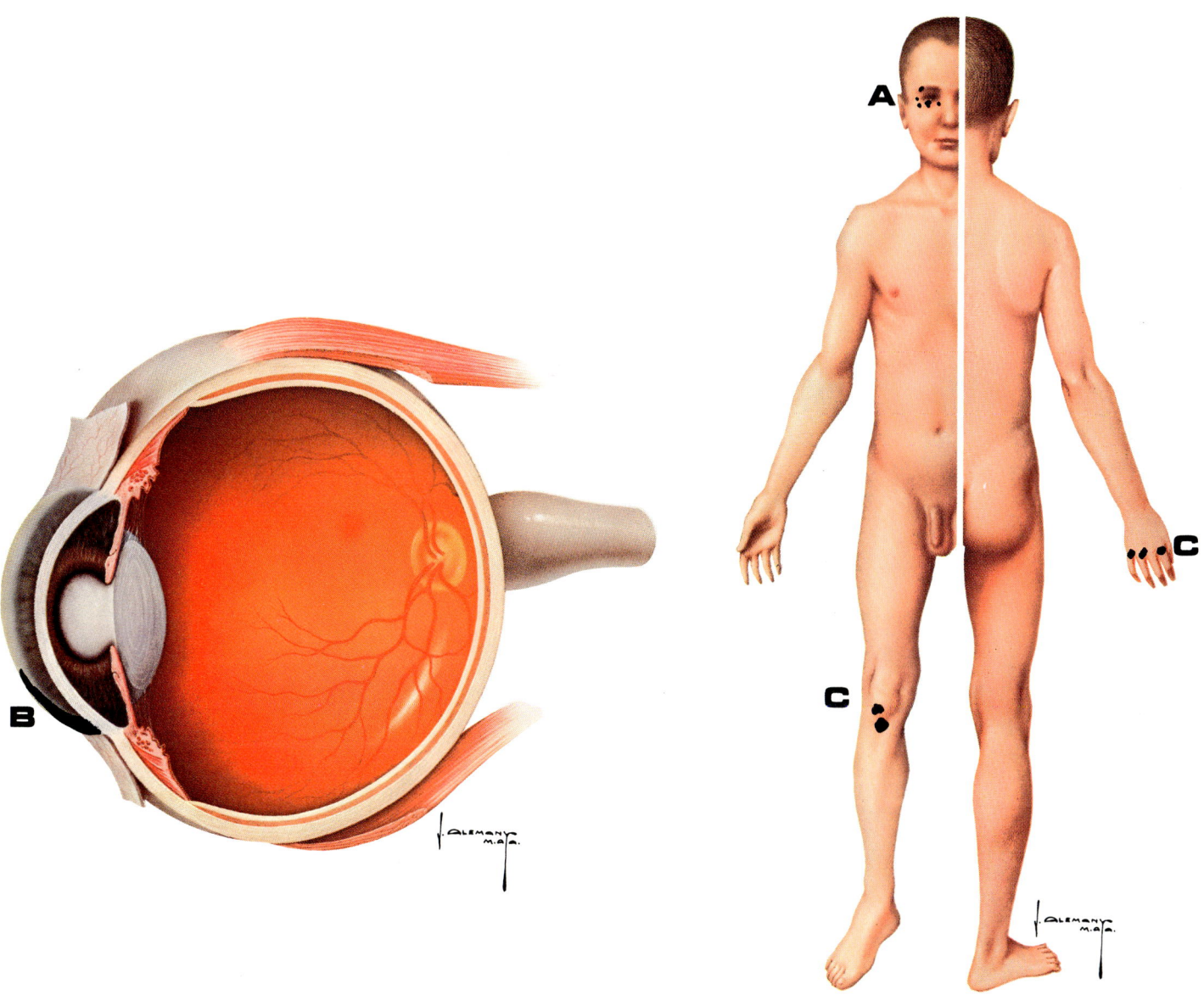

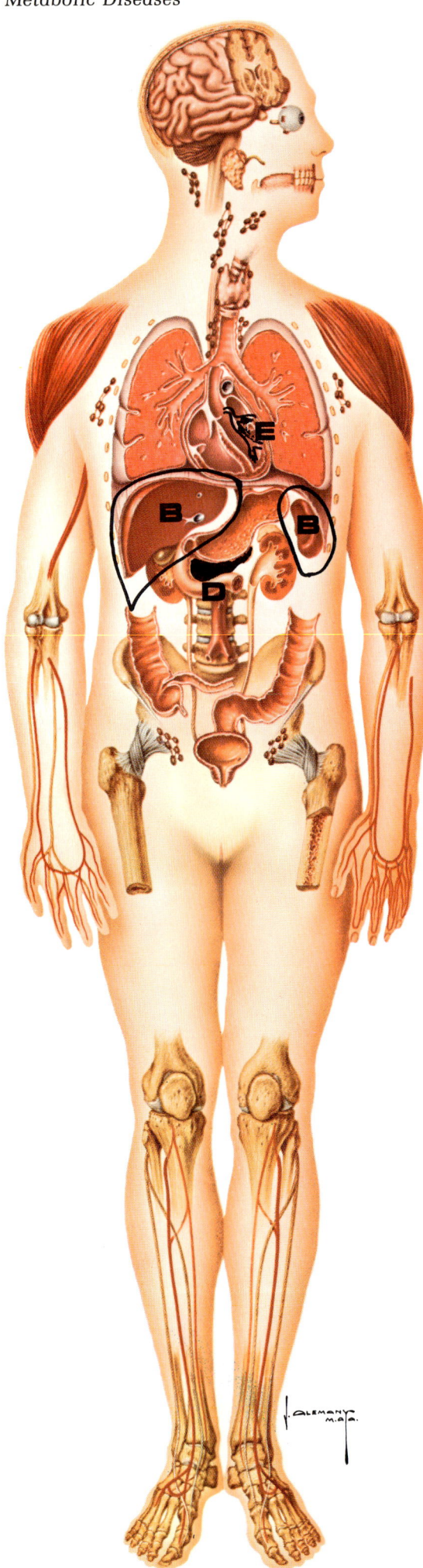

Essential Hypertriglyceridemia

A 13-year-old white female developed acute midepigastric pain and was brought to the emergency room. She had had attacks of abdominal pain in the past. One sibling was known to have hypertriglyceridemia.

Physical examination revealed lipemia retinalis (A), hepatosplenomegaly (B), eruptive xanthomas on the buttocks and elbows (C), and guarding, palpable tenderness and rebound tenderness throughout the abdomen, indicating pancreatitis (D).

Laboratory examination revealed an elevated serum amylase and lipase but, more important, a very high triglyceride and moderate elevation of the serum cholesterol and phospholipids.

Treatment with a low-fat diet was very successful in lowering the serum lipids.

Differential Diagnosis:
1. Essential hypercholesterolemia
2. Diabetes mellitus
3. Gaucher's disease
4. Hypothyroidism
5. Nephrotic syndrome
6. Primary biliary cirrhosis
7. Xanthomatosis, idiopathic

Clinical Note. This is the juvenile type, in which hepatosplenomegaly and abdominal pain are common. The adult form presents more frequently with diabetes and coronary artery disease (E). The cause of the abdominal pain is usually not discernible. In contrast to essential hypercholesterolemia, xanthelasmas and tendon xanthomas are absent. Occasionally a low-carbohydrate diet is more effective than a low-fat diet.

Pathology. Microscopic examination of the xanthomas and bone marrow reveal lipid-laden foam cells.

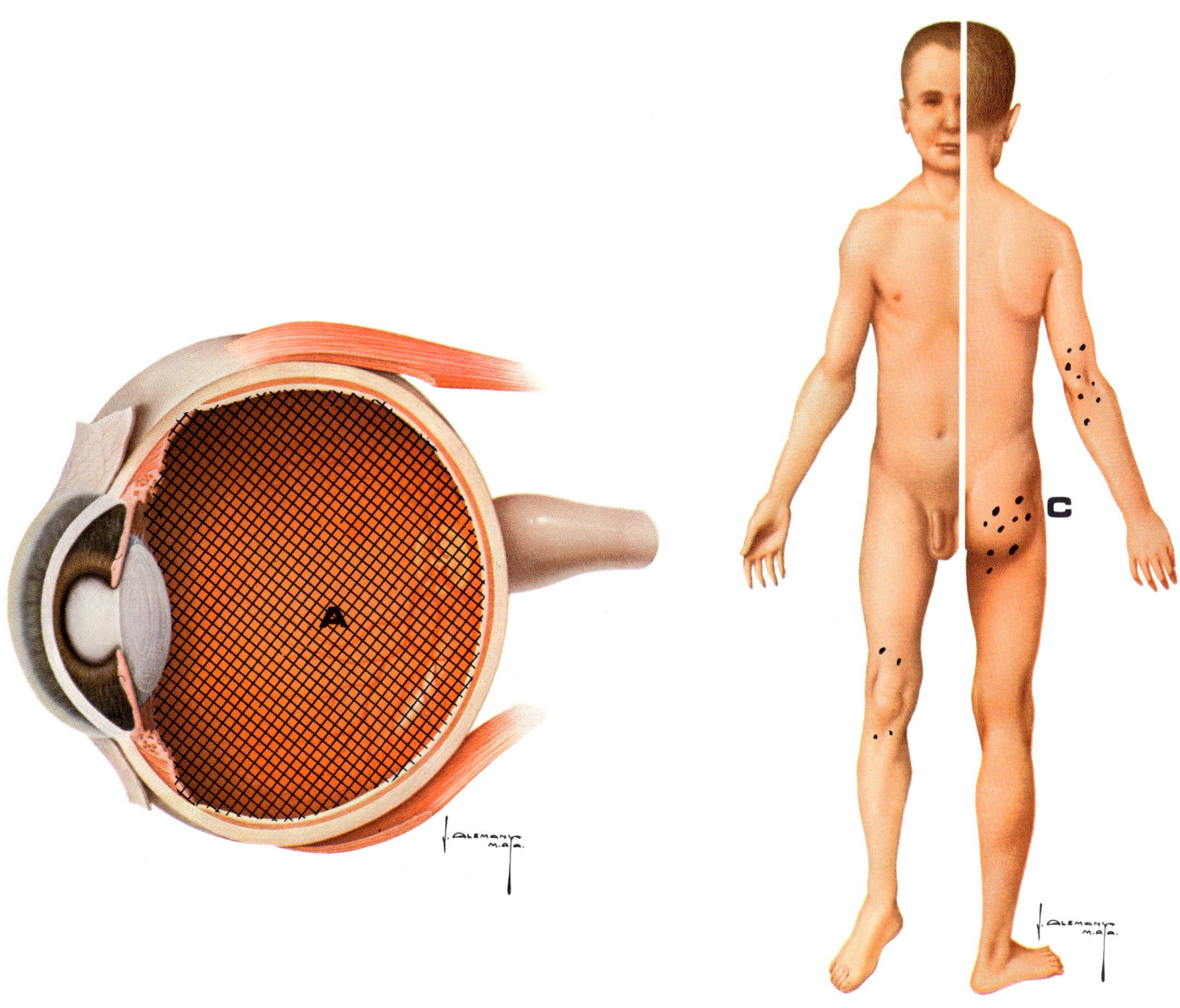

214 · *Metabolic Diseases*

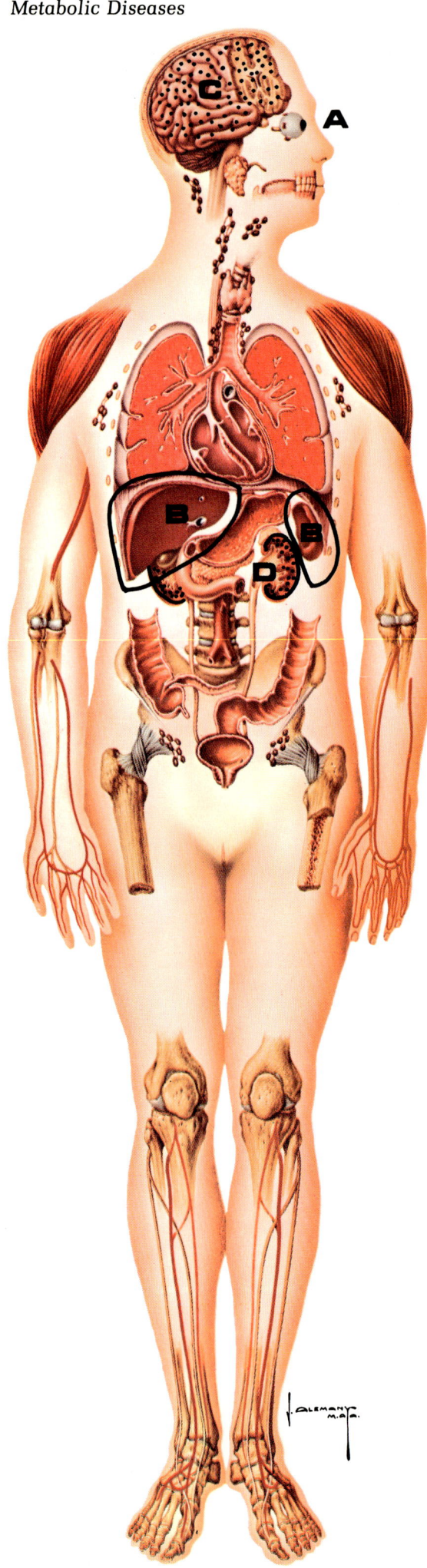

Galactosemia

A 3-month-old white female was admitted to the pediatric service with vomiting, diarrhea, and weight loss for some time. Jaundice had been noted 1 week prior to admission.

Physical examination revealed icteric sclera, bilateral cataracts (A), and hepatosplenomegaly (B).

Laboratory examination revealed galactosuria, proteinuria, amino-aciduria, and abnormal liver function tests. Enzyme assay of red cells revealed a deficiency of galactose-1-phosphate uridyl transferase.

Treatment by exclusion of milk and other lactose- and galactose-containing foods was helpful.

Differential Diagnosis:
1. Glycogen storage disease
2. Cytomegalic inclusion disease
3. Biliary atresia
4. Juvenile diabetes mellitus
5. Idiopathic hypoglycemia
6. Hepatitis
7. Maple syrup urine disease
8. Niemann-Pick disease
9. Erythroblastosis fetalis

Clinical Note. The presence of cataracts in half of these children helps to differentiate this from other causes of jaundice in the newborn. Enzyme assay has obviated the necessity of the galactose tolerance test.

Pathology. In addition to cataracts and cirrhosis of the liver due to the deposits of galactose-1-phosphate, there is *brain damage* (C) related to a disturbance of galactolipid biosynthesis. The galactose-1-phosphate is deposited in the renal tubules (D), causing the tubular reabsorptive defects.

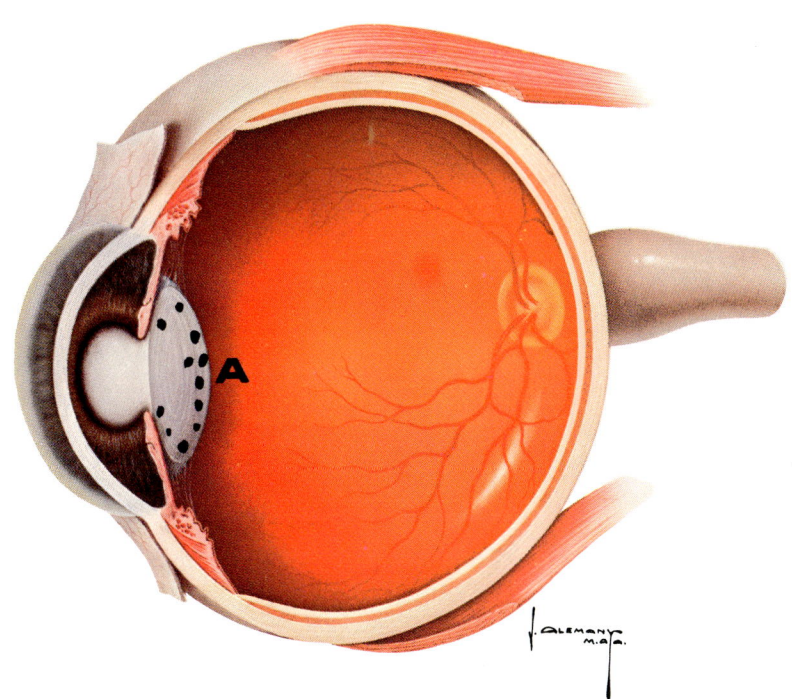

Metabolic Diseases

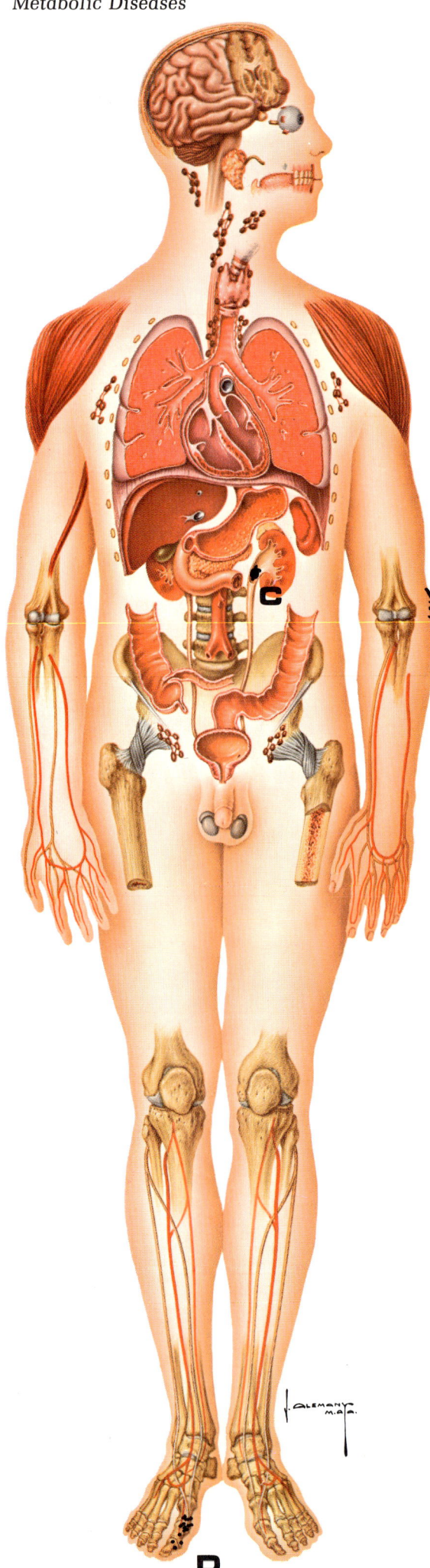

Gout

A 47-year-old white male complained of sudden, severe colicky left flank pain and vomiting. History revealed he had been treated for pain in his right big toe 3 years before. His father had suffered from gout.

Physical examination revealed tophaceous deposits of both ears (A), enlarged olecranon bursae (B), and marked tenderness in the left flank.

Laboratory examination revealed a serum uric acid of 9.3 mg. per cent, and urate crystals were numerous in the urine.

X-ray examination revealed a nonopaque calculus at the left ureteropelvic junction (C) on intravenous pyelography, and punched-out areas of the right big toe (D).

Treatment. Surgical removal of the stone was performed, and he was subsequently started on a combination of colchicine and probenecid for prophylaxis.

Differential Diagnosis:
1. Hyperparathyroidism
2. Ochronosis
3. Rheumatoid arthritis
4. Gonococcal arthritis
5. Tuberculosis
6. Reiter's disease
7. Secondary gout (due to leukemia, etc.)

Gout · 217

Clinical Note. Only 10 to 20 per cent of the cases of gout develop with nephrolithiasis, but in some a stone may have been passed before arthritic symptoms appear. In late stages the kidney may be infiltrated with urate deposits, and there is associated arteriolar sclerosis and pyelonephritis leading to hypertension. The great toe is the most common site of arthritis; but the knee, elbows, and even the metacarpophalangeal joints may also be involved. The response to colchicine aids in the differential diagnosis when joints other than the big toe are involved. A family history is found in up to 20 per cent of cases, and only 5 per cent of cases are females. Note the similarity of this disease to hyperparathyroidism, page 90, which may also manifest with renal calculi.

Pathology. There may be deposits of the urates in the joints, synovia, tendon sheaths, heart valves, and kidney as well as the ears. There is little inflammatory reaction to the deposits.

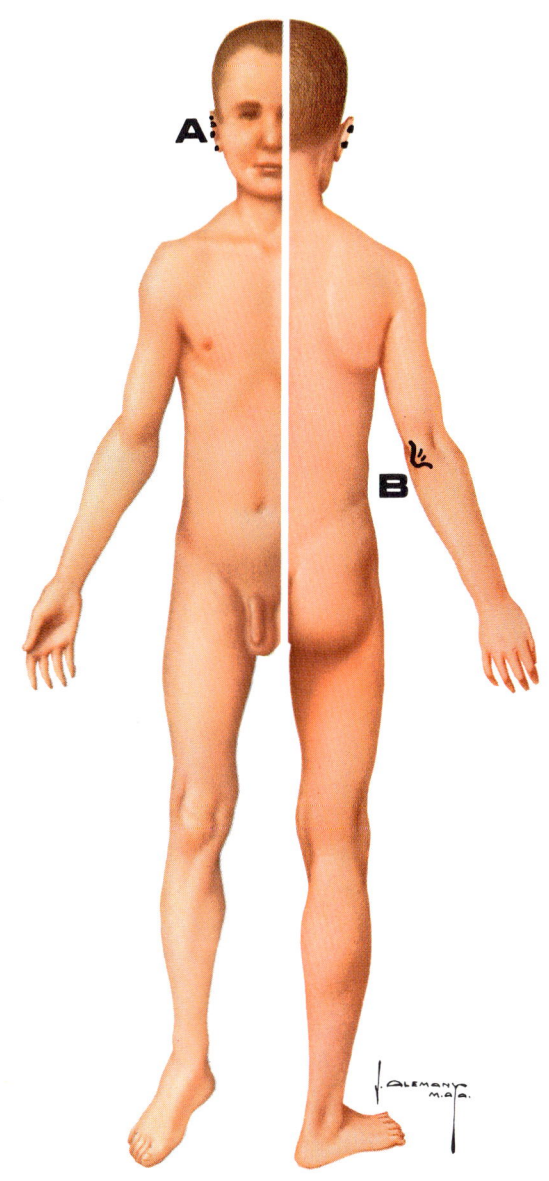

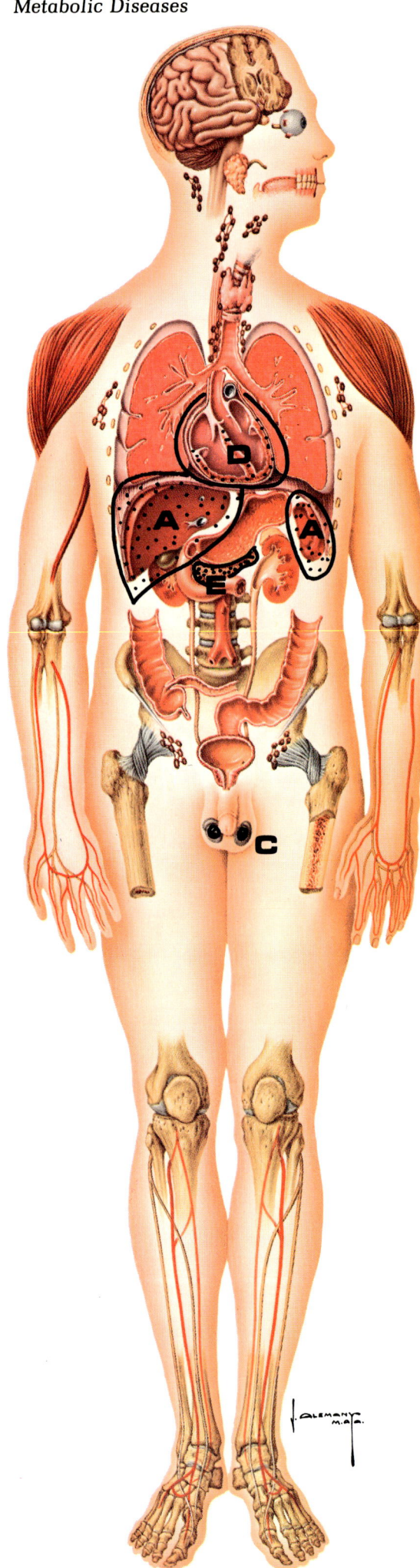

Idiopathic Hemochromatosis

A 46-year-old white male was found to have glycosuria on a routine annual physical examination. On questioning, it was found that he had had occasional attacks of right upper quadrant pain, but cholecystograms had been unremarkable. One brother had hemochromatosis.

Physical examination revealed hepatosplenomegaly (A), bronzing of the skin, particularly in areas exposed to light (B), but no jaundice; testicular atrophy (C), and cardiomegaly (D).

Laboratory examination revealed a blood sugar of 175 mg. per cent and a high serum iron and iron-binding capacity. Liver biopsy revealed the iron deposits in the hepatic parenchyma.

Treatment with frequent phlebotomies was begun. Later desferrioxamine was tried.

Differential Diagnosis:
1. Diabetes mellitus
2. Cirrhosis of the liver
3. Wilson's disease
4. Cholecystitis
5. Chronic pancreatitis
6. Carcinoma of the pancreas
7. Metastatic carcinoma of the liver

Clinical Note. This diagnosis should be considered in any case of early diabetes. The excess iron in the body is due to a primary genetic defect in the intestinal absorptive mechanism in this type. It may also be due to massive intake of iron, too many transfusions, or poor utilization of iron in certain anemic states. As suggested by the case history, a third of the siblings have the disease. There is no jaundice until late in the disease, as in Wilson's disease.

Pathology. The iron deposits in the parenchyma of the various organs but is greatest in the liver and pancreas (E) and, to a lesser degree, in the endocrine glands, heart muscle, and skin. Very little extra is found in the urine. There is a fibrotic reaction in most organs secondary to the iron deposits.

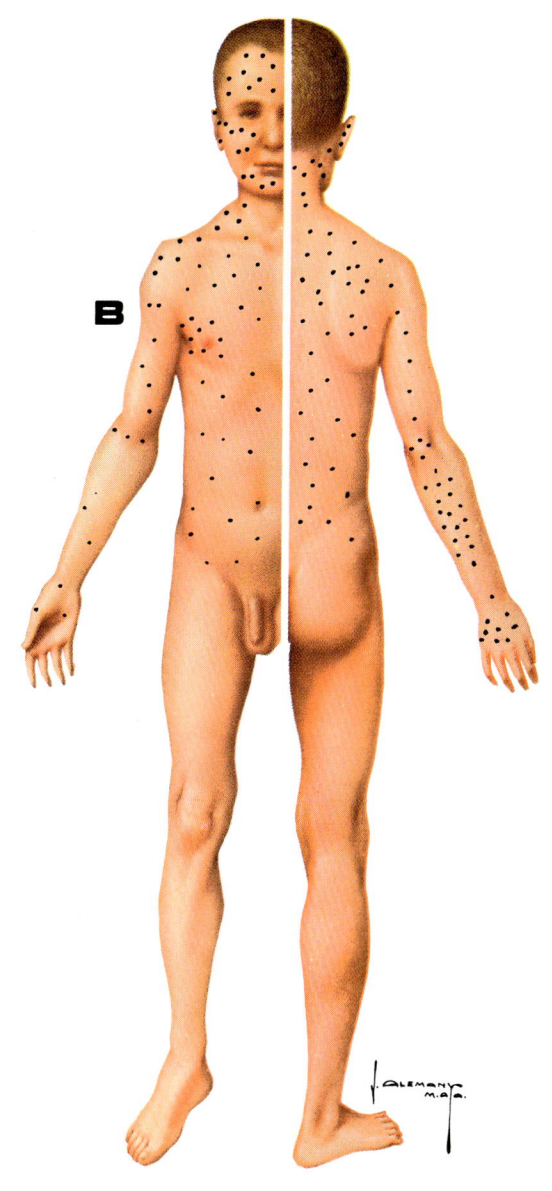

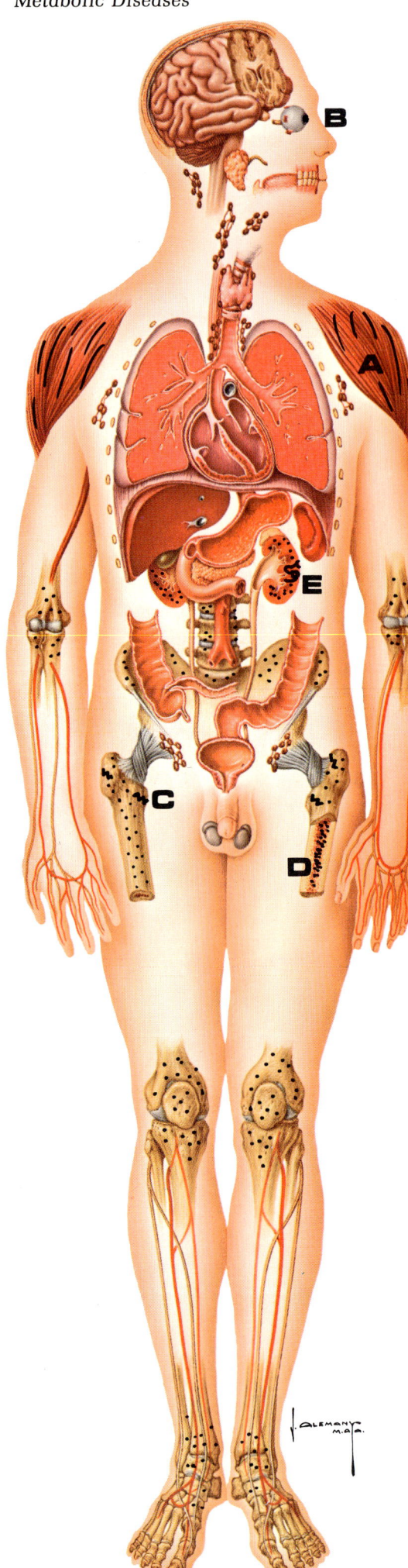

Lignac-Fanconi Syndrome (Cystinosis)

A 5-year-old was brought to the pediatric clinic because of retarded growth and development. His parents had complained frequently to their family doctor about the boy's muscle weakness, which at times was extreme.

Physical examination revealed muscular hypotonia and reduced reflexes throughout all 4 extremities (A), tenderness on palpation of the left femur, and crystal (cystine) deposits in the cornea bilaterally (B).

Laboratory examination revealed a normal BUN and a normal blood calcium but low blood phosphate, uric acid, bicarbonate, and potassium. There were amino-aciduria and glycosuria but no cystinuria.

X-ray examination revealed symmetrical infractions in the pelvis and femurs (Milkman's syndrome) (C) and diffuse osteomalacia. There was no evidence of nephrocalcinosis.

Treatment. The child seemed to respond well to an alkalinizing regimen, vitamin D, and calcium tablets.

Differential Diagnosis:
1. Renal tubular acidosis
2. Rickets (vitamin D deficiency)
3. Hyperparathyroidism
4. Chronic renal failure of whatever cause
5. Heavy metal poisoning
6. Wilson's disease
7. Hypophosphatasia

Clinical Note. Routine examination of the urine for amino-aciduria is becoming a very important test not only for children with stunted growth but for the mentally retarded and adults who work in a heavy metal industry. A quick dipstick test should be developed as soon as possible. Although this is primarily a disease of children (transmitted by recessive gene), adult cases, both hereditary and acquired, are now being recognized.

Pathology. There is deposition of cystine crystals in all the organs of the reticuloendothelial system but very little in the urine. This picture presents a contrast to that in cystinuria, in which deposits are rare in the tissues, including the cornea, but much cystine appears in the urine, and cystine stones are common. In Lignac-Fanconi syndrome bone marrow aspiration may reveal the cystine deposits (D) in the reticuloendothelial system. The proximal segment of the convoluted tubules is shortened and joined to the glomerulus by an elongated "swan neck" (E).

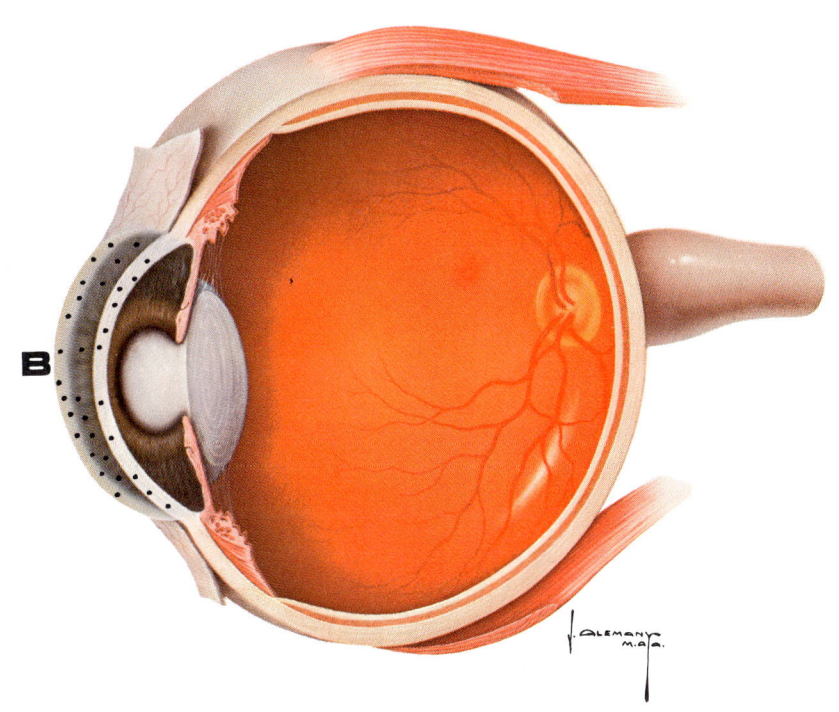

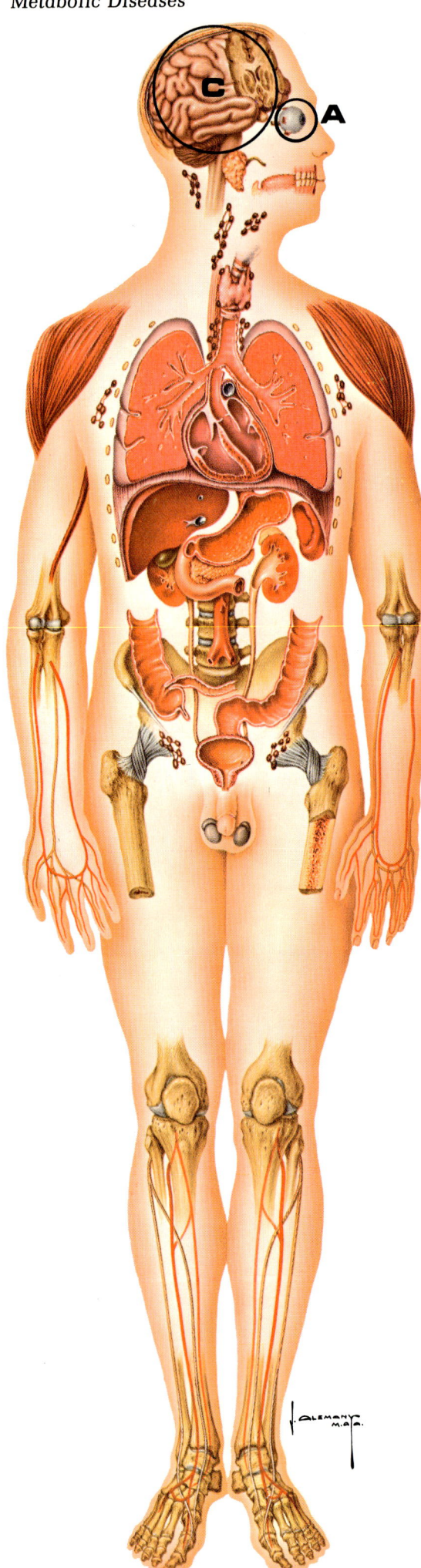

Phenylpyruvic Oligophrenia

A 4-year-old white male was brought to the state hospital for evaluation of grand mal convulsions. One sibling had already been institutionalized for mental retardation.

Physical examination revealed blue eyes (A), light skin with some eczema (B), and an I.Q. of 49, verbal scale, indicating mental retardation (C).

Laboratory examination revealed large amounts of phenylpyruvic acid, phenyllactic acid, and phenylalanine in the urine. The blood levels of phenylalanine were also high.

Treatment with a phenylalanine-deficient diet led to some improvement.

Differential Diagnosis:
1. Idiopathic mental retardation
2. Mental retardation due to birth trauma or anoxia
3. Schilder's disease
4. Degenerative encephalopathy
5. Pellagra
6. Space-occupying lesion of the brain

Clinical Note. Only a quarter or less of these patients present with seizures or eczema. Two thirds have blonde hair and blue eyes. The mental retardation is usually severe, but will be preventable now that screening of urine of infants is performed in many clinics. The phenylalanine and phenylpyruvic acid do not form stones.

Pathology. Because of the absence of phenylalanine hydroxylase, phenylalanine cannot be converted to tyrosine and thus accumulates in the blood and urine; a large portion is converted to phenylpyruvic acid by transaminations. The brain shows very little gross or microscopic changes, and other organs appear normal.

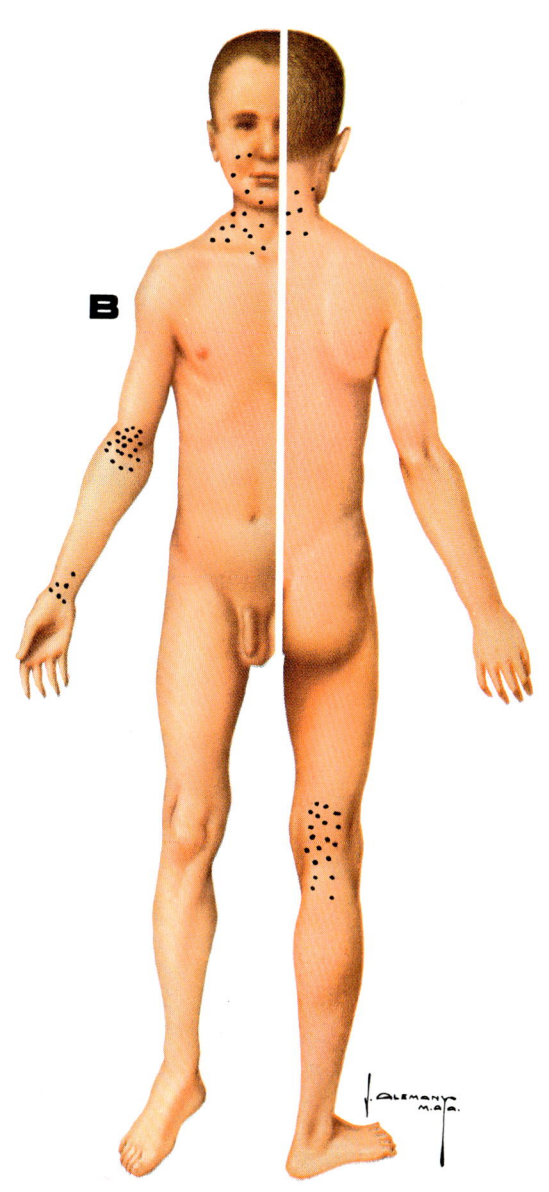

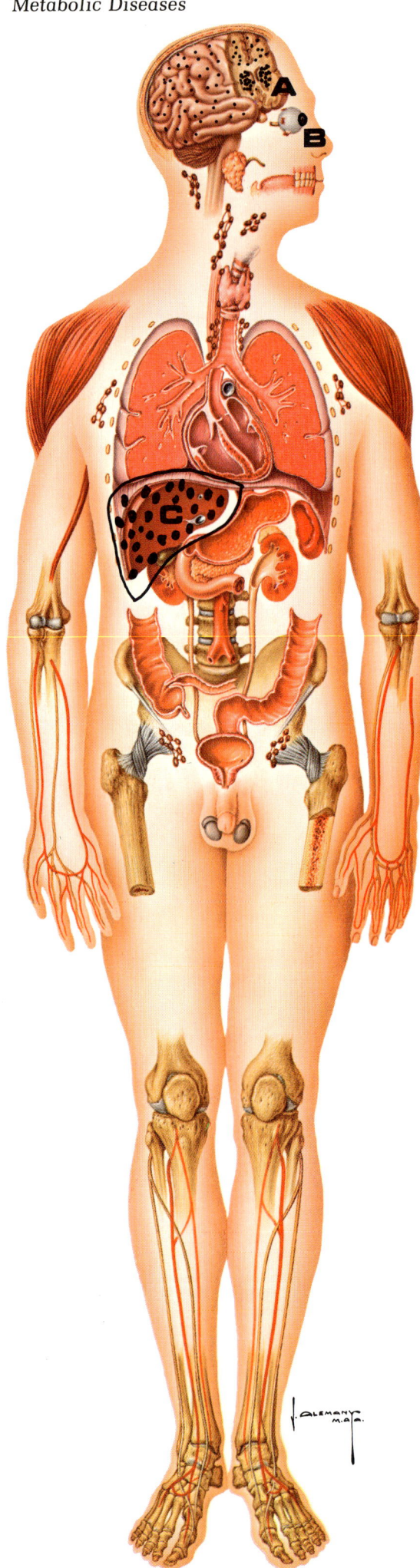

Wilson's Disease

A 20-year-old white male had been troubled with an increasing tremor and beating movements of his arms for 1 year prior to admission. A year ago he had had an episode of high temperature just before the onset of the tremors, and the local physician had attributed his tremors at that time to an "encephalitis." An aunt had died at the age of 25 of a similar ailment.

Physical examination revealed dysarthric speech, tremor, rigidity, and rhythmic choreiform movements (A) of both upper extremities. A Kayser-Fleischer ring (B) was noted on slit-lamp examination. Palpation of the abdomen revealed a coarsely nodular, enlarged liver (C).

Laboratory examination revealed aminoaciduria and an elevated urine copper.

Differential Diagnosis:
1. Phenothiazine toxicity
2. Postencephalitic parkinsonism
3. Huntington's chorea
4. Sydenham's chorea
5. Laennec's cirrhosis with hepatic failure

Clinical Note. Although this is the most common form of the disease, another type appears later in life. It is fruitful to consider this condition in all cases of "Parkinsonism," especially since therapy in the form of diet restrictions and penicillamine is now available. No kidney lesion has been found to explain the aminoaciduria.

Pathology. The corpus striatum is involved by increased copper, astrocytic proliferation, and often cavitation. There are frequently areas of focal degeneration throughout the cortex. The liver reveals multilobular cirrhosis with fibrous septa that are less heavily collagenous than in Laennec's cirrhosis. Parenchymal regeneration is intense. The cornea reveals copper-containing granules in Decemet's membrane. Skeletal changes occur in about two thirds of the cases.

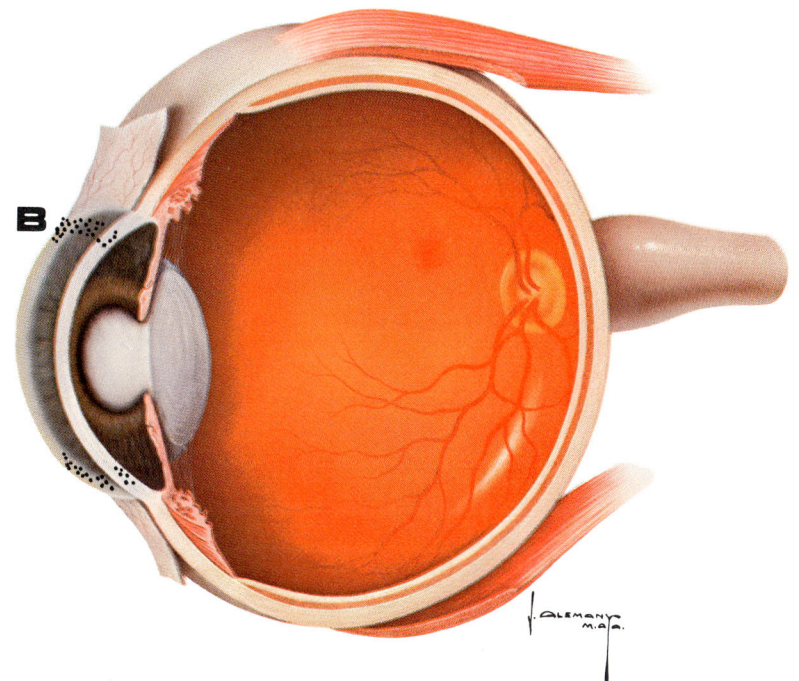

Chapter 9

Neoplasms

Neoplasms are one of the commonest systemic diseases seen today. They present as systemic disease in three different ways: (1) by metastasis to distant organs; (2) by the secretion of various hormones which produce systemic symptoms; and (3) by being a primary tumor of the blood cells (then involvement of multiple organs is evident at the outset).

The etiology of neoplasms is still uncertain, but certain chemicals, viruses (in animals), chronic trauma, radiation, and hormones have been found to be carcinogenic. Many tumors are first recognized by metastasis to a distant site. The lungs and liver are the most frequent sites, probably because of their abundant supply of blood and lymphatics. Certain tumors have peculiar preferences for certain metastatic sites. For example, solid tumors of the thyroid commonly metastasize to bone.

X-ray, radioisotopes, biopsy, and exploratory surgery have become the most important tools in the diagnosis of neoplasms. Needle biopsy can be successfully performed for almost any organ of the body and eliminates the need for exploratory surgery in many cases. Radiation and chemotherapy have markedly improved the life-span of most patients with these tumors.

228 · Neoplasms

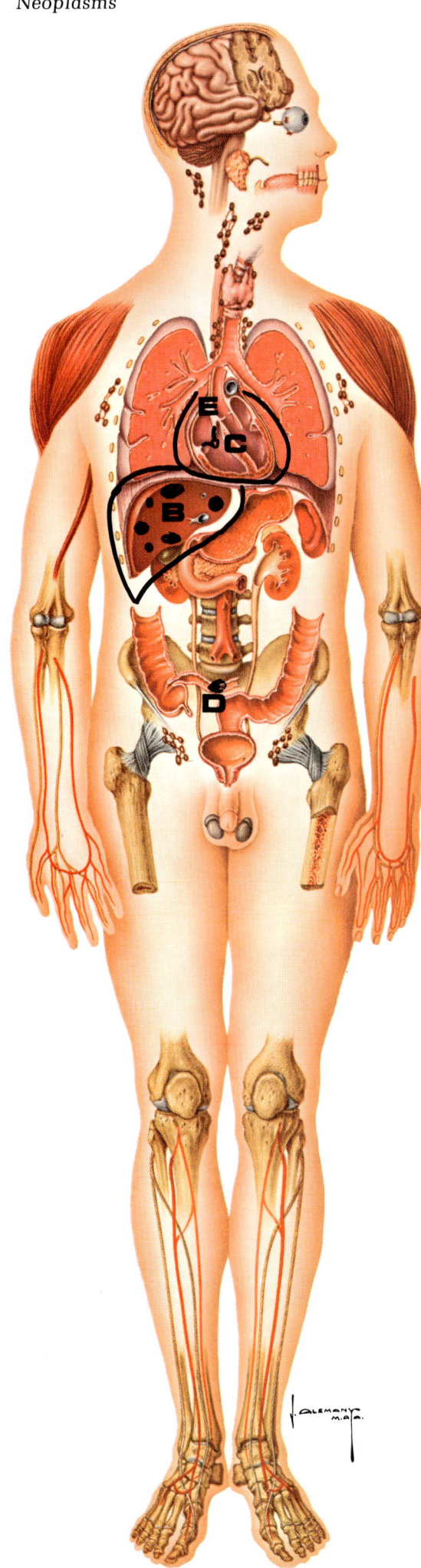

Carcinoid Syndrome

A 59-year-old white male had had intermittent abdominal cramps and diarrhea for 4 years. Two previous hospital work-ups failed to reveal a cause for this condition. He had lost 10 pounds of weight. For 1 year prior to this admission he had experienced recurrent flushing of his face and neck. For 2 months prior to admission he had had a hacking nonproductive cough.

Physical examination revealed a violaceous flush of his face and neck (A) and, to a lesser degree, the rest of his body. There was hepatomegaly (B). There were sibilant rales throughout the chest.

Laboratory examination revealed a 24-hour urine 5-hydroxyindoleacetic acid of 58 mg.

X-ray examination of the chest revealed cardiomegaly (C).

At exploratory laparotomy a malignant carcinoid of the terminal ileum (D) with liver metastasis was found.

Differential Diagnosis:
1. Intestinal parasites
2. Salmonellosis
3. Ulcerative colitis
4. Regional enteritis
5. Sprue

6. Zollinger-Ellison syndrome
7. Neoplasms of the large and small bowels
8. Pheochromocytoma
9. Polycythemia vera
10. Menopause syndrome
11. Rheumatic heart disease
12. Bronchial asthma
13. Pellagra

Clinical Note. The intestinal, vasomotor, respiratory, and cardiac involvement must each be taken into consideration separately in the differential diagnosis. Serotonin, secreted in large amounts by the metastasis, causes contraction of the smooth muscle in the small blood vessels, the intestines, and bronchioles, causing most of the symptoms. It is not certain what causes the pulmonary and tricuspid valve lesions (E), but it is probably also due to chronic effects of serotonin. The tumor swallows up much of the dietary tryptophan to form serotonin, causing a deficiency of this amino acid and a "pellagra" syndrome. These patients are often labeled neurotic for years before objective findings appear. Then it's too late to save them.

Pathology. The tumor was grossly yellow and on microscopic examination revealed nests of argentaffin-positive epithelial cells set in a fibrous stroma. The tumors may occur also in the appendix, stomach, rectum, bronchi, or ovary. The liver is enlarged because of the metastasis, and the tricuspid and pulmonary valves are fibrosed and thickened.

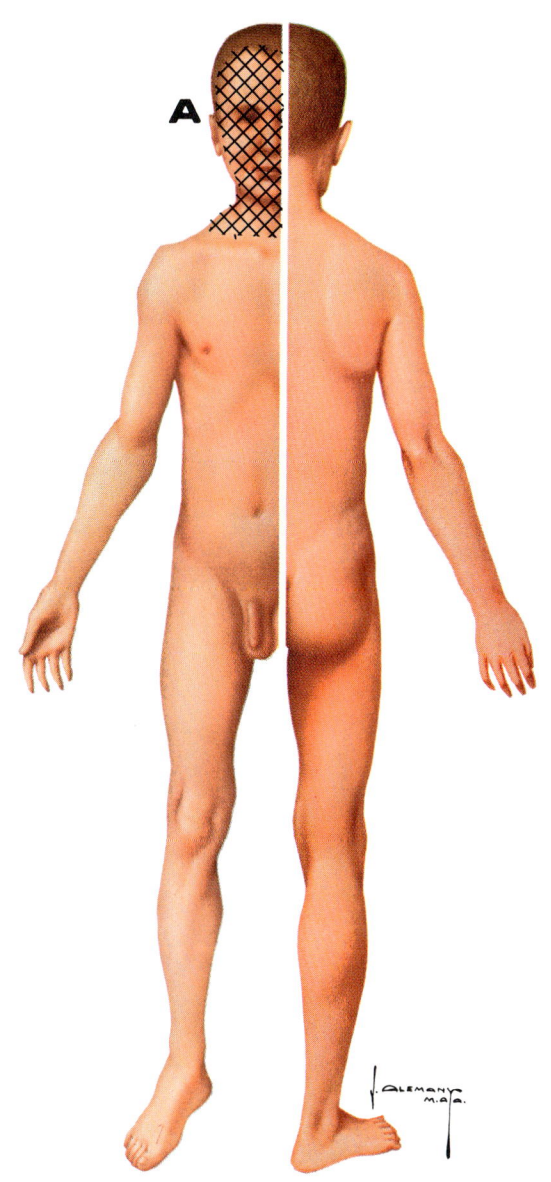

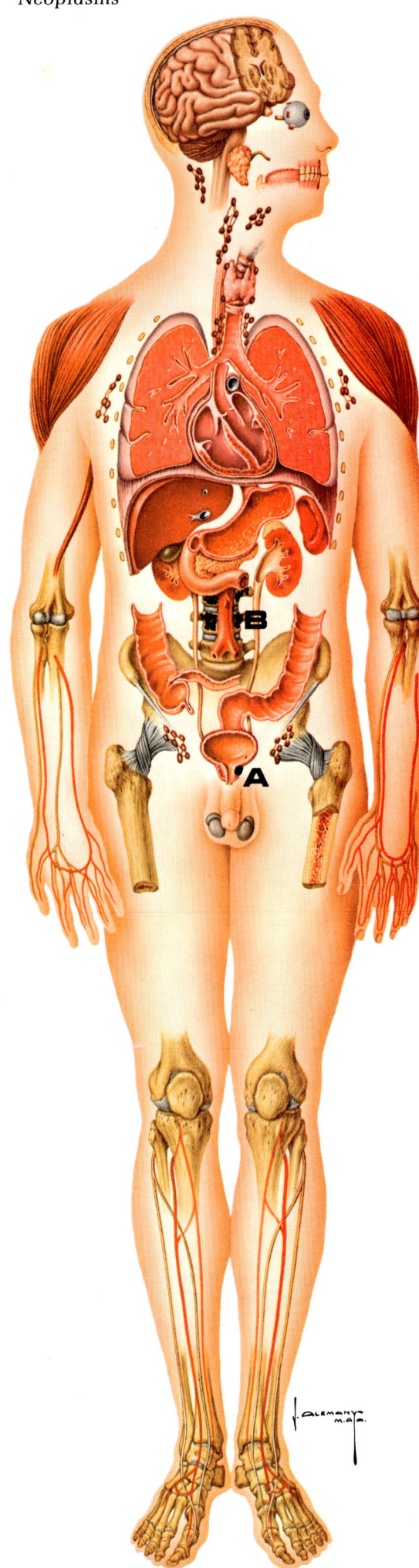

Metastatic Carcinoma, Case 1

A 72-year-old white male developed severe low back pain 2 weeks prior to admission. A review of systems revealed he had had difficulty in voiding and intermittent hematuria for 6 months prior to admission.

Physical examination revealed a firm nodule in the left lobe of the prostate (A).

Laboratory examination revealed an acid phosphatase of 14.6 King-Armstrong units and an alkaline phosphatase of 28 King-Armstrong units.

X-ray examination of the lumbosacral spine revealed radiopaque densities in the L-3 and L-4 vertebrae (B).

Treatment with a transurethral resection, bilateral orchiectomy, and 5 mg. of stilbestrol daily was helpful.

Differential Diagnosis:
1. Herniated nucleus pulposus
2. Multiple myeloma
3. Tuberculosis of the spine
4. Spondylolisthesis
5. Cauda equina tumor
6. Rheumatoid spondylitis
7. Osteoarthritis

Clinical Note. Prostatic carcinoma often presents with bony metastasis before obstructive uropathy. This is a typical example of how carcinomas may present as a systemic disease. As in other systemic conditions, there may be a variety of presentations, only a few of which will be discussed in this book. All patients with low back pain of a persistent nature should be x-rayed even though one gets tired of so many negative reports.

Pathology. The cords of cuboidal or polygonal cells are identified as malignant by their invasiveness and not by anaplastic changes, which are frequently not present. The increased bony density is due to osteoblastic proliferation in the involved bone.

Metastatic Carcinoma, Case 2

A 63-year-old white female complained of intermittent diarrhea and abdominal cramps for 6 months prior to admission. Occasionally the diarrhea was mixed with blood.

Physical examination revealed a right lower quadrant mass (A), and an enlarged nodular liver (B) without jaundice.

X-ray examination of the large bowel by a barium enema revealed an adenocarcinoma of the ascending colon, confirmed by needle biopsy of the liver.

Differential Diagnosis:
1. Appendiceal abscess
2. Ovarian tumor
3. Ectopic pregnancy
4. Retroperitoneal sarcoma
5. Amoebic dysentery
6. Ulcerative colitis

Clinical Note. Tumors of the large intestinal tract commonly metastasize to the liver but may also spread to the lungs. Only 1 per cent metastasize to the brain. They may spread by direct extension to the bladder and ureters or the stomach (in transverse colon carcinomas). Metastases are not the only systemic manifestation of tumors of the gastrointestinal tract. Acanthosis nigricans and polymyositis have been found. Pancreatic tumors may produce thrombophlebitis and emotional disturbances.

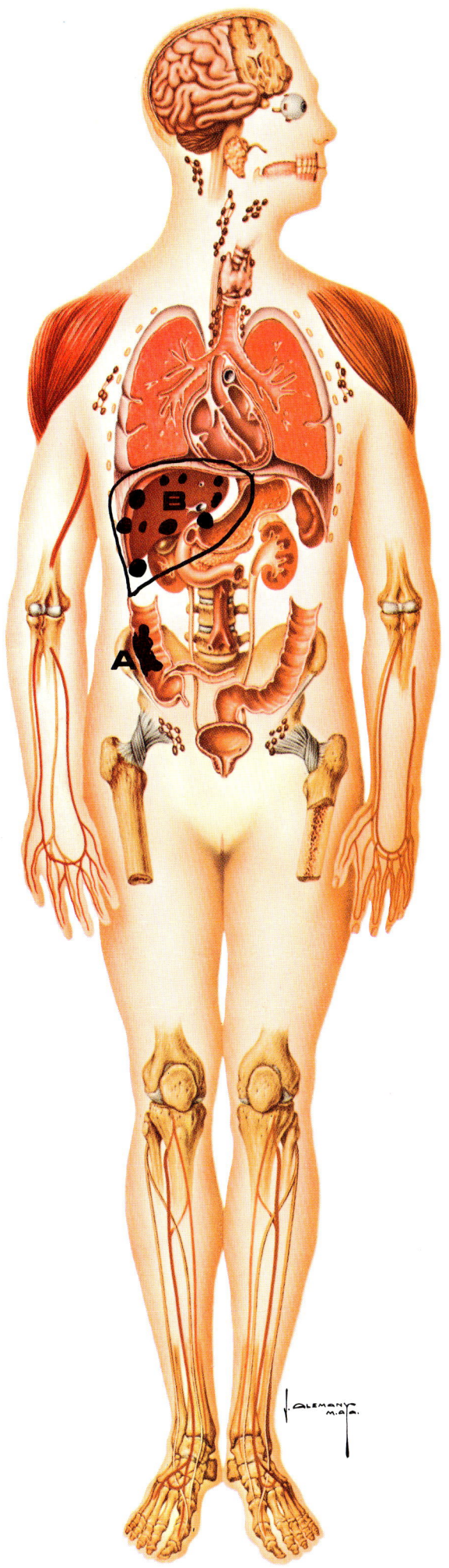

232 · Neoplasms

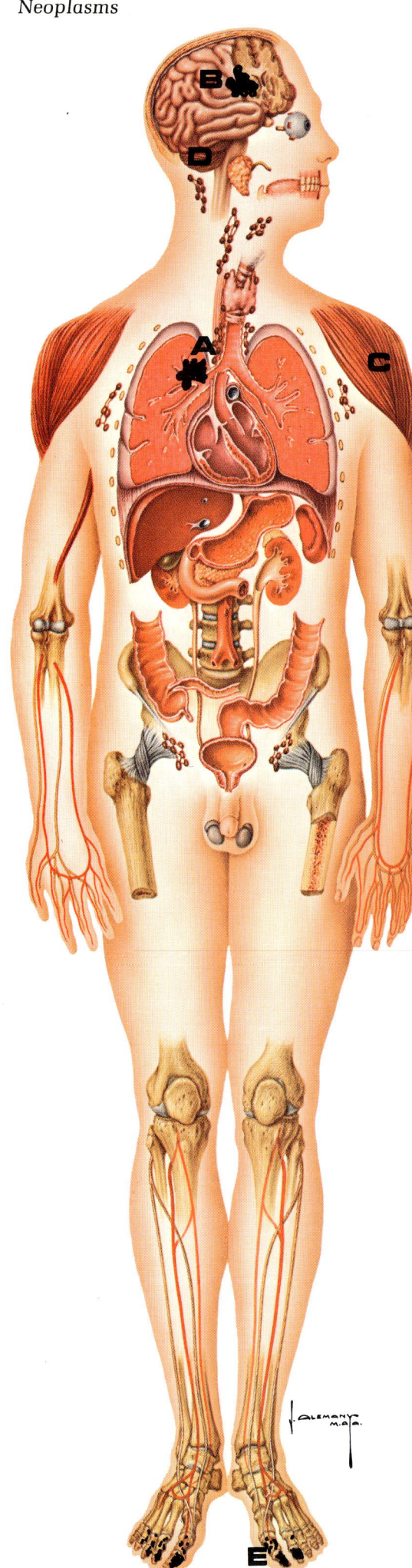

Metastatic Carcinoma, Case 3

A 50-year-old white male sustained a sudden left-sided convulsion. His wife stated that he had been a chain smoker for several years and in the past few months had complained of a chronic cough and bloody sputum.

Physical examination revealed a left-sided hemiplegia.

X-ray examination of the chest revealed a right hilar mass lesion (A). Right carotid angiography revealed a space-occupying lesion of the right cerebral hemisphere (B), which on biopsy proved to be a bronchogenic carcinoma.

Differential Diagnosis:
1. Meningioma
2. Hodgkin's disease
3. Tuberculosis
4. Cryptococcosis
5. Cerebral embolism
6. Bacterial meningitis
7. Periarteritis nodosa

Clinical Note. These tumors may also present with hepatomegaly; and so, when a gastrointestinal work-up is negative, do not forget a chest x-ray. These tumors may also have systemic manifestations without metastasis, among them muscular atrophy (C), cerebellar ataxia (D), and osteoarthropathy (E). By direct extension they may involve other organs in the mediastinum such as the esophagus and heart.

Hodgkin's Disease

This 36-year-old white male with a 5-year history of Hodgkin's disease was readmitted for therapy because he had had recurrent morning chills and fever and increasing swelling in the left side of his neck for 3 months.

Physical examination revealed 3 large, rubbery nontender lymph nodes (A) in left posterior cervical triangle, several similar nodes in both axilla, and a hard spleen (B) 8 cm. below the left subcostal margin.

Laboratory Examination. A biopsy of the left cervical node had previously confirmed Hodgkin's disease.

A chest x-ray revealed bilateral hilar adenopathy (C).

Treatment. He responded well to a course of nitrogen mustard.

Differential Diagnosis:
1. Chronic lymphocytic leukemia
2. Congestive splenomegaly
3. Chronic infections (tuberculosis, etc.)
4. Infectious mononucleosis
5. Sarcoidosis
6. Gaucher's disease
7. Myeloid metaplasia
8. Hemolytic anemias

Clinical Note. The lymph node enlargement and splenomegaly in this case present a clinical picture remarkably similar to that described by Thomas Hodgkin in 1832. The fever usually occurs in waves of several days separated by normothermic periods (Pel-Ebstein type). Although anemia, eosinophilia, and other changes in the blood picture occur, no laboratory study is typical or consistent, and diagnosis depends on biopsy. Other systems involved with significant frequency are the skin (25% of cases) (D), the nervous system (usually the spinal cord and peripheral nerve) (E), and bone (F).

Pathology. Microscopically the lymph node contains the characteristic Reed-Sternberg cell, a giant cell with a multilobulated nucleus, coarse chromatin, and prominent nucleoli. There are distortion of architecture, necrosis, and lymphoid and reticular hyperplasia.

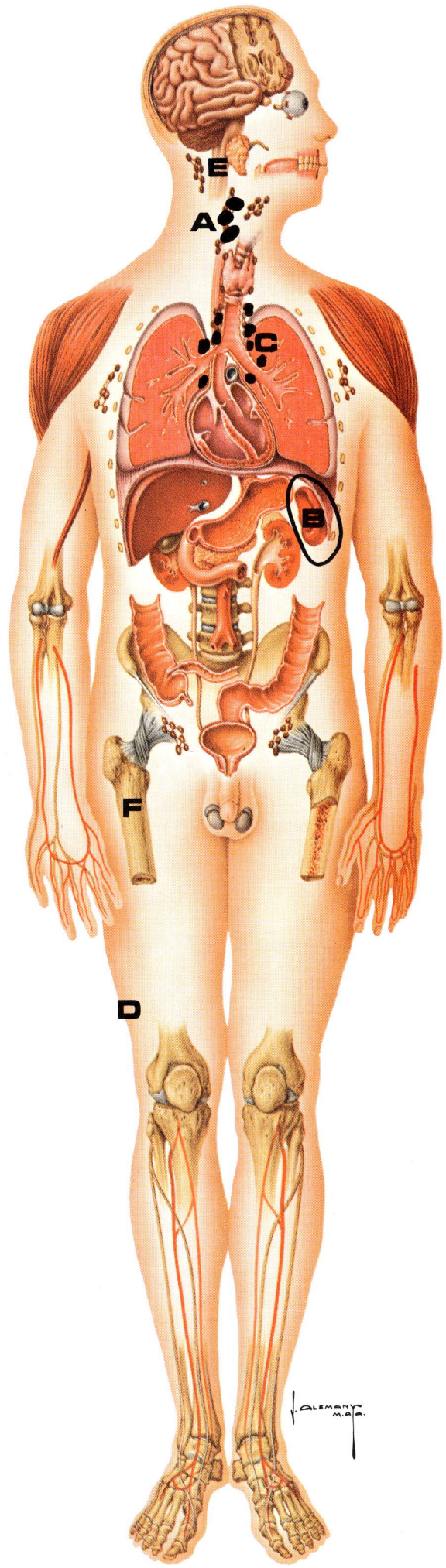

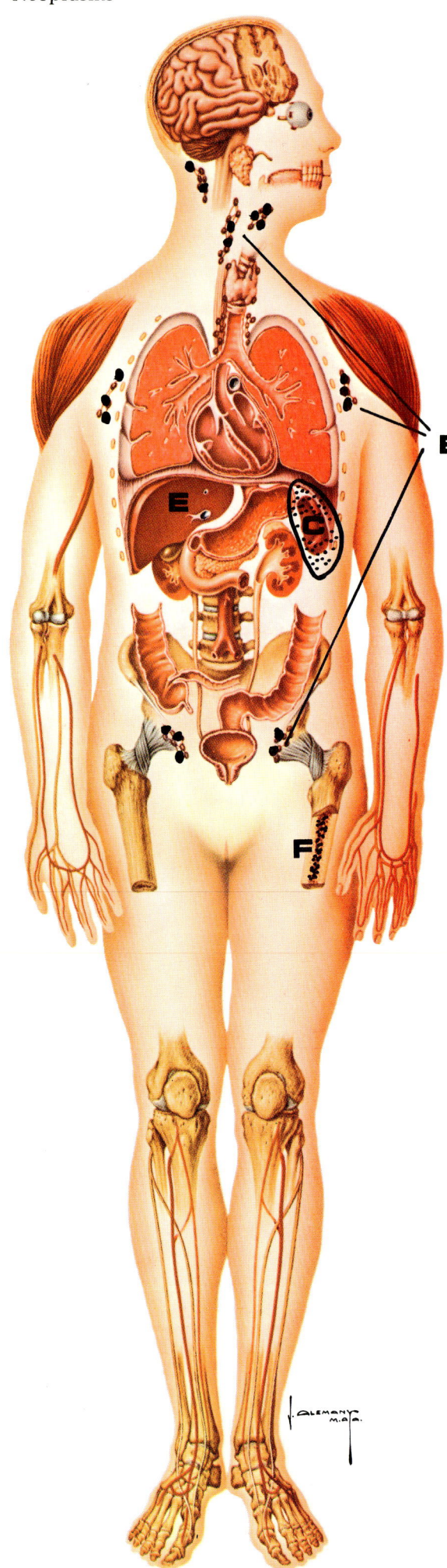

Acute Lymphatic Leukemia

This 4-year-old white female was admitted to the hospital after several days of antibiotic therapy had failed to alleviate an upper respiratory infection and a spiking temperature.

Physical examination revealed injected ulcerated tonsils and oropharynx (A), generalized lymphadenopathy (B), splenomegaly (C), and large purpuric lesions over both lower extremities (D).

Laboratory examination revealed a white count of 25,600 cells/cu. mm., 85 per cent of which were lymphoblasts, a platelet count of 35,000/cu. mm., and a hemoglobin of 8 gm. per cent.

Bone marrow examination revealed almost 95 per cent lymphocytes and lymphoblasts.

Treatment with prednisone and methotrexate brought about temporary remission.

Differential Diagnosis:
1. Infectious mononucleosis
2. Hodgkin's disease
3. Metastatic neuroblastoma
4. Agranulocytosis
5. Collagen disease
6. Brucellosis

7. Histoplasmosis
8. Typhoid fever
9. Sarcoidosis
10. Tuberculosis
11. Infectious hepatitis
12. Sickle cell anemia

Clinical Note. Any infection, particularly of the respiratory tract, which fails to respond to antibiotics should bring this diagnosis to mind. The diagnosis is not always so clear as in this case. There may be only a few blast cells in the peripheral blood (aleukemic type). Even in this variety the bone marrow is severely infiltrated. Leukemic infiltrates may involve any organ of the body, but the liver (E), spleen, and lymph nodes are most commonly involved. The bones and joints may be involved so severely that the condition simulates rheumatic fever. There may be central and peripheral nervous system involvement, even meningitis. Pulmonary infiltrates may simulate bronchopneumonia.

Pathology. The lymph nodes show poorly preserved architectural patterns with partial obliteration of follicular architecture and cells predominantly of the lymphocyte series. The spleen and liver are also infiltrated with lymphocytes and lymphoblasts. Bone marrow and bone are severely infiltrated with lymphoblasts (F), and the erythroid and megakaryocytic elements are markedly reduced.

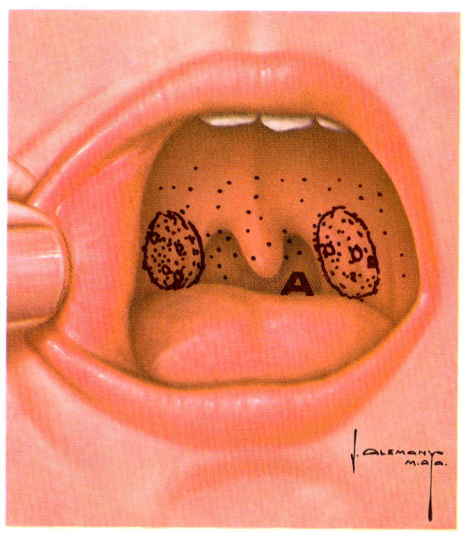

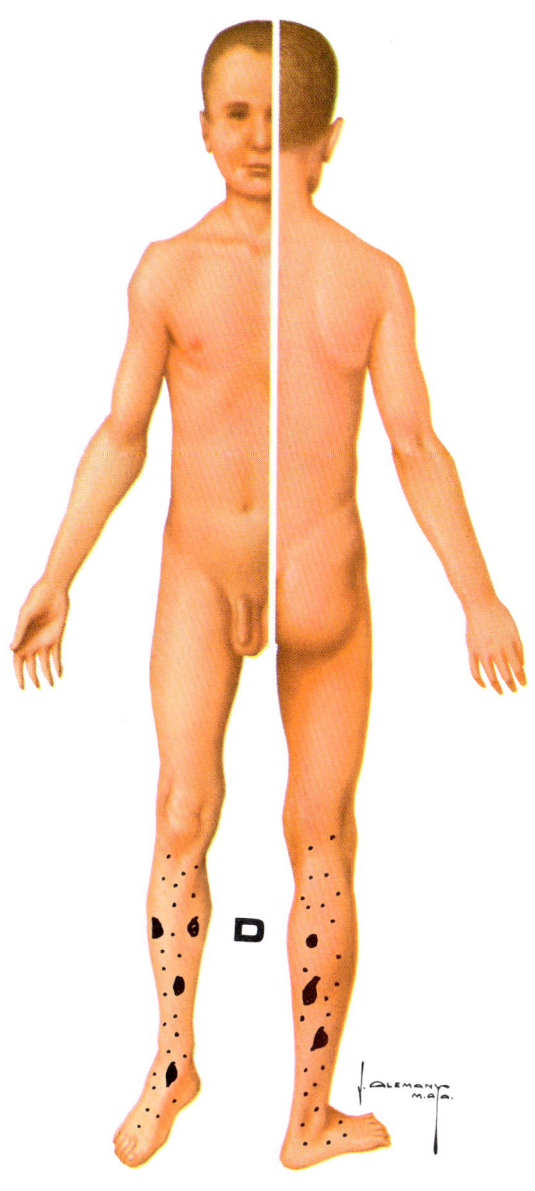

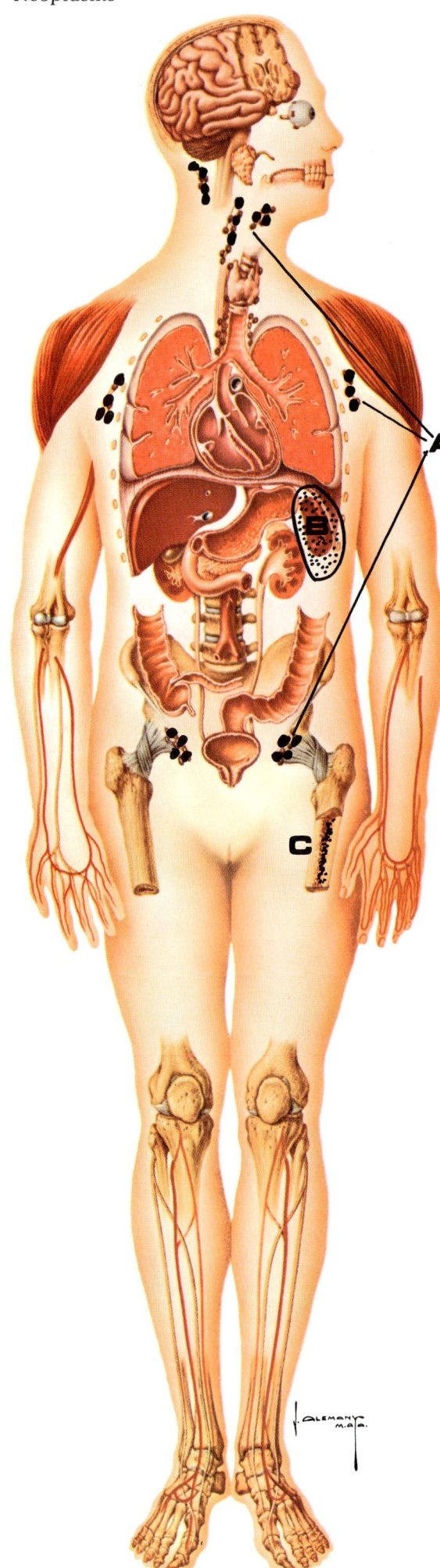

Chronic Lymphatic Leukemia

A 68-year-old white female complained of increasing anorexia and weight loss for 6 months prior to admission. On the day of admission she developed a nosebleed which she could not stop.

Physical examination revealed hemorrhages and exudates of the eye grounds, generalized lymphadenopathy (A), and splenomegaly (B).

Laboratory examination revealed a white cell count of 280,000, 90 per cent of which were lymphocytes; and lymphoblasts could not be recognized. There was also a hemolytic anemia and thrombocytopenia.

Bone marrow examination revealed extensive replacement with lymphocytes and some lymphoblasts (C).

Treatment with chlorambucil was effective.

Differential Diagnosis:
1. Chronic myelogenous leukemia
2. Infectious mononucleosis
3. Reticuloendotheliosis
4. Hodgkin's disease
5. Myelofibrosis with myeloid metaplasia
6. Tuberculosis
7. Brucellosis
8. Kala-azar

Clinical Note. Here is another disease that manifests with lymphadenopathy and splenomegaly. However, it is almost always in the elderly and has a very insidious onset. Chronic myelogenous leukemia does not often manifest with lymphadenopathy, but the spleen is larger. Skin involvement is rare in chronic myelogenous leukemia, also, in contrast to the lymphatic form, in which herpes zoster and exfoliative dermatitis abound. Both conditions are associated with anemia, but the anemia of chronic lymphatic leukemia is often hemolytic, of the autoimmune variety, and responds to corticosteroids. These patients are very susceptible to infection.

Pathology. In addition to bone marrow infiltration, there are abundant lymphocytes in the lymph nodes, lumbar vertebrae, liver, spleen, and kidneys.

Chronic Myelogenous Leukemia

A 36-year-old white male was admitted to the hospital for a herniorrhaphy. Routine CBC, performed on admission, revealed a white count of 93,000 cells per cu. mm. The patient was otherwise totally asymptomatic. Family history revealed that his father had died of myelogenous leukemia 5 years previously.

Physical examination revealed a massive splenomegaly (A) but no lymphadenopathy.

Laboratory examination revealed numerous myelocytes, promyelocytes, and occasional myeloblasts on peripheral smear. There were eosinophilia and basophilia. There was an elevated serum B_{12} level, and the neutrophils did not stain for alkaline phosphatase. BMR was elevated.

Treatment with busulfan was very successful.

Differential Diagnosis:
1. Other leukemias
2. Myelofibrosis with myeloid metaplasia
3. Metastatic carcinoma
4. Hodgkin's disease
5. Tuberculosis
6. Hyperthyroidism
7. Portal vein thrombosis
8. Hypersplenism, of various causes

Clinical Note. The absence of lymphadenopathy distinguishes this disease clinically from lymphatic leukemia. The absence of alkaline phosphatase in the neutrophils distinguishes this from myeloid metaplasia. This case illustrates the value of routine laboratory tests for screening.

Pathology. The bone marrow is replaced by leukemic cells (B). The leukemic cells may infiltrate any other organ in the body.

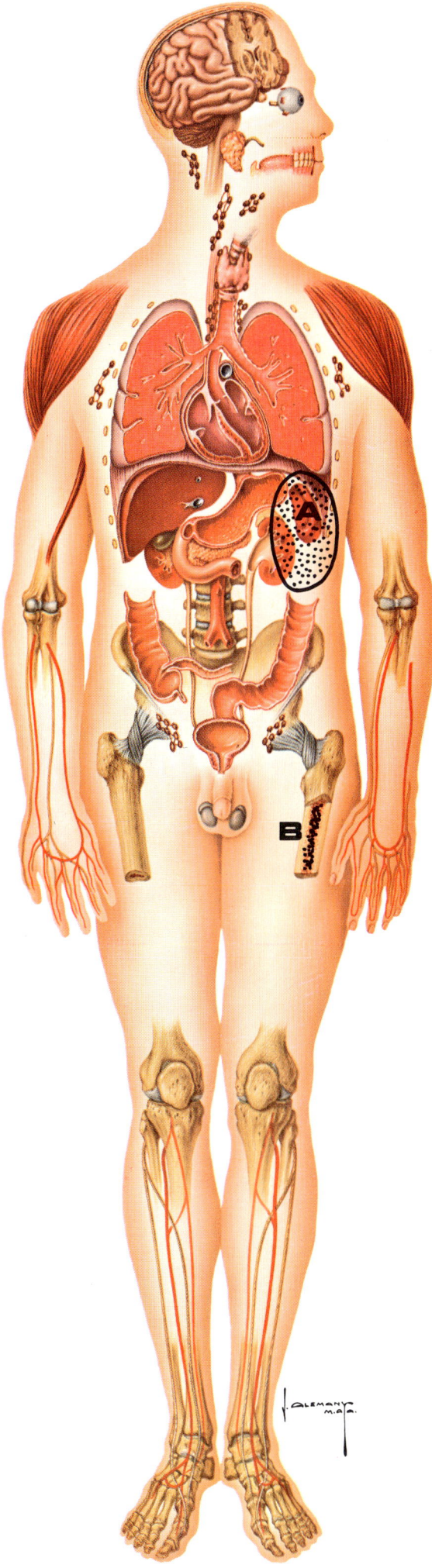

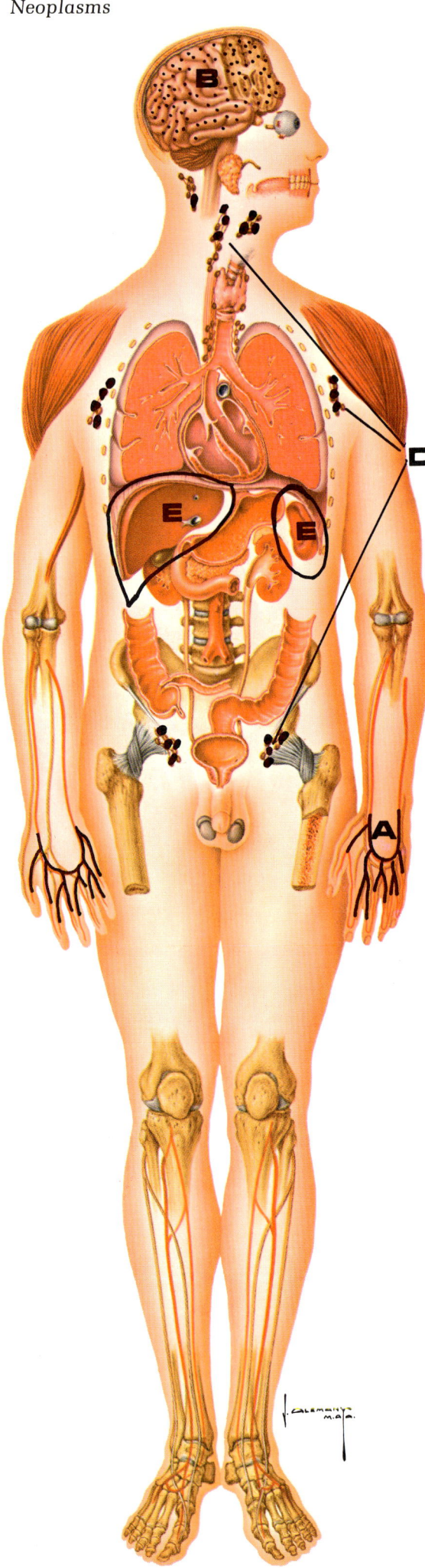

Macroglobulinemia

A 59-year-old white male was admitted to the hospital because of recurrent epistaxis and bleeding gums. For the past 6 months he had been severely fatigued and had noted that his hands would become blue and cold periodically (Raynaud's sign) (A). His family had observed that he was irritable and depressed at times (B).

Physical examination revealed engorgement and segmentation of the retinal veins, retinal hemorrhages (C), diffuse lymphadenopathy (D), hepatosplenomegaly (E).

Laboratory examination revealed a hemoglobin of 7.8 gm., positive Rumpel-Leede test, positive rouleaux formation on blood smear, and a narrow-based protein peak in the gamma globulin range which was indistinguishable from the pattern in multiple myeloma; ultracentrifugation showed a peak in the 19 S range (multiple myeloma shows a peak in the 7 S range). Bone marrow revealed marked infiltration by small lymphocytes.

Treatment with chlorambucil and plasmapheresis failed to alter the course significantly.

Differential Diagnosis:
1. Multiple myeloma
2. Purpura hyperglobulinemica
3. Leukemia
4. Hodgkin's disease
5. Infectious mononucleosis
6. Subacute bacterial endocarditis
7. Collagen diseases
8. Histoplasmosis
9. Cirrhosis of the liver
10. Kala-azar

Clinical Note. Although both multiple myeloma and macroglobulinemia may present with anemia and fatigue, multiple myeloma causes symptoms from bone infiltration in 90 per cent, and there are usually x-ray findings to explain these symptoms. X-rays rarely show anything more than osteoporosis in macroglobulinemia. Renal symptoms and those of hypercalcemia are rare in this disease, too. The bleeding tendency in this disease is due to interference of coagulation by the abnormal proteins, but the abnormal proteins may also cause vascular thrombosis by coating the red cells and increasing blood viscosity.

Pathology. The lymphadenopathy and hepatosplenomegaly can be explained by the marked infiltration and proliferation of small lymphocytes in these organs as well as in the bone marrow.

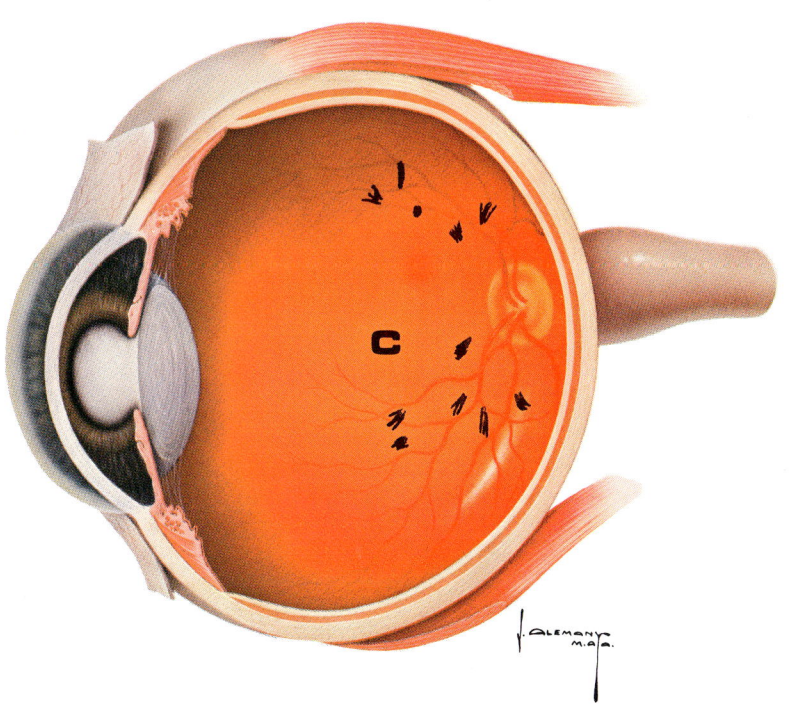

Myelofibrosis With Myeloid Metaplasia

A 48-year-old white female complained of fatigue, weight loss, and shortness of breath for several months. She was especially intolerant to heat.

Physical examination revealed massive hepatosplenomegaly (A) but no significant lymphadenopathy. There were petechiae (B) in the lower extremities.

Laboratory examination revealed a hemoglobin of 8.5 gm., a WBC of 43,000 cells per cu. mm., most of which were mature neutrophils, but a few myelocytes and promyelocytes were noted. The neutrophils stained heavily with the alkaline phosphatase stain. There was a thrombocytopenia. Tear-drop-shaped red cells were noted on the smear. There was a "dry tap" on bone marrow aspiration, but a trephine biopsy of the bone revealed characteristic fibrosis (C).

X-ray examination revealed osteosclerosis throughout the long bones.

Differential Diagnosis:
1. Chronic myelogenous leukemia
2. Gaucher's disease
3. Kala-azar
4. Cirrhosis of the liver
5. Diabetes mellitus
6. Hyperthyroidism
7. Hodgkin's disease
8. Subacute bacterial endocarditis
9. Metastatic carcinoma
10. Tuberculosis

Clinical Note. Very few conditions (chronic myelogenous leukemia and Gaucher's disease among them) produce such a massive spleen. These patients may present with thrombophlebitis when the platelet count is high, or with bleeding from the skin or intestinal tract when the platelets are low. There is still a question of whether the extramedullary erythropoiesis is a reaction to the myelofibrosis or part of a neoplastic process.

Multiple Myeloma

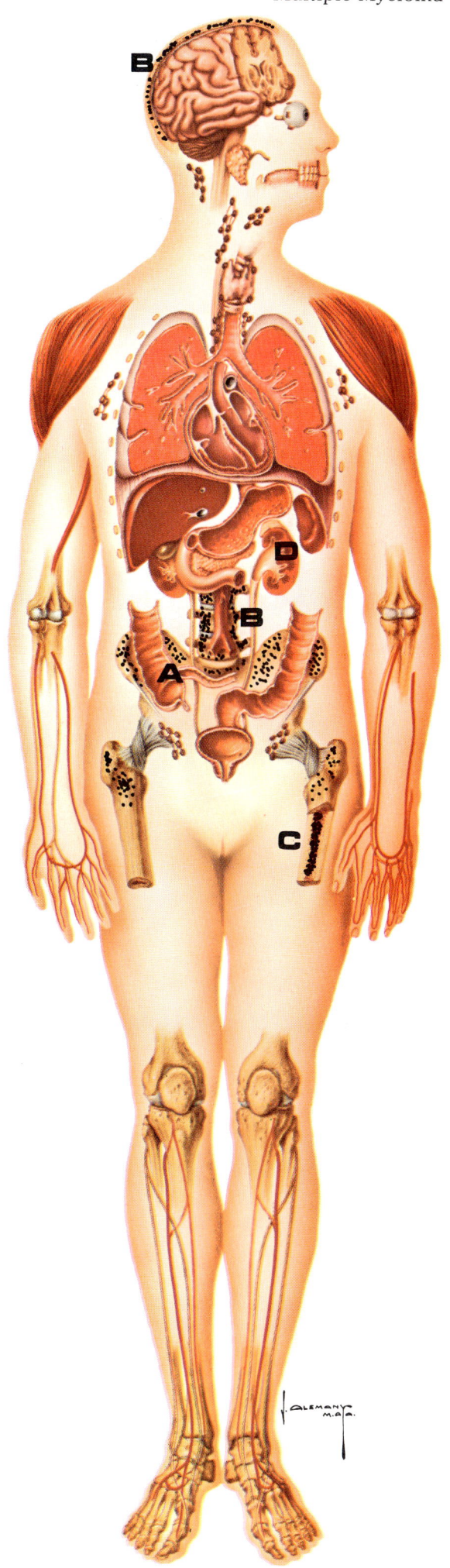

A 53-year-old Negro female had been suffering from fatigue, anorexia, intermittent nausea, and constipation (A) for the past 3 months. She had had increasing low back pain for the past month; and when she developed paralysis and loss of sensation in her lower extremities, she was admitted to the hospital for evaluation.

Physical examination revealed pale nails and conjunctivae, paralysis of the lower extremities, a sensory level at T-12 bilaterally, and exquisite tenderness of T-10 and T-11 vertebrae (B).

Laboratory examination revealed a rapid sedimentation rate, rouleaux formation, a normocytic, normochromic anemia, a near gamma globulin peak on paper electrophoresis, Bence-Jones proteinuria, and increased plasmocytes and plasmoblasts on bone marrow examination (C). Blood calcium and uric acid were elevated.

X-ray examination revealed a pathologic fracture of T-12, L-1, and L-2 vertebrae and punched-out radiolucent lesions of the skull and spine (B).

Treatment with radiation and urethan was begun.

Differential Diagnosis:
1. Spinal cord tumors
2. Metastatic carcinoma
3. Pernicious anemia
4. Guillain-Barré syndrome
5. Tuberculosis of the spine
6. Hodgkin's disease
7. Macroglobulinemia
8. Hyperparathyroidism
9. Herniated thoracic disk
10. Pancreatic carcinoma

Clinical Note. The combination of anemia, bone pain, and gastrointestinal symptoms is seldom seen in any other entity except metastatic carcinoma. Whereas both multiple myeloma and macroglobulinemia involve the nervous system, the spinal cord and peripheral nerves are more frequently involved in multiple myeloma. The renal involvement (D) is due to deposition of Bence-Jones protein in the nephron.

Pathology. The bone and bone marrow are infiltrated with atypical plasma cells having abundant vacuolated cytoplasm and an eccentric nucleus. These may contain 1 or more nucleoli. The abnormal proteins, such as para-amyloid, may infiltrate kidneys or nerves.

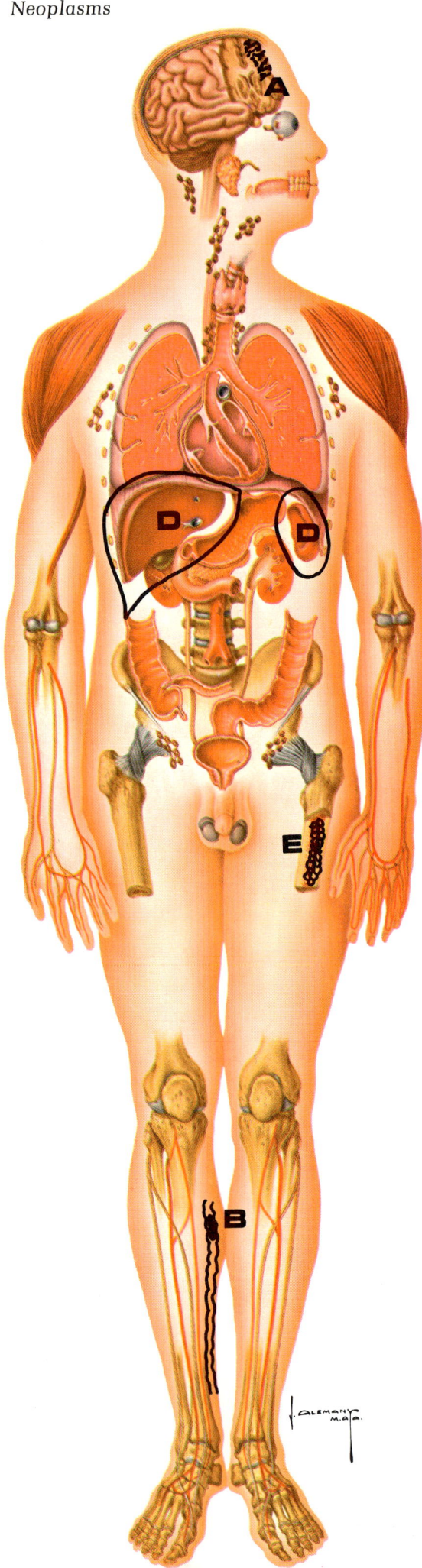

Polycythemia Vera

A 55-year-old white male was brought to the emergency room because of sudden onset of left-sided hemiplegia (A). Past history revealed that he had had 2 previous admissions to the hospital for thrombophlebitis (B). He also had complained of frequent nosebleeds.

Physical examination revealed engorged retinal veins (C), hepatosplenomegaly (D), and weakness and hypoactive reflexes of the left extremities, with a positive Babinski sign on the left.

Laboratory examination revealed a red cell count of 6.2 million cells/cu. mm., WBC of 14,000 cells/cu. mm., and a platelet count of 625,000/cu. mm. A bone marrow examination revealed increased numbers of all elements, particularly the megakaryocytes. M and E ratio was normal. No abnormalities in the coagulation tests could be found. Arterial oxygen, carbon dioxide, and prothrombin time were normal. Blood volume was increased greatly.

Treatment with frequent phlebotomies and later the use of ^{32}P was very successful.

Differential Diagnosis:
1. Cerebral thrombosis due to atherosclerosis
2. Cerebral hemorrhage due to essential hypertension
3. Pulmonary emphysema and fibrosis
4. Congenital heart disease with venous to arterial shunting
5. Chronic myelogenous leukemia
6. Other blood dyscrasias
7. Other causes of secondary polycythemia
8. Cushing's syndrome and unilateral renal disease
9. Methemoglobinemia

Clinical Note. Most cases of polycythemia vera are asymptomatic for years until a thrombophlebitis, bleeding episode, or cerebrovascular accident occurs. This disorder is differentiated from secondary polycythemia by the normal arterial oxygen saturation. This condition should always be considered in determining the etiology of a CVA.

Pathology. Other than the hyperplastic marrow (E) and hyperplasia of the spleen, there are no distinct findings.

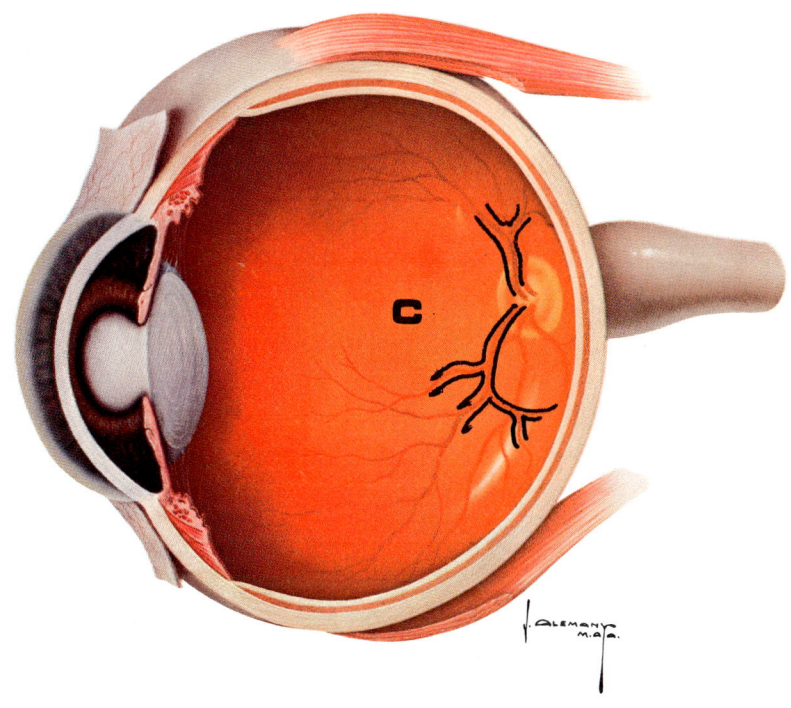

Chapter 10

Organ Failure

This chapter introduces a new concept of organ failure—that is, failure of any one of the principal organs (heart, lungs, kidneys) of the body to fulfill its physiologic or metabolic functions adequately results in a systemic disease. For example, failure of the lungs to eliminate carbon dioxide or absorb oxygen causes disease in many organs. The uremia of kidney failure results in coma, pericarditis, uremic ulcers, and skin lesions. Heart failure results in congestion of the lungs, liver, and extremities as well as uremia. The first clue to each one of these types of organ failure may be involvement of a remote organ. For example, hepatomegaly may be the first sign of heart failure. The clinician should have at his fingertips the battery of laboratory tests necessary to diagnose each type of organ failure. Table VII lists these. It should not be necessary to emphasize to the reader after he reads this chapter that no organ of the body is independent of any other organ.

246 · Organ Failure

Chronic Pulmonary Emphysema

A 62-year-old white male was admitted to the hospital in a comatose state. There was a history of long-standing pulmonary emphysema.

Physical examination revealed a comatose white male with carbon dioxide narcosis, indicating central nervous system suppression (A); tachypnea, tachycardia, distended neck veins, and pitting edema as signs of right-sided heart failure (B); hepatomegaly (C); sibilant and sonorous rales throughout the chest, and prolonged expiration.

Laboratory examination revealed polycythemia, indicating bone marrow stimulation (D) by the chronic anoxia; increased arterial blood carbon dioxide and decreased arterial oxygen saturation; increased carbon dioxide combining power and a pH of 7.1.

X-ray examination revealed pulmonary emphysema and fibrosis in the chest (E) with cardiomegaly. An EKG revealed right ventricular hypertrophy and P-pulmonale.

Differential Diagnosis:
1. Barbiturate intoxication
2. Diabetic coma
3. Insulin shock
4. Hepatic coma
5. Meningitis
6. Uremia
7. Encephalitis
8. Cerebrovascular accident
9. Cerebral concussion
10. Epilepsy

Clinical Note. In its late stages, pulmonary emphysema affects many organs. The right heart is enlarged by pulmonary hypertension, and fails. There is chronic passive congestion of the liver, and eventually liver function studies may change. There is carbon dioxide narcosis, which may at first lead only to an organic psychosis. The reduced cardiac output and anoxia may cause renal insufficiency (F) with an elevated BUN. Hypertrophy of the bones (G) may develop (pulmonary osteoarthropathy). There may be papilledema as well.

Pathology. The alveoli are replaced by larger air sacs transversed by fibrous bands, and there is associated interstitial fibrosis. The capillary beds are destroyed. These tissue changes may be interspersed with normal lung tissue. The bronchi and bronchioles may be dilated, chronically inflamed, and their walls weakened.

Chronic Congestive Heart Failure

A 54-year-old white female complained of increasing shortness of breath and swelling of her legs.

Physical examination revealed distended neck veins (A), crepitant rales over both lower lobes posteriorly, cardiomegaly (B), hepatomegaly (C), splenomegaly (D), and 4+ pitting edema of both lower extremities (E).

Laboratory examination revealed an increased blood volume, reduced arterial oxygen saturation with a normal arterial pCO_2, increased circulation time, and a decreased vital capacity.

X-ray examination of the chest revealed pulmonary edema (F).

Differential Diagnosis:
1. Pulmonary emphysema
2. Myocardial infarction
3. Subacute bacterial endocarditis
4. Cirrhosis of the liver
5. Glomerulonephritis
6. Myxedema
7. Beriberi
8. Hyperthyroidism
9. Anemia of various causes
10. Rheumatic fever
11. Collagen diseases
12. Leukemia
13. Amyloidosis
14. Hemochromatosis

Clinical Note. Congestive heart failure is a disease of many organs. The lungs are engorged and edematous; the liver shows chronic passive congestion, and occasionally the spleen is congested, as in this case. There may be congestion of the abdominal viscera, causing nausea and vomiting. When cardiac output is markedly reduced, there is renal failure (G). Irritability, restlessness, and even stupor may result from reduced cerebrovascular perfusion. Thus congestive heart failure may have to be considered in the differential diagnosis of symptoms arising from any organ.

Pathology. The heart muscle is hypertrophied, and there may be areas of fibrosis and necrosis. Other pathological changes of the heart depend on the etiology of the failure. Microscopically, the lungs show engorgement of the capillaries, thick alveolar septa, and perivascular mononuclear cells containing hemosiderin (ingested erythrocytes). The liver shows changes of chronic passive congestion.

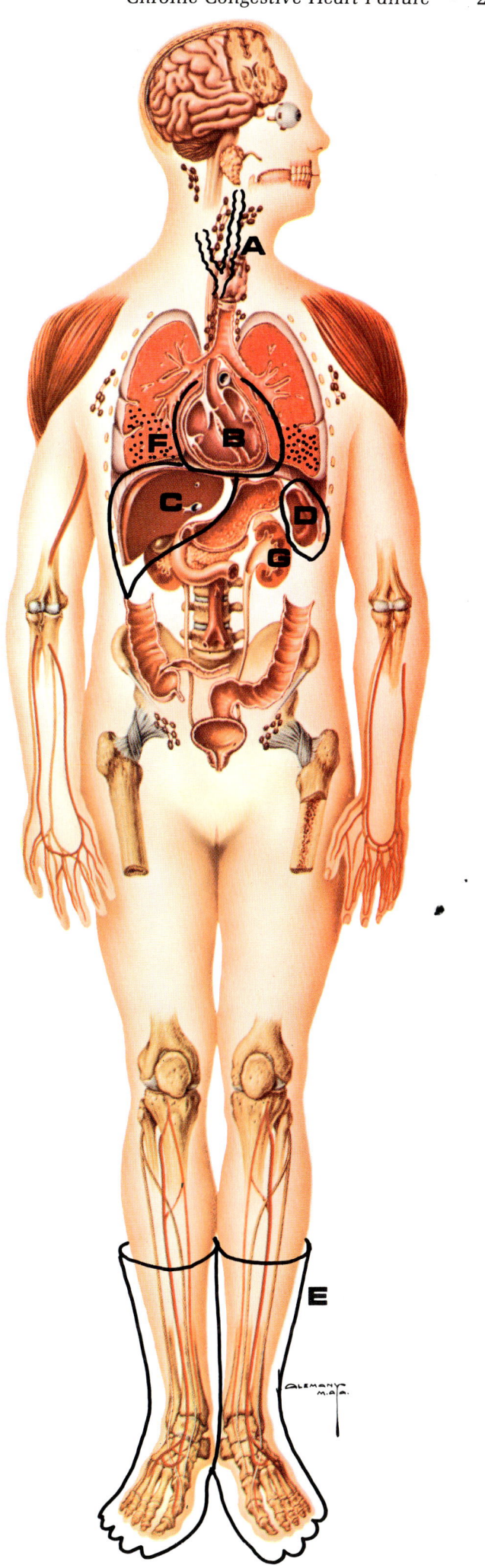

248 · Organ Failure

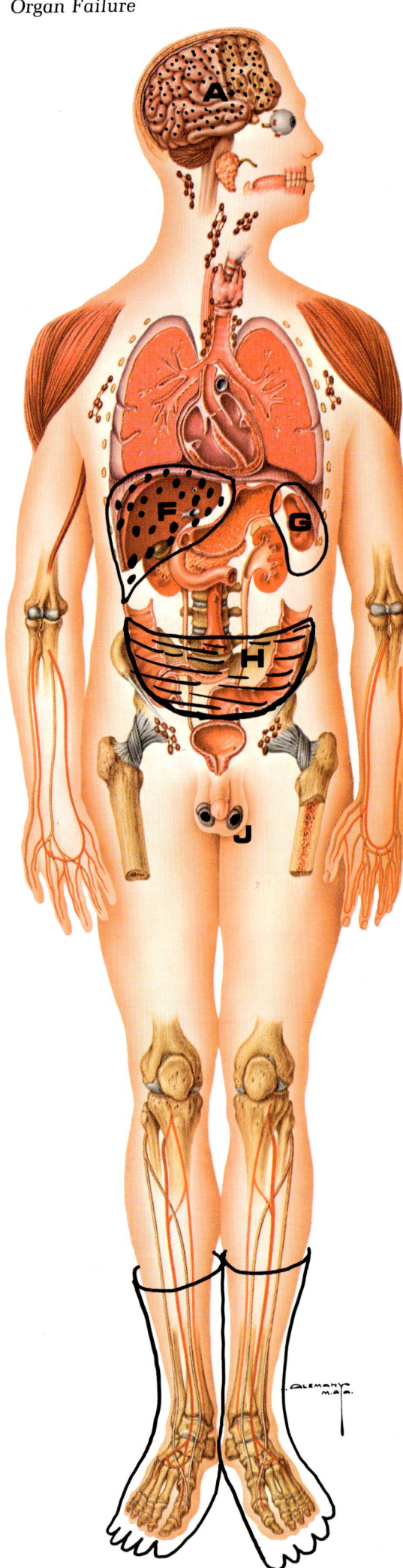

Chronic Hepatic Failure

A 56-year-old white male known alcoholic was brought to the emergency room in a comatose state.

Physical examination revealed, in addition to the coma, a flapping tremor of the hands, indicating central nervous system involvement (A), spider angiomas (B), loss of hair on the chest and genitalia (C), gynecomastia (D), palmar erythema (E), hepatomegaly (F), splenomegaly (G), ascites (H), pitting edema of the lower extremities (I), and testicular atrophy (J).

Laboratory examination revealed a high blood ammonia level, a total bilirubin of 5.4 mg. per cent with a 3.8 mg. per cent direct bilirubin, increased serum transaminase, and a low serum albumin. There were a macrocytic anemia and a high prothrombin time.

X-ray examination of the esophagus at a later date revealed esophageal varices.

Treatment with a low protein diet, neomycin, and peritoneal dialysis was helpful.

Differential Diagnosis:
1. Hemochromatosis
2. Viral hepatitis
3. Carbon tetrachloride poisoning
4. Hyperthyroidism
5. Uremia
6. Congestive heart failure

7. Chronic pulmonary emphysema
8. Phenothiazine toxicity
9. Leptospirosis
10. Schistosomiasis
11. Collagen disease
12. Hemolytic anemias
13. Cushing's syndrome
14. Pernicious anemia

Clinical Note. The involvement of the central nervous system, skin, blood, gastrointestinal tract, endocrine system, and spleen makes it rather obvious that this is a systemic disease. Renal function is often impaired by secondary aldosteronism and reduced renal blood flow from the hypovolemia. The anemia may be due to excessive blood loss (i.e., in bleeding esophageal varices), reduced blood formation (inhibition of folic acid utilization by the alcohol), or excessive destruction of red cells (by the congested spleen). Gastrointestinal bleeding also results from peptic ulcers. The spleen may be sufficiently enlarged to cause a pancytopenia. Prior to the coma the central nervous system involvement may be recognized by personality changes and memory loss. Since the liver manufactures plasma proteins that bind hormones (transcortin, thyroxin-binding protein, etc.), it is understandable why these patients may appear cushingoid or hypothyroid. Androgen and estrogen metabolism are altered as well.

Pathology. Microscopy reveals fat-laden cells in some places and banners of fibrous tissue radiating out into the lobules from the portal areas. Later the fibrous tissue increases to the point that lobular architecture is lost.

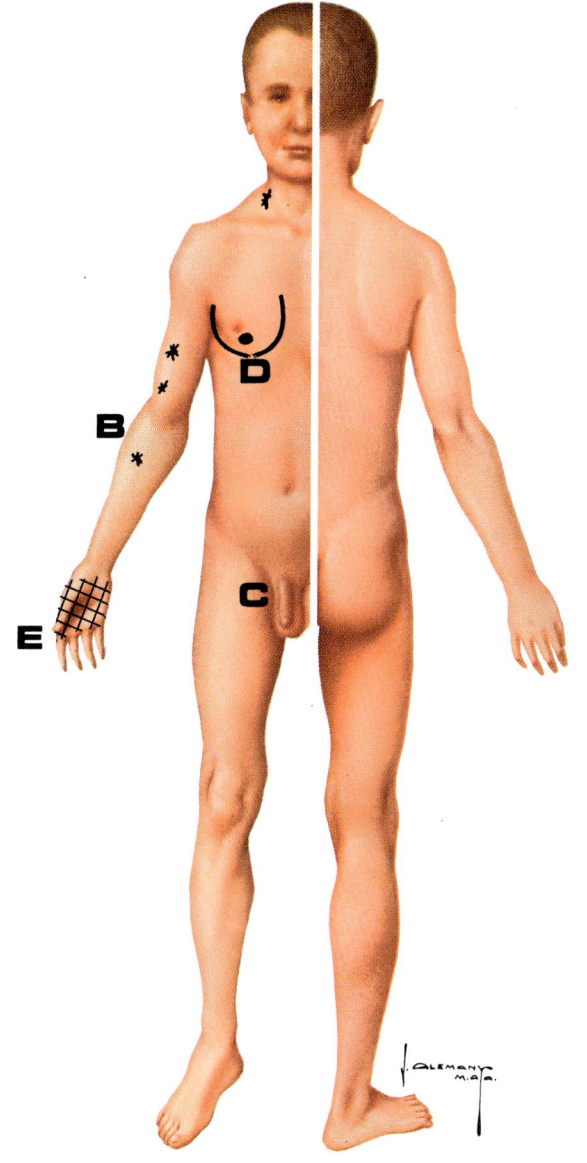

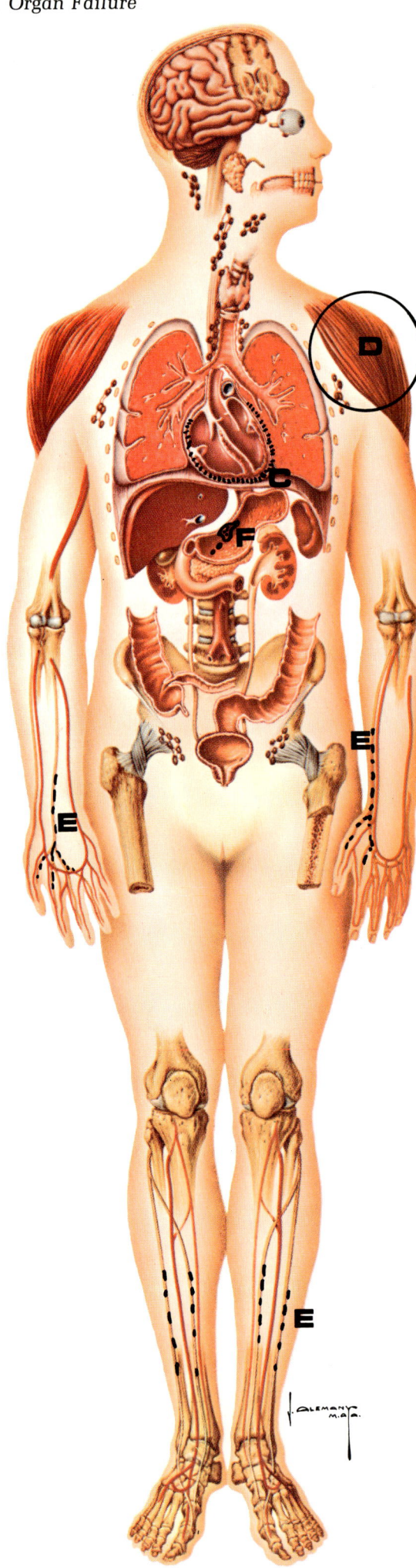

Chronic Renal Failure

A 14-year-old white female with a known history of chronic pyelonephritis had complained of nausea and vomiting for some time. On the day of admission she sustained a generalized convulsion.

Physical examination revealed "uremic frost" of the face (A), petechiae and excoriations of the distal portions of all 4 extremities (B), a pericardial friction rub, indicating pericarditis (C), pitting edema of the extremities, twitching and tremor of the extremities as evidence of neuromuscular involvement (D), and glove and stocking hypesthesia and hypalgesia with atrophy of the small hand muscles bilaterally, indicating a peripheral neuropathy (E).

Laboratory examination revealed a normocytic anemia, a BUN of 108 mg. per cent, a creatinine of 4.5 mg. per cent, a low serum potassium and calcium, and a high serum phosphorus and pyuria.

Treatment with renal dialysis and digitalization was helpful.

Differential Diagnosis:
1. Cirrhosis of the liver
2. Congestive heart failure
3. Chronic pulmonary emphysema
4. Alcoholism
5. Obstructive uropathy

6. Diabetes mellitus
7. Insulin shock
8. Hypopotassemia
9. Hypoparathyroidism
10. Phenothiazine toxicity
11. Collagen disease
12. Thrombocytopenia purpura
13. Hyperparathyroidism
14. Aldosteronism
15. Pellagra
16. Carbon tetrachloride poisoning

Clinical Note. This case demonstrates the involvement of the nervous system, blood, gastrointestinal system, heart, and skin in this disorder. There may be a "uremic lung" as well. In some cases congestive heart failure develops secondary to the circulatory overload produced by the low urinary output. The petechiae may be due to a frank thrombocytopenia or platelet dysfunction. Anemia may develop from bone marrow depression or hemorrhagic diathesis associated with bleeding peptic ulcers (F). The neuromuscular symptoms may be due to tetany or the low serum potassium. Other symptoms may develop, depending on the etiology of the renal failure.

Pathology. There is replacement of renal tubules and glomeruli by fibrous tissue, and usually a mononuclear reaction occurs. Occasionally, large numbers of interstitial neutrophils are found, indicating an acute exacerbation of the pyelonephritis. The lungs may show a fibrinous exudate in the alveolar spaces and an interstitial pneumonitis. The pericardium also shows a fibrinous exudate which is sterile.

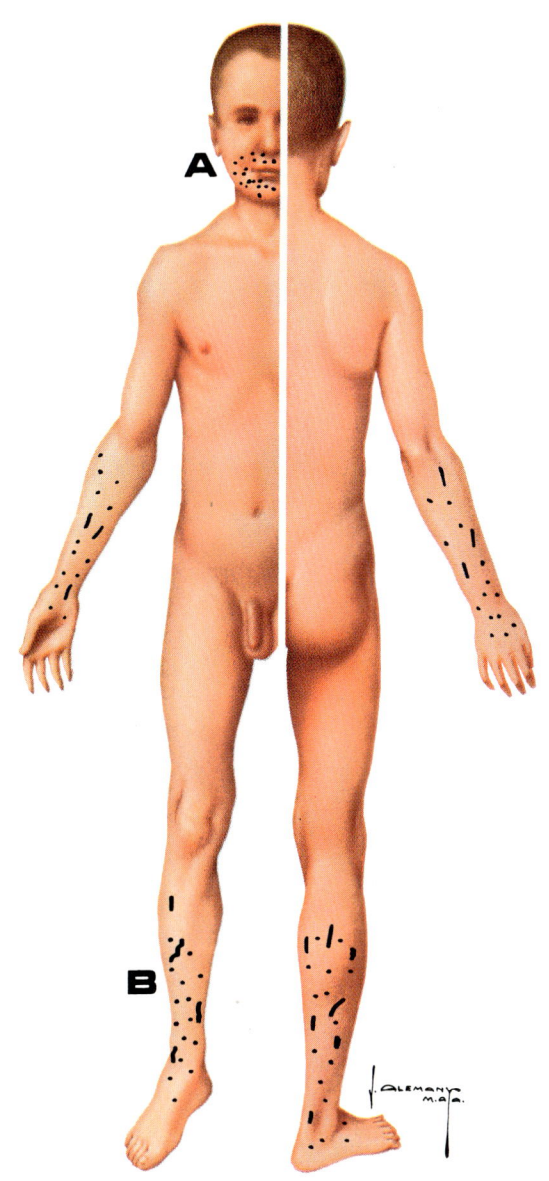

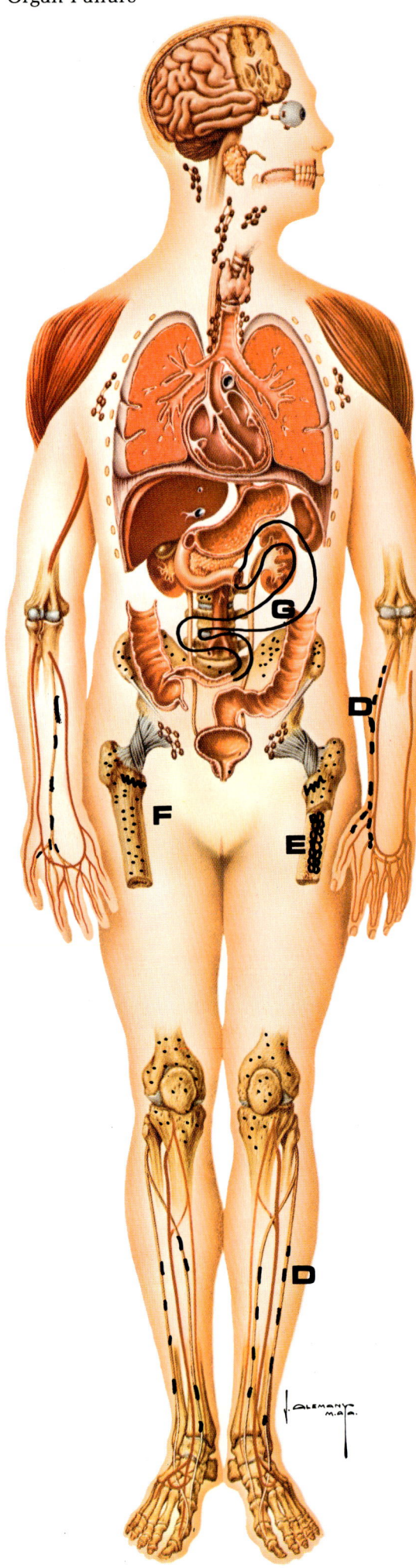

Malabsorption Syndrome

A 54-year-old white female fractured her right femur in an apparently minor fall. Careful questioning revealed that she had suffered from marked weight loss and bulky, foul-smelling stools for several months.

Physical examination revealed atrophy of the filiform papillae (A), cheilosis (B), hyperkeratosis follicularis and ecchymosis of the skin (C), diminished vibratory and position sense and hypesthesia of the distal portion of all 4 extremities, indicating a peripheral neuropathy (D), and a positive Trousseau phenomenon.

Laboratory examination revealed an elevated plasma prothrombin time; macrocytic, hyperchromic anemia; low serum cholesterol, albumin, calcium, potassium, and a flat oral glucose tolerance test. Radioactive triolein and oleic acid uptakes were low, and there was an increase in 5-hydroxyindoleacetic acid in the urine. Jejunal mucosal biopsy was diagnostic. A bone marrow examination revealed megaloblasts and hyperplasia (E).

X-ray examination of the skeleton revealed osteomalacia (F) with Milkman's fractures. A small bowel series revealed dilated loops of small bowel (G) and scattering of the barium.

Differential Diagnosis:
1. Chronic pancreatitis
2. Hypoparathyroidism
3. Rickets
4. Pernicious anemia
5. Alcoholism
6. Pellagra
7. Diabetes mellitus
8. Whipple's disease
9. Amyloidosis
10. Carcinoid syndrome
11. Ulcerative colitis
12. Amebiasis

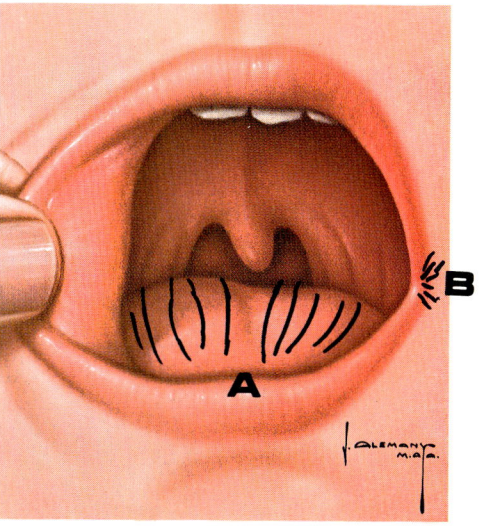

Clinical Note. Here we have involvement of the nervous system, blood, skin, and bone secondary to disease of the intestinal mucosa (G). Involvement of each organ is due to deficient absorption of one or more substances vital to its metabolism. Thus the production of blood cells is reduced because of poor absorption of iron, B_{12}, or folic acid. Osteomalacia results from poor absorption of calcium and vitamin D. Skin changes may result from poor vitamin A absorption. Muscle weakness results from hypokalemia, and hyponatremia may lead to cramps and hypotension.

Pathology. In adult celiac disease the jejunal mucosa shows flattening of the intestinal mucosa without distinct villi, a dense mononuclear cell infiltrate, and a sparse brush border. Other causes of the malabsorption syndrome have a varied pathology.

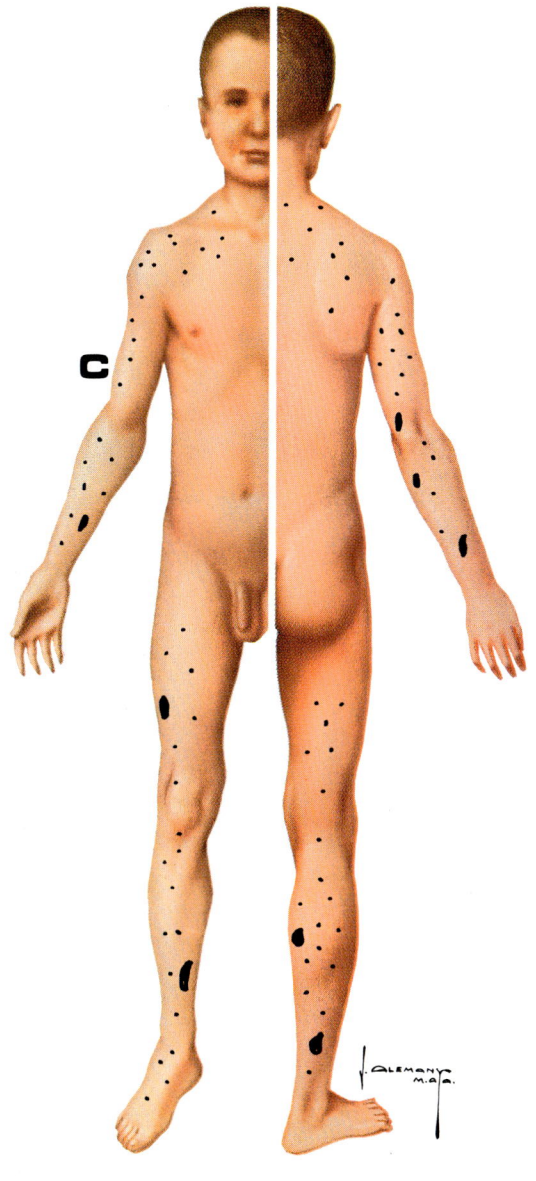

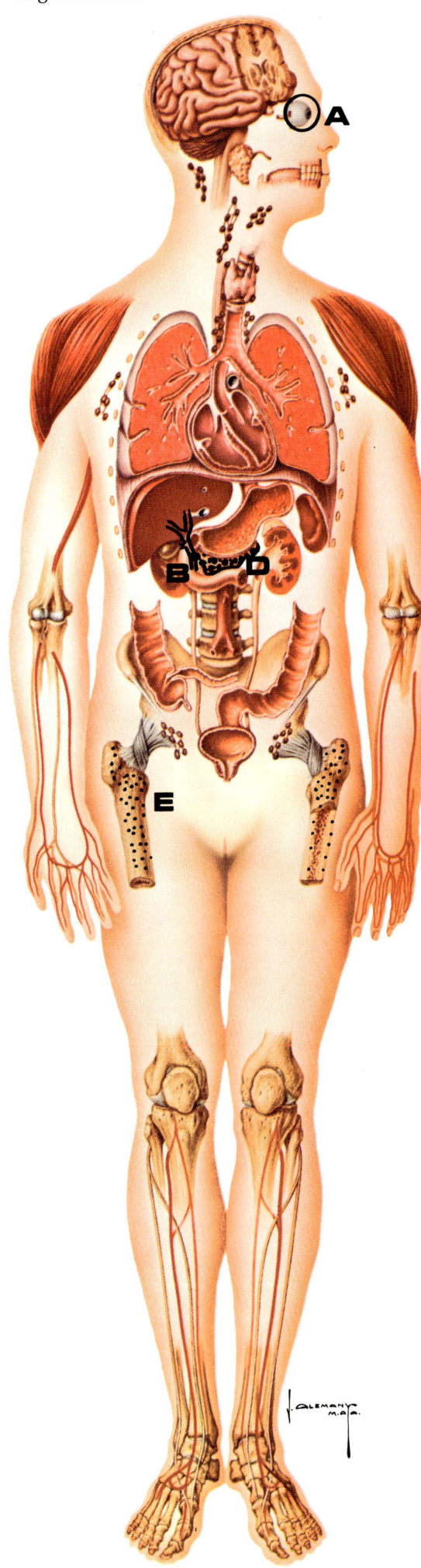

Chronic Pancreatitis

A 43-year-old white female was admitted to the hospital with severe generalized abdominal pain. She had had several attacks of similar abdominal pain for the past 5 years, and in the past 6 months her stools became bulky and foul-smelling, and she had lost 40 pounds. Years ago her aunt had been diagnosed as having pancreatitis.

Physical examination revealed icteric sclera (A) and jaundice, indicating common bile duct obstruction (B), generalized abdominal tenderness and rebound tenderness with hypoactive bowel sounds, and diabetic retinopathy (C).

Laboratory examination revealed a serum amylase of 632 units, a lipase of 3.5 cc. (elevated), a FBS of 250 mg. per cent, and a serum bilirubin of 3.5 mg. per cent. Duodenal drainage at a later date revealed low bicarbonate and pancreatic enzymes in the duodenal juice.

X-ray examination revealed calcifications of the pancreas (D) and early osteomalacia of both femurs (E).

Treatment with insulin, intravenous fluids, intubation, and intestinal rest was effective.

Differential Diagnosis:
1. Diabetic neuropathy
2. Porphyria
3. Cholecystitis

4. Ruptured peptic ulcer
5. Intestinal obstruction
6. Appendicitis
7. Celiac disease
8. Whipple's disease
9. Common duct stone
10. Pneumonia
11. Sickle cell anemia
12. Periarteritis nodosa
13. Carcinoma of the pancreas
14. Fibrocystic disease
15. Hyperparathyroidism
16. Hemochromatosis

Clinical Note. This is another example of how failure of function in the organ may lead to involvement of many other organs. Pressure on the common bile duct by the diseased pancreas causes hepatic involvement; fibrosis of the pancreas causes islet cell destruction and diabetes mellitus; failure of enzyme secretion leads to a malabsorption syndrome (p. 252) and its systemic complications. Not all cases of chronic pancreatitis are due to alcoholism, as is demonstrated by this case. The disease may be transmitted as a mendelian autosomal dominant gene in certain families. Nor do all cases present with recurring abdominal pain. The first symptom may be steatorrhea or diabetes mellitus. A pancreatic pseudocyst may develop and lead to intestinal obstruction.

Pathology. The acinar and islet cells are replaced by fibrosis, and calcium deposits are noted in the main duct and intralobular ducts.

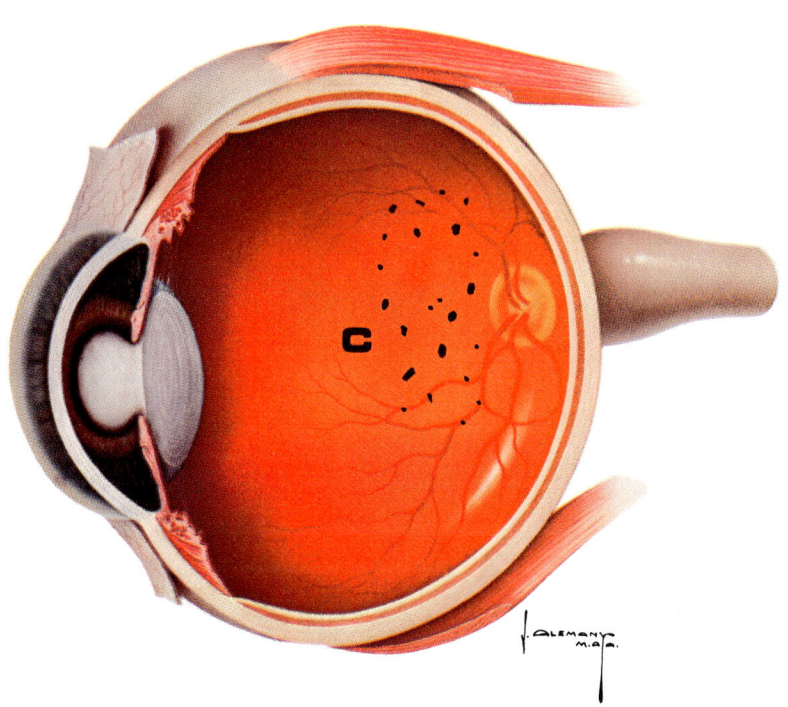

Chapter 11

The Reticuloendothelioses

Reticuloendothelial tissue is found in all organs. Thus the diseases listed here involve many organs, only a few of which may manifest clinically in individual cases. The diseases may be classified not only by the organs that show physical signs but also by the type of lipid that appears in the reticuloendothelial cells. Thus in Hand-Schüller-Christian disease there are cholesterol esters, in Gaucher's disease there is kerasin, and in Niemann-Pick disease there is sphingomyelin. Gaucher's disease and Niemann-Pick disease are hereditary, but Hand-Schüller-Christian disease is not. Diagnosis is established by biopsy of the involved tissue and analysis of its lipid content.

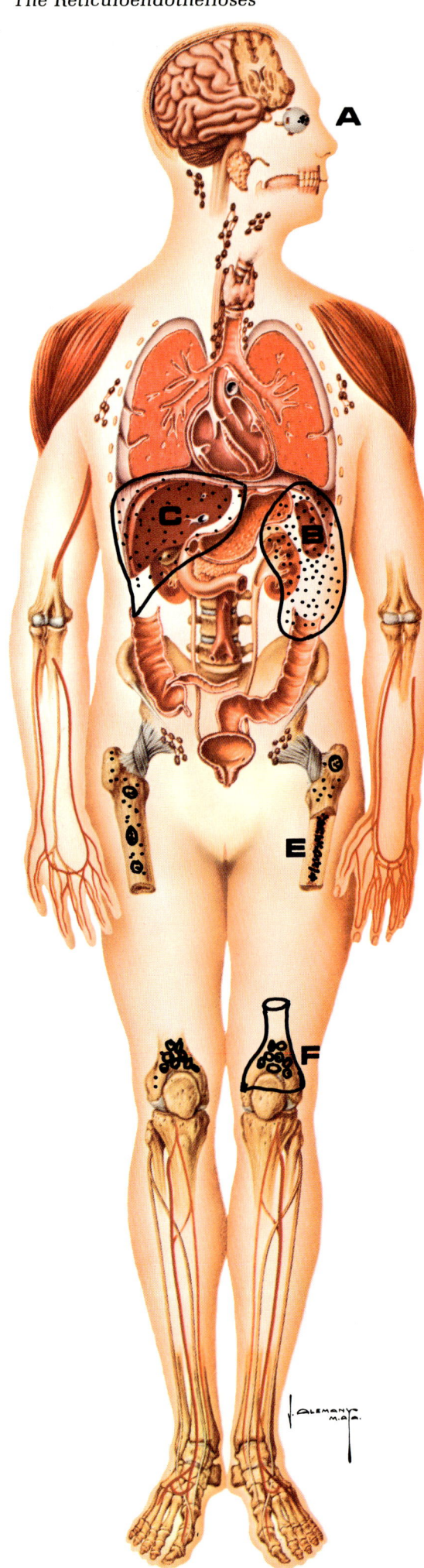

Gaucher's Disease

A 28-year-old white female complained of increasing protuberance of her belly and feeling a lump in her left side.

Physical examination revealed bilateral pingueculae of the bulbar conjunctiva (A), massive splenomegaly (B), hepatomegaly without jaundice (C), and hyperpigmentation of the skin (D) in areas exposed to light.

Laboratory examination revealed an elevated serum acid phosphatase, anemia, leukopenia, and thrombocytopenia.

Bone marrow examination revealed infiltration by the Gaucher cell (E): large round reticulum cells having a small eccentrically placed nucleus and wrinkled cytoplasm with a network of fibrils and filled with the cerebroside kerasin.

X-ray examination of the femurs revealed radiolucent cystic changes in the proximal and distal portions (F) with the characteristic Erlenmeyer flask appearance.

Differential Diagnosis:
1. Hodgkin's disease
2. Chronic myelogenous leukemia
3. Myeloid metaplasia
4. Cirrhosis of the liver
5. Hemachromatosis
6. Von Gierke's disease
7. Felty's syndrome
8. Infectious mononucleosis

Clinical Note. Unlike many conditions associated with splenomegaly, there is rarely any lymphadenopathy of the peripheral nodes. However, abdominal and thoracic lymph nodes may be infiltrated by the Gaucher cells. Infiltration of the bone may lead to pathologic fractures. The severe pancytopenia may require splenectomy. In infants there may be extensive infiltration of the brain, as in certain cases of glycogen storage disease.

Pathology. Any organ of the body may be infiltrated with Gaucher cells; but except for the spleen, marrow, lungs, and bone, functional impairment is rare in adults.

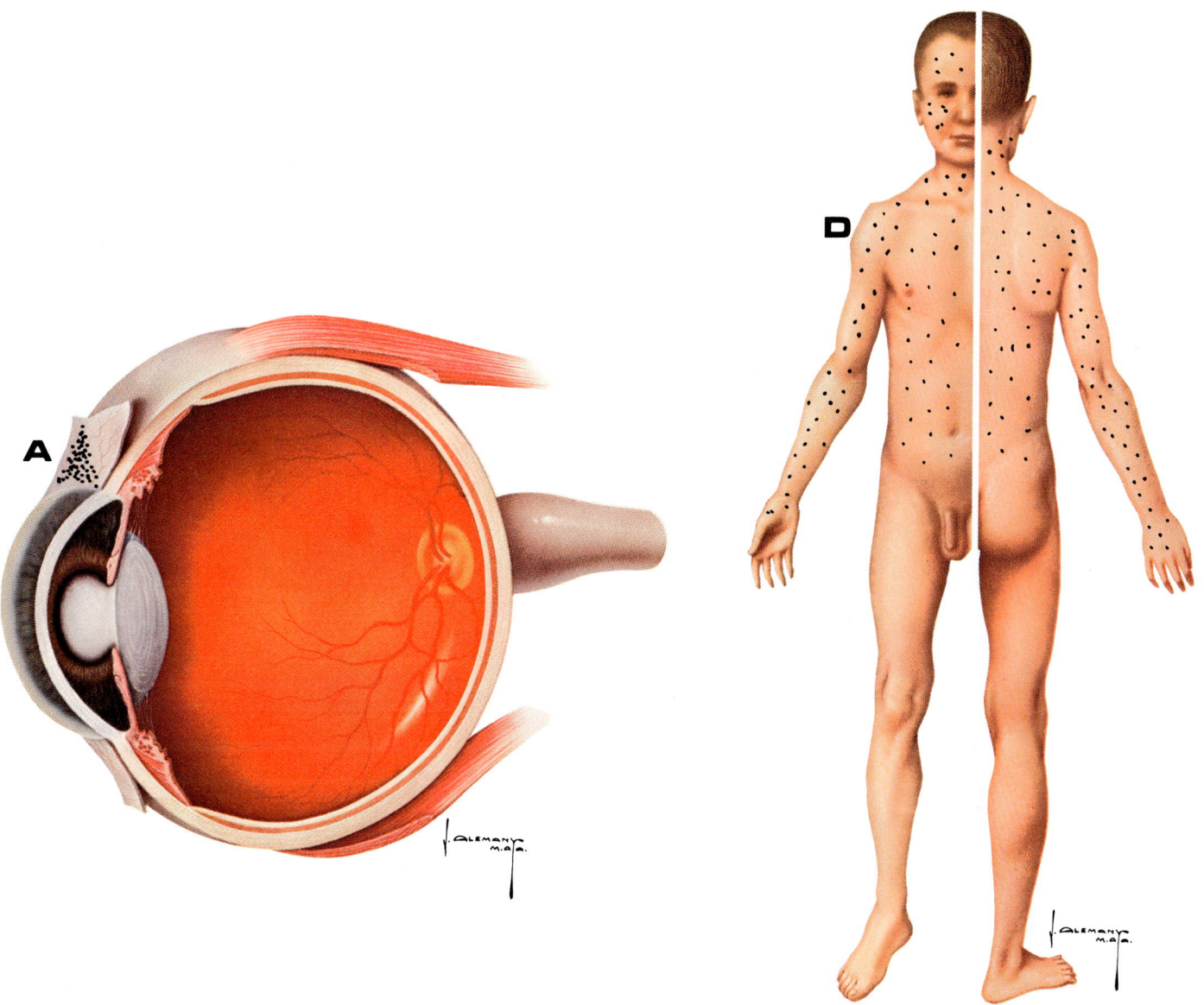

Histiocytosis X: Hand-Schüller-Christian Disease

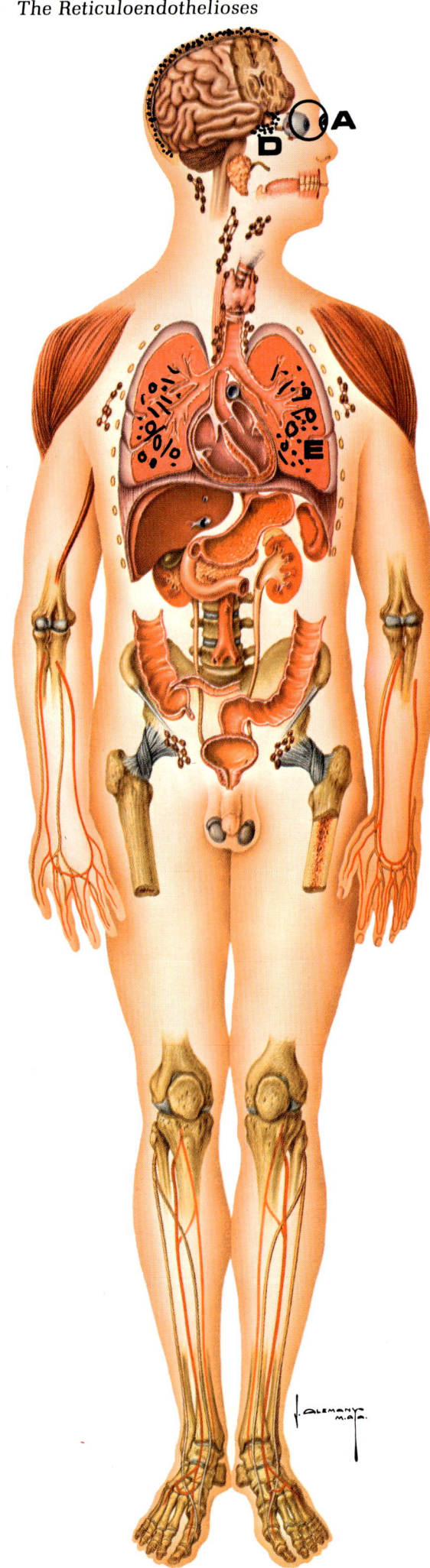

A 14-year-old white male complained of severe thirst and frequency of urination.

Physical examination revealed dehydration, bilateral exophthalmos (A), a maculopapular rash of the trunk and extremities (B), and soft-tissue nodules of the scalp (C).

Laboratory examination showed a 24-hour urine volume of 10,000 ml. and specific gravity of 1.003. The Hickey-Hare test was positive.

X-ray examination of the skull revealed numerous round and oval lytic lesions, particularly in the area of the sella turcica (D).

Bone biopsy revealed the characteristic cholesterol-laden histiocytes of this disease.

Treatment. Corticosteroids and x-ray therapy were of some benefit.

Differential Diagnosis:
1. Pituitary adenoma
2. Tuberculum sellae meningioma
3. Craniopharyngioma
4. Metastatic carcinoma
5. Tuberculosis

Clinical Note. The classic triad of this disease, diabetes insipidus, exophthalmos, and osteolytic lesions of the skull, is due to disease at one point—in and about the sella turcica. It is not well-known that involvement of the visceral organs may occur, particularly in the lungs. The lungs show both reticular and nodular infiltration and polycytic areas (E) on x-ray, and there may be severe alveolar-capillary block and emphysema terminally. In this more benign histiocytosis anemia and thrombocytopenia are uncommon. Neurologic involvement is almost unknown. In contrast to Gaucher's disease and Niemann-Pick disease, this is not a hereditary disorder.

Pathology. The lipid within the reticuloendothelial cells is cholesterol. There may be a granulomatous reaction, as indicated by the presence of eosinophils and giant cells.

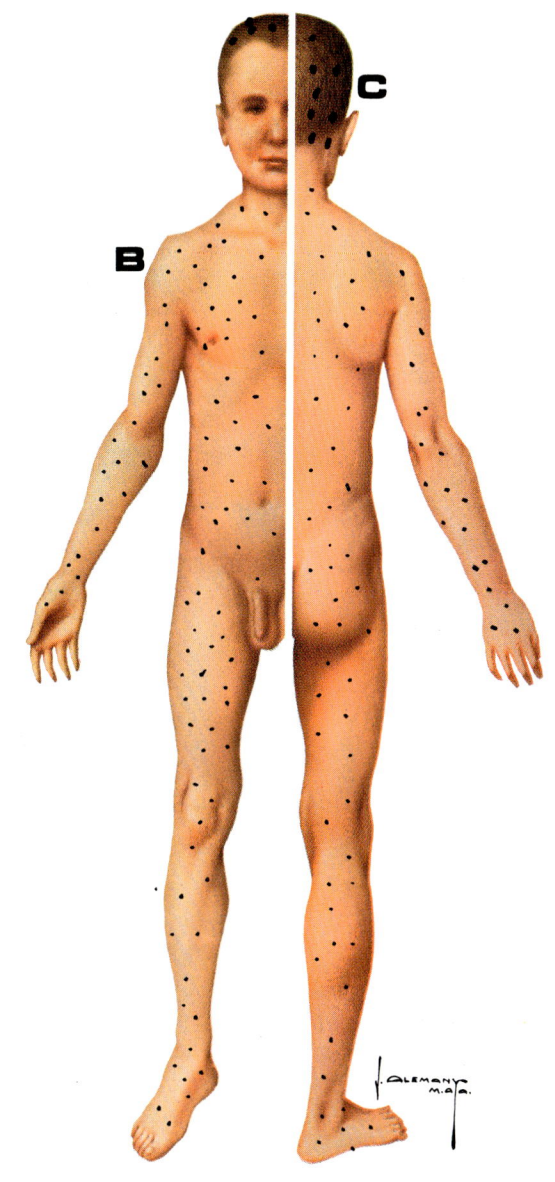

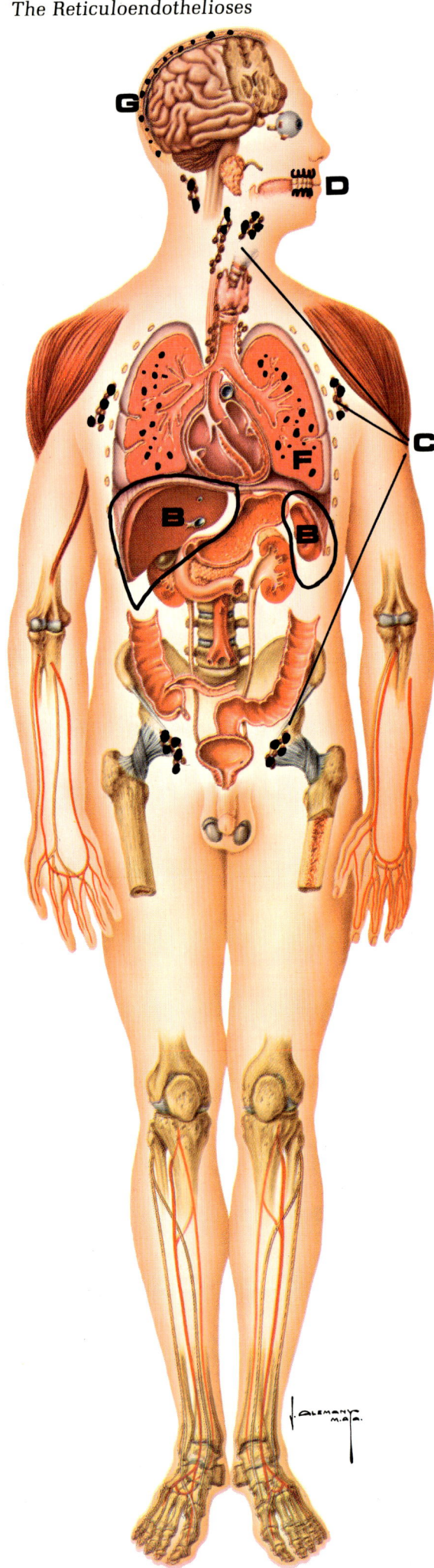

Histiocytosis X: Letterer-Siwe Disease

A 22-year-old white male was admitted to the hospital because of generalized erythematous purpuric rash (A) and fever.

Physical examination revealed, in addition to the rash, hepatosplenomegaly (B), lymphadenopathy (C), hyperplasia of the gums (D), and ulcers of the mouth (E).

Laboratory examination revealed a pancytopenia with normoblasts in the peripheral blood. Bone marrow and lymph node biopsy helped to establish the diagnosis.

X-ray examination revealed diffuse nodular infiltration of the lungs (F) and osteolytic lesions of the skull (G).

Treatment with corticosteroids gave some dramatic improvement for a short time.

Differential Diagnosis:
1. Gaucher's disease of infancy
2. Niemann-Pick disease
3. Acute leukemia
4. Miliary tuberculosis
5. Von Gierke's disease
6. Galactosemia
7. Amyloidosis
8. Idiopathic thrombocytopenia purpura
9. Kala-azar

Clinical Note. Here again is a disease with almost the identical organ infiltration of Niemann-Pick disease except that there are no nervous system involvements. The presentation of severe rash, often with purpura and fever, is more consistent with Letterer-Siwe disease. Also the involvement of the skull should suggest Letterer-Siwe. Bone marrow examination reveals here no foam cells laden with sphingomyelin but merely reticulum cell hyperplasia.

Pathology. There is a histiocytic infiltration in many visceral organs, but these histiocytes do not contain cholesterol or other lipids.

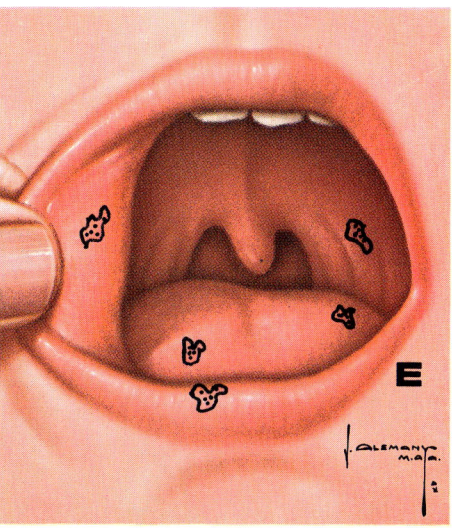

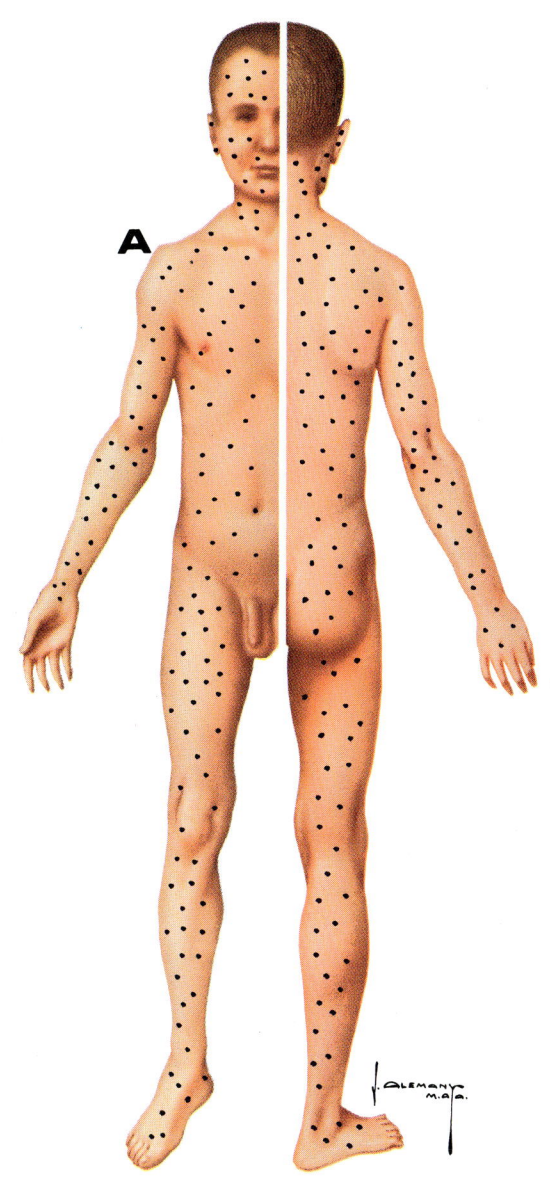

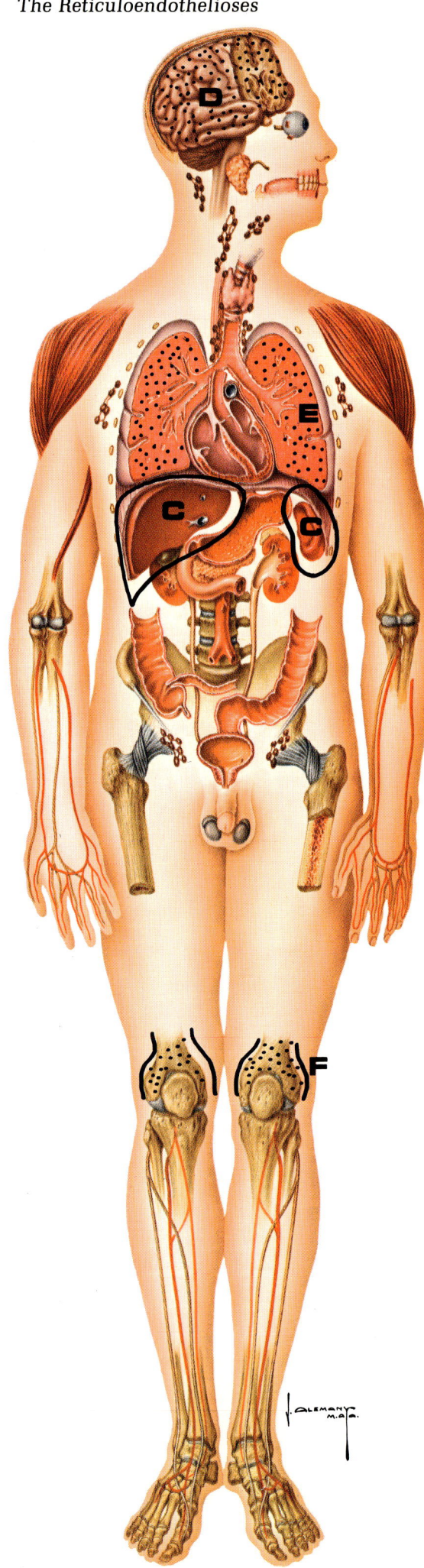

Niemann-Pick Disease

A 15-month-old white male was brought for evaluation because of both physical and mental retardation.

Physical examination revealed cherry-red spots of both maculae (A), yellow skin with eruptive xanthomas (B), and hepatosplenomegaly (C). The child could not walk or sit up alone, could not talk, and failed to show much spontaneity. All these signs indicated involvement of the central nervous system (D).

Laboratory examination revealed slight anemia and thrombocytopenia, but liver function tests were normal. *Bone marrow examination* revealed foam-laden reticuloendothelial cells which contained a large amount of *sphingomyelin*.

X-ray examination revealed diffuse fine nodular infiltrates throughout both lung fields (E) and diffuse demineralization and widening of the metaphysis of the distal femurs bilaterally (F).

Differential Diagnosis:
1. Gaucher's disease of infancy
2. Letterer-Siwe disease
3. Leukemia, acute
4. Von Gierke's disease

5. Galactosemia
6. Amyloidosis
7. Mediterranean anemia
8. Malabsorption syndrome
9. Kala-azar
10. Amaurotic familial idiocy
11. Miliary tuberculosis

Clinical Note. Here we have a disease with hepatosplenomegaly associated with central nervous system and lung involvement. Miliary tuberculosis may cause this. Boeck's sarcoid can cause this combination of involvement, but usually occurs in adults and has a slower course. Von Gierke's disease may cause central nervous system involvement, but there is no splenomegaly. The cherry-red spot on both maculae may suggest amaurotic familial idiocy, but the latter is not associated with hepatosplenomegaly. Bone and lung involvement help to differentiate Niemann-Pick disease from the other conditions in the differential list. Although the bone marrow findings are similar to those in Gaucher's disease, the chemical determination of sphingomyelin pins down the diagnosis.

Pathology. The lipid-laden reticuloendothelial cells may be found anywhere in the body. The lipid may also accumulate in the parenchymal cells of many organs. In the nervous system there is patchy destruction of ganglion cells and demyelinization.

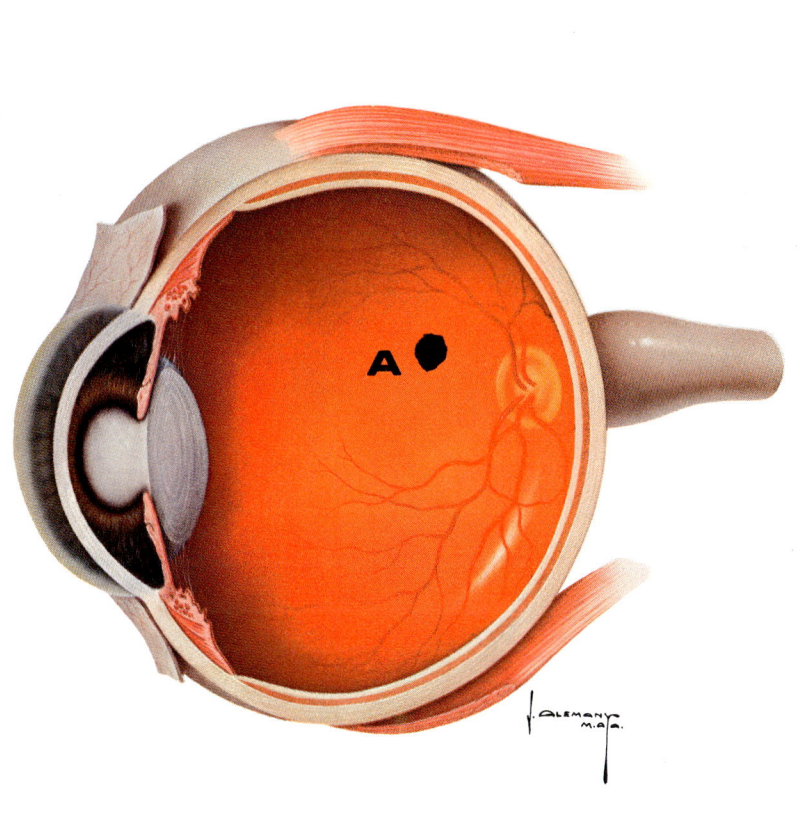
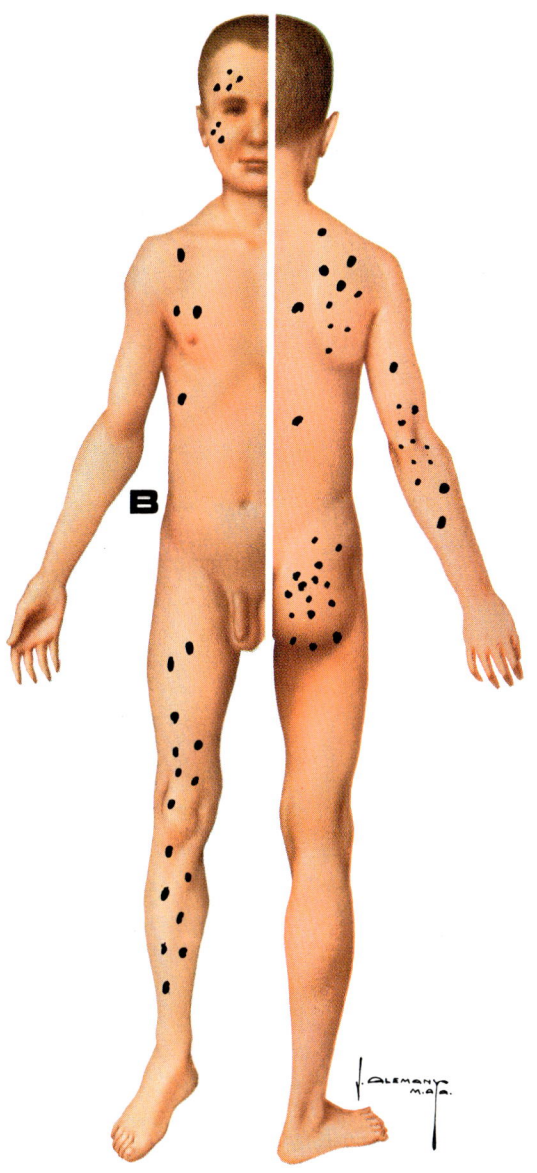

Chapter 12

Toxic Diseases

Physicians should maintain a high index of suspicion for these disorders because they are common, they are treatable, and in some cases our drugs are responsible for them. An occupational history is more essential than ever today. Environmental pollution, a major political issue today, will have to be faced head on by the medical profession. Just what effects chronic exposure to such chemicals as carbon monoxide has on our bodies remains to be determined.

Most of the diseases listed here typically affect certain specific organs. The blood, liver, and nervous system are the organs most commonly affected by toxins. The diagnosis is usually determined by the history, but confirmation by the laboratory is possible in most cases.

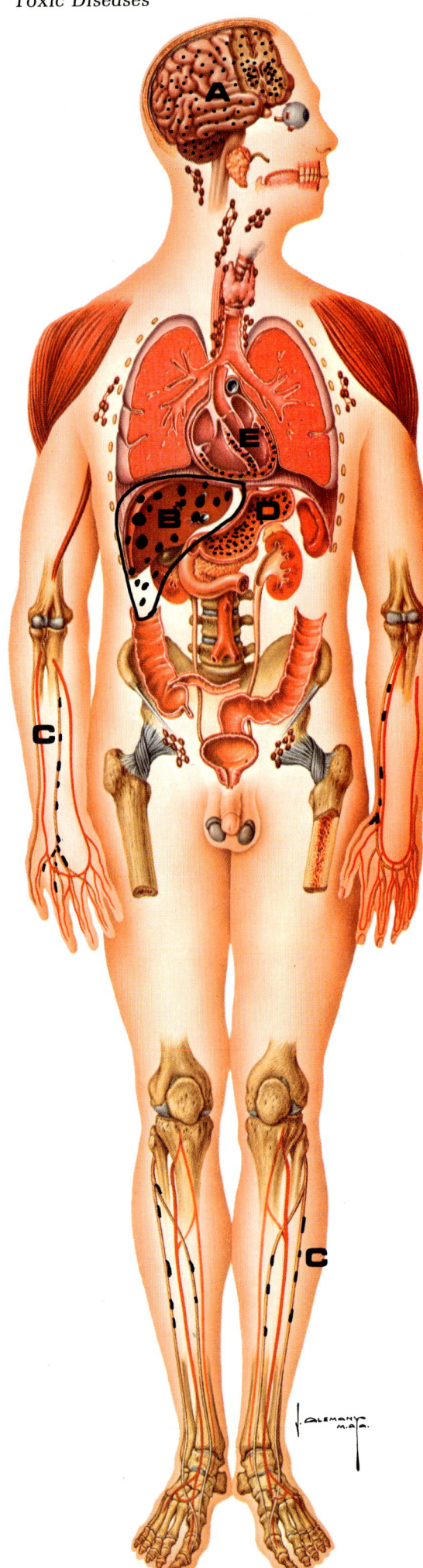

Alcoholism

A 39-year-old white male known alcoholic sustained a grand mal convulsion and was brought to the emergency room in a confused state.

Physical examination revealed a stuporous, disoriented white male with tremor and dyskinesia of all 4 extremities, indicating central nervous system involvement (A), and hepatomegaly (B) with jaundice. Neurologic examination a few days later also revealed evidence of a peripheral neuropathy (C).

Laboratory examination revealed a bilirubin of 4.8 mg. per cent, about half of which was the indirect type; an elevated transaminase, alkaline phosphatase, and prothrombin time; and a low serum albumin.

Treatment with vitamins, tranquilizers, and anticonvulsants was effective.

Differential Diagnosis:
1. Porphyria
2. Lead intoxication
3. Digitalis intoxication
4. Uremia
5. Insulin shock
6. Pellagra
7. Pernicious anemia
8. Leptospirosis
9. Wilson's disease
10. Phenothiazine intoxication
11. Carbon tetrachloride poisoning
12. Infectious mononucleosis
13. Salicylate intoxication

Clinical Note. Here again note the marked similarity to porphyria, lead intoxication, and phenothiazine toxicity. What looks like a "drunk" may not always be a "drunk." The central and peripheral nervous system is involved as well as the liver. In acute intoxication a severe hemorrhagic gastritis (D) develops. An alcoholic myocardopathy (E) has also been described. Although the organic mental syndrome induced by acute alcoholic intoxication is transient, permanent damage to the brain develops from repeated use of alcohol in large quantities. Delirium tremens develops from abstinence from alcohol and is transient. Methyl alcohol causes a similar *disturbance* but frequently affects the optic nerves, resulting in blindness.

Pathology. There are fatty infiltration and cirrhotic changes in the liver. The brain shows midbrain, subarachnoid, and subdural hemorrhages and patchy gliosis throughout. The peripheral nerves show axonal degeneration in various stages, with loss of myelin sheaths. The gastric mucosa becomes congested and inflamed.

Hypokalemia

A 64-year-old white male cardiac complained of increasing depression, irritability, muscle weakness, and abdominal pain.

Physical examination revealed a pulse rate of 48/min., hypoactive reflexes on all 4 extremities, indicating neuromuscular involvement (A), and distended abdomen with hypoactive bowel sounds (B).

Laboratory examination revealed a serum potassium of 2.2 mEq./L. An EKG showed a prolonged QT interval, inverted T-waves, and depressed ST segments in most leads, indicating myocardial involvement (C).

Treatment with an intravenous infusion of potassium brought about immediate relief of symptoms.

Differential Diagnosis:
1. Porphyria
2. Diabetic acidosis
3. Uremia
4. Pellagra
5. Digitalis intoxication
6. Alcoholism
7. Periarteritis nodosa
8. Trichinosis
9. Syphilis
10. Malabsorption syndrome
11. Pernicious anemia
12. Hypothyroidism
13. Adrenal insufficiency
14. Hyperthyroidism
15. Familial periodic paralysis

Clinical Note. The involvement of the central and peripheral nervous system, muscle, heart, and intestinal tract presented here is quite typical. In addition, there may be renal tubular degeneration (D) and a reduced glucose tolerance. Hypopotassemia may develop from prolonged use of diuretics, as in this case, as well as from chronic diarrhea and vomiting, celiac disease, renal tubular acidosis, aldosteronism, and pyelonephritis.

Pathology. The muscle may show Zenker's waxy degeneration, myocardial necrosis, and vacuolation of the epithelial cells of the proximal convoluted tubules.

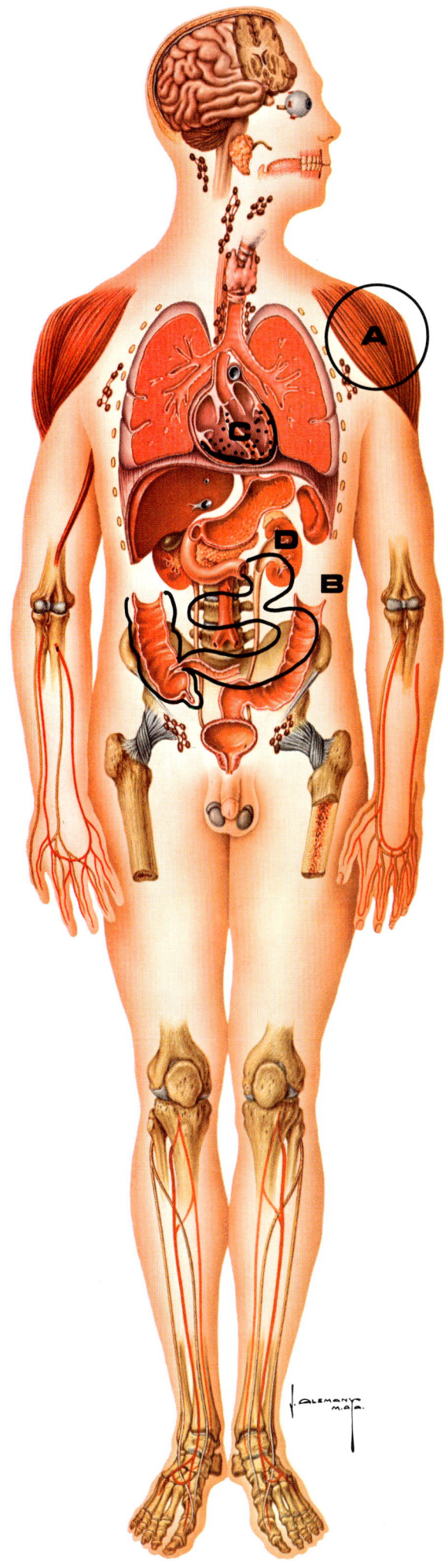

270 · Toxic Diseases

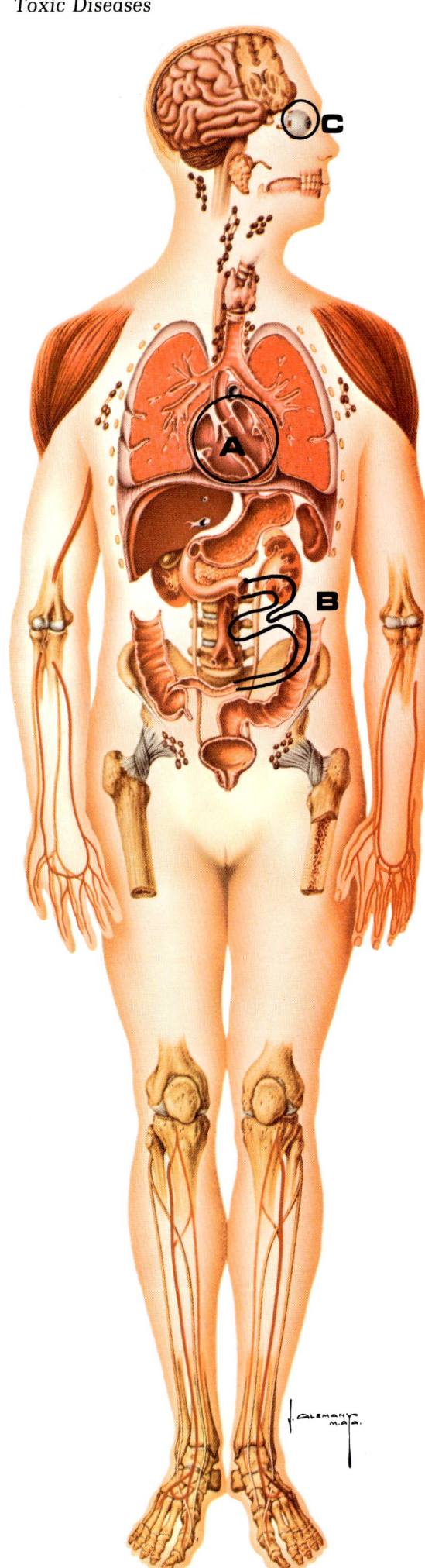

Digitalis Intoxication

A 54-year-old white female known cardiac complained of intermittent nausea and vomiting, headaches and fatigue, and blurred vision for some time. Objects had at times appeared green. On the day of admission she developed an irregular heart beat.

Physical examination revealed bigeminal rhythm (A) and a generalized abdominal tenderness, indicating intestinal involvement (B).

Laboratory examination revealed a BUN of 44 mg. per cent and a creatinine of 3.2 mg. per cent.

Treatment with the rapid infusion of potassium chloride eliminated the extrasystoles.

Differential Diagnosis:
1. Hypertensive encephalopathy
2. Uremia
3. Hypopotassemia
4. Aspirin intoxication
5. Alcoholism
6. Pellagra
7. Porphyria
8. Lead intoxication
9. Chagas' disease
10. Periarteritis nodosa
11. Rheumatic fever
12. Sickle cell anemia
13. Leukemia
14. Hyperthyroidism

Clinical Note. This case illustrates that increasing renal failure, which is common in cardiacs, may precipitate digitalis intoxication without any alteration in the dose. Diuretics which lead to hypokalemia may do the same. The effects of digitalis on the nervous system, gastrointestinal tract, eyes (C), and heart are illustrated by this history.

Pathology. Large doses of digitalis given intravenously have produced myocardial infarction and hemorrhage in animals.

Phenothiazine Intoxication

A 24-year-old white female schizophrenic complained of sudden onset of yellow skin and eyes, and dark urine.

Physical examination revealed icteric sclera (A), jaundiced skin, hepatomegaly (B), and tremor and cogwheel rigidity of the extremities, indicating involvement of the basal ganglia (C).

Laboratory examination revealed a bilirubin of 10.8 mg. per cent, most of which was of the indirect type, a serum transaminase of 120 units (5-40 units was normal), and a high alkaline phosphatase. Liver biopsy was helpful in diagnosis.

Treatment with Cogentin intravenously relieved the tremor and rigidity, and the jaundice gradually subsided after withholding chlorpromazine therapy.

Differential Diagnosis:
1. Cirrhosis of the liver
2. Wilson's disease
3. Hyperthyroidism
4. Porphyria
5. Carbon tetrachloride poisoning
6. Metastatic carcinoma
7. Leptospirosis
8. Infectious mononucleosis
9. Obstructive jaundice of other causes
10. Infectious hepatitis
11. Pernicious anemia
12. Alcoholism

Clinical Note. Involvement of the liver and the extrapyramidal system is common in this disorder, but the two do not usually occur together. Often the central nervous system involvement is much more severe, with extreme tremor and rigidity and opisthotonus. Spasmodic torticollis and other tics may occur. The immediate relief of extrapyramidal symptoms after administering Cogentin is a useful diagnostic test. Relief of jaundice after a course of corticosteroids is likewise helpful in differentiating this disorder from other causes of obstructive jaundice. Phenothiazines may also cause orthostatic hypotension and convulsive seizures.

Pathology. Microscopically, the liver shows dilated bile canaliculi with bile plugs, bile-stained parenchymal cells, and periportal mononuclear and eosinophilic reaction. Occasionally, there is centrilobular necrosis of the liver cells. Sections of the brain are unremarkable.

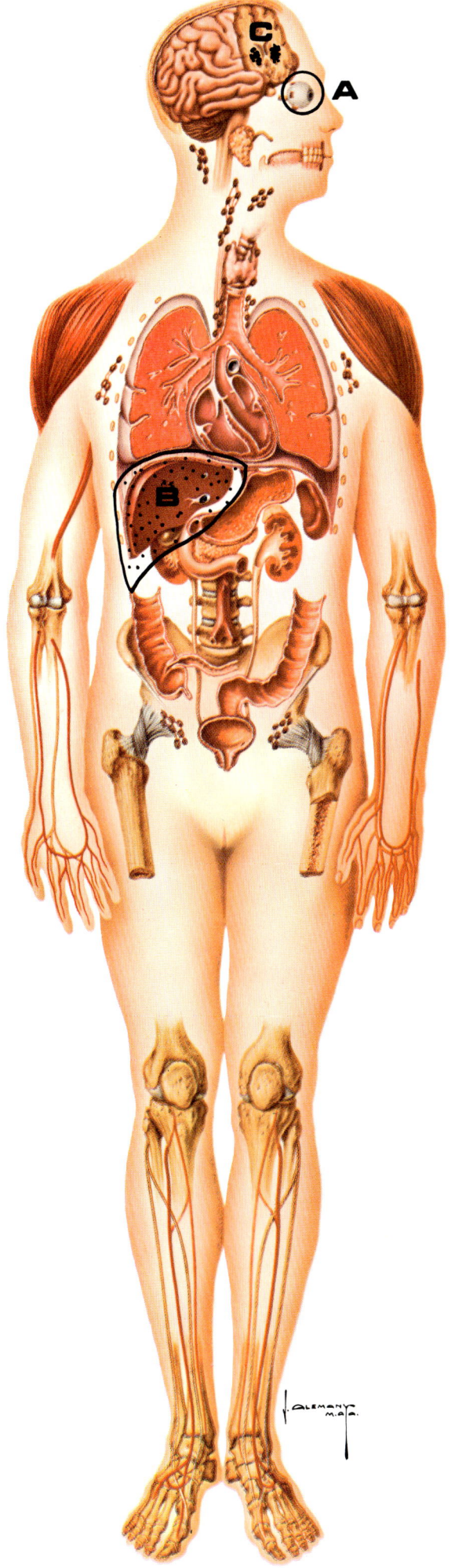

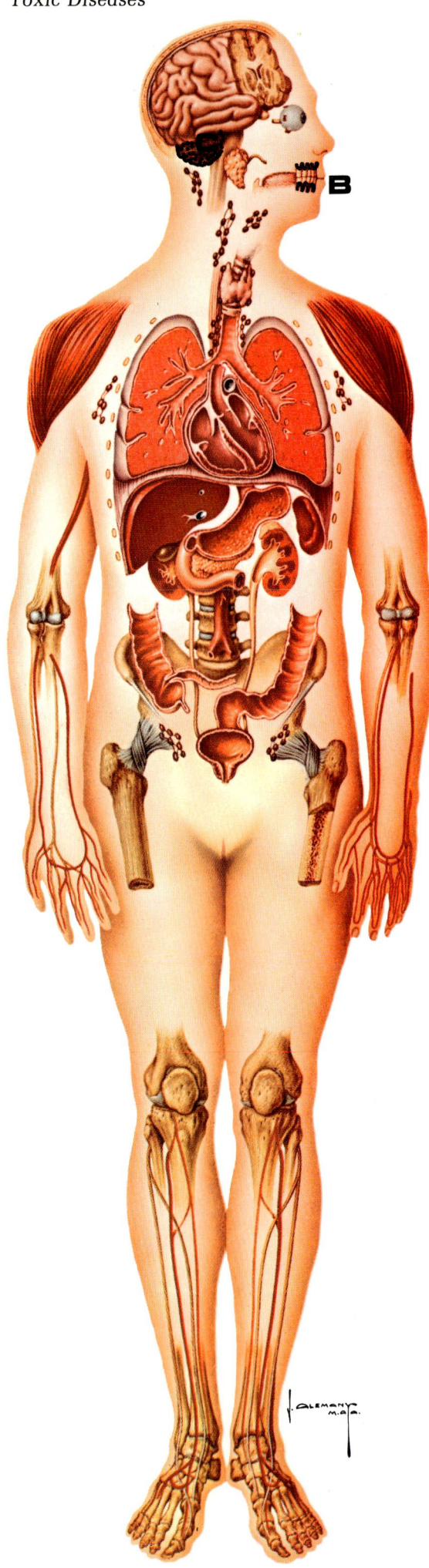

Dilantin Intoxication

A 29-year-old white female epileptic complained of increasing incoordination and dizziness since her dose of Dilantin had been increased.

Physical examination revealed acne of the face and upper thorax (A), hypertrophy of the gums (B), and bilateral horizontal nystagmus and ataxic gait as evidence of cerebellar involvement (C).

Laboratory examination was unremarkable.

Differential Diagnosis:
1. Friedreich's ataxia
2. Cerebellar tumor
3. Tuberous sclerosis
4. Lupus erythematosus
5. Syphilis
6. Serum sickness
7. Leukemia
8. Hodgkin's disease
9. Tuberculosis
10. Cushing's syndrome
11. Diabetes mellitus
12. Pellagra
13. Scurvy

Pathology. The drug is believed to affect the Purkinje cells of the cerebellum and possibly the labyrinth.

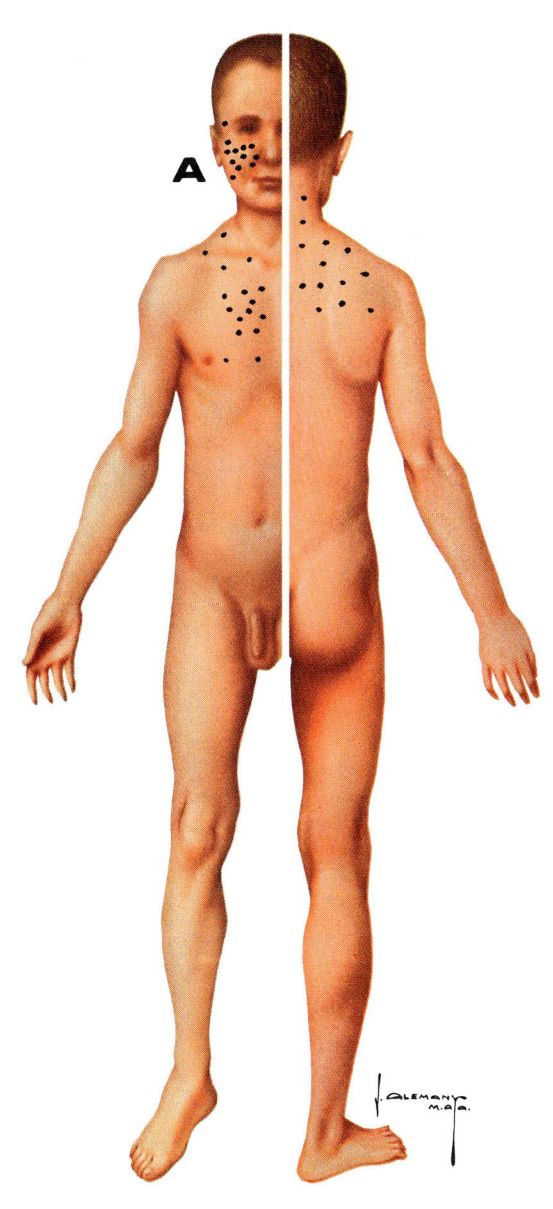

274 · Toxic Diseases

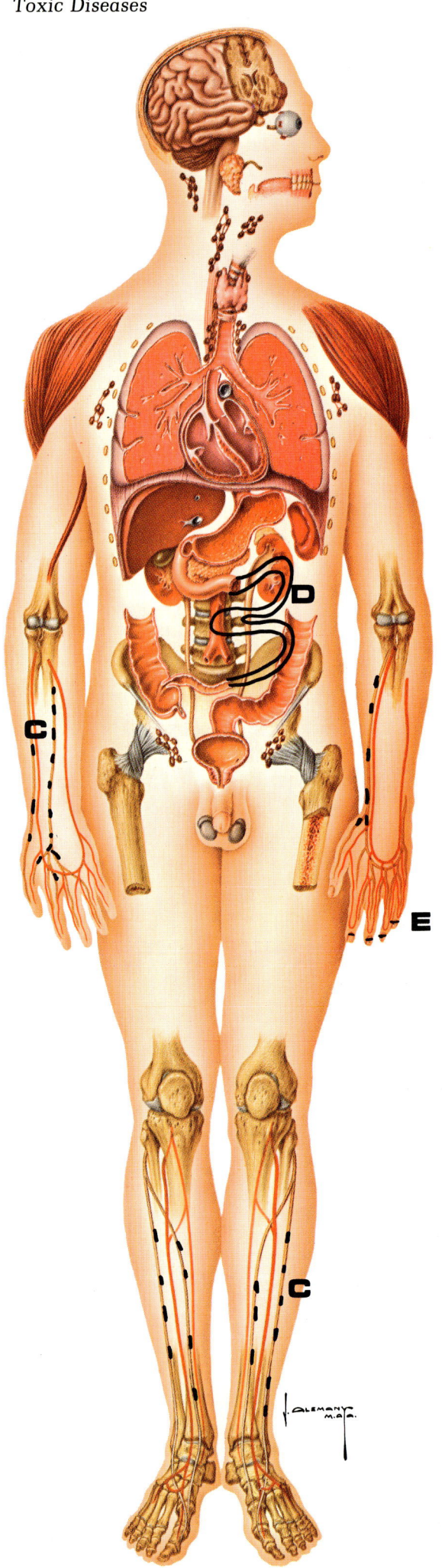

Arsenic Poisoning

A 32-year-old white male chemical factory worker complained of recurrent abdominal cramps and numbness and tingling in his hands and feet.

Physical examination revealed pigmentation and scaling of the skin (A), hyperkeratosis of the palms and soles (B), and glove and stocking hypesthesia and hypalgesia and weakness of dorsiflexion of the wrists and feet, as evidence of a peripheral neuropathy (C).

Laboratory examination revealed elevated arsenic content in the urine and hair samples.

Treatment with dimercaprol (BAL) was of some help.

Differential Diagnosis:
1. Lead poisoning
2. Periarteritis nodosa
3. Porphyria
4. Diabetes mellitus
5. Sickle cell anemia
6. Pellagra
7. Trichinosis
8. Alcoholic neuropathy
9. Serum sickness

Clinical Note. The skin, peripheral nerve, and gastrointestinal involvement (D) demonstrated here is typical and very suggestive of porphyria. Industrial exposure is now rare, and homicidal poisoning is declining in popularity. BAL is not useful in treatment of the chronic form of this disease as the damage usually is done. Half these cases have white transverse striae of the fingernails (Mees' stripes) (E).

Pathology. The peripheral nerves show myelin degeneration and swelling of the axis cylinders. Hyperkeratosis may undergo malignant changes.

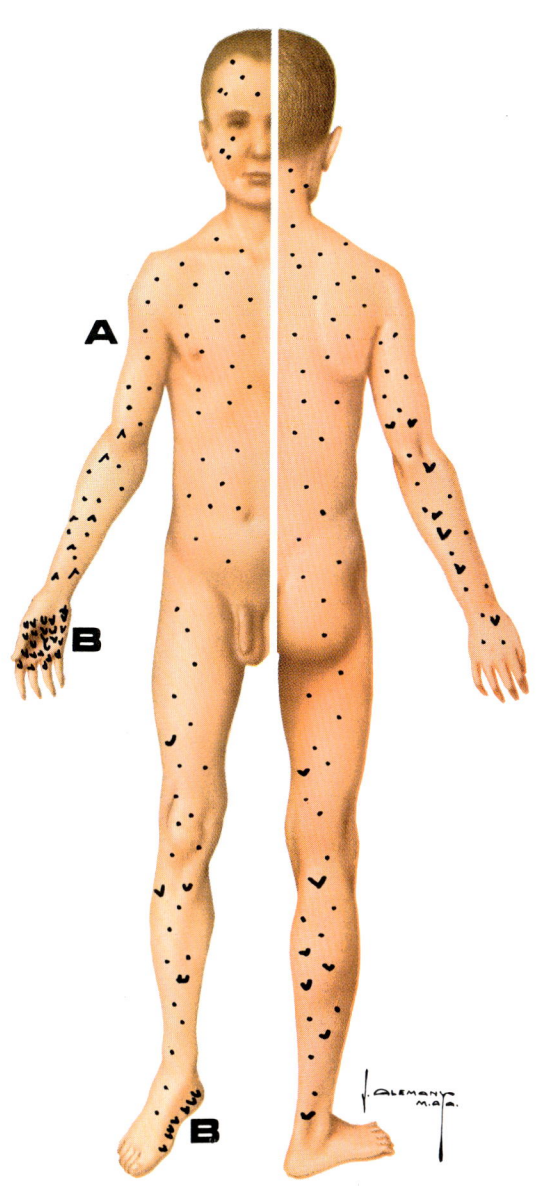

276 · Toxic Diseases

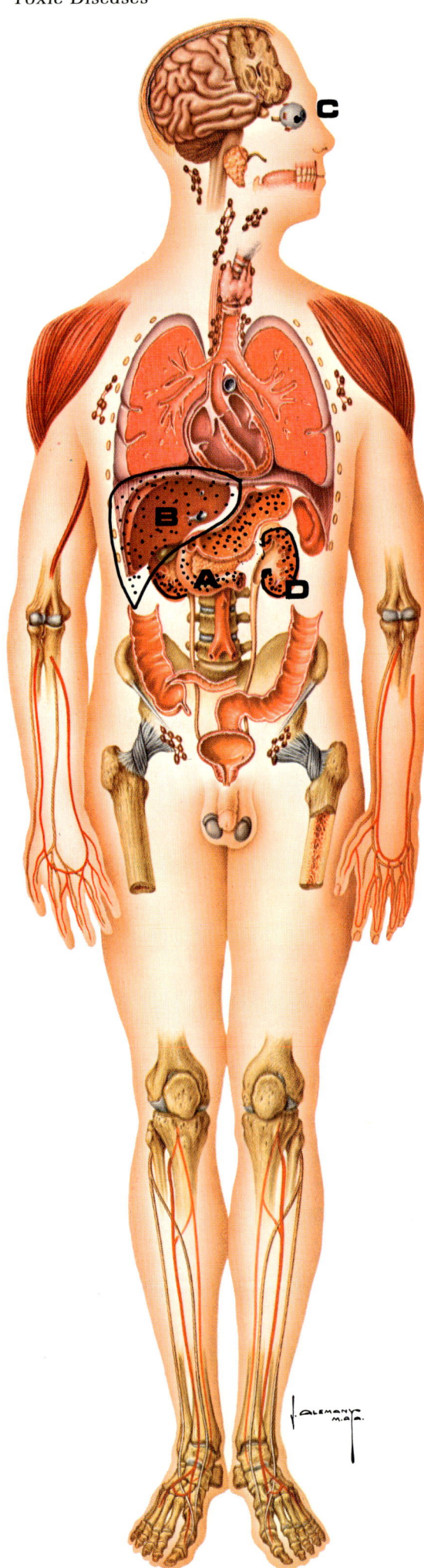

Carbon Tetrachloride Poisoning

A 4-year-old boy was brought to the emergency room with acute nausea and vomiting, indicating gastrointestinal involvement (A), and lethargy. His mother had discovered that a bottle of household cleaner had been opened that afternoon.

Physical examination revealed no significant findings other than the lethargy. Three days later, however, a *repeat physical examination* revealed jaundice, hepatomegaly (B), and a right subconjunctival hemorrhage (C). He also had oliguria, indicating renal involvement (D).

Laboratory examination revealed a serum bilirubin of 7.8 mg. per cent, with equal elevation of the indirect and direct bilirubin, increased urine urobilinogen, elevated transaminase and thymol turbidity, a BUN of 80 mg. per cent, and granular casts in the urine.

Treatment with renal dialysis allowed a complete recovery.

Differential Diagnosis:
1. Viral gastroenteritis
2. Acute appendicitis
3. Cholecystitis
4. Peptic ulcer

5. Infectious hepatitis
6. Leptospirosis
7. Sickle cell anemia
8. Metastatic carcinoma
9. Acute leukemia
10. Glycogen storage disease
11. Porphyria
12. Pellagra
13. Periarteritis nodosa
14. Acute glomerulonephritis
15. Yellow fever

Clinical Note. Since the onset of the hepatorenal syndrome is delayed, there may be no evidence of carbon tetrachloride ingestion when the patient presents, and a diagnosis of glomerulonephritis or infectious hepatitis is mistakenly made. It is sometimes difficult to get a history of carbon tetrachloride ingestion in suicidal adults. Small industries may have a significant amount of this chemical in the air, which may lead to milder symptoms. Note the similarity of the involvement to that in leptospirosis (p. 164).

Pathology. Microscopically the liver shows centrilobular necrosis and hemorrhage and associated mononuclear cell reaction. The proximal convoluted tubules of the kidney are involved initially with swelling, granularity, and vacuolation. Later the basement membranes of the glomeruli are thickened, and the tufts are congested.

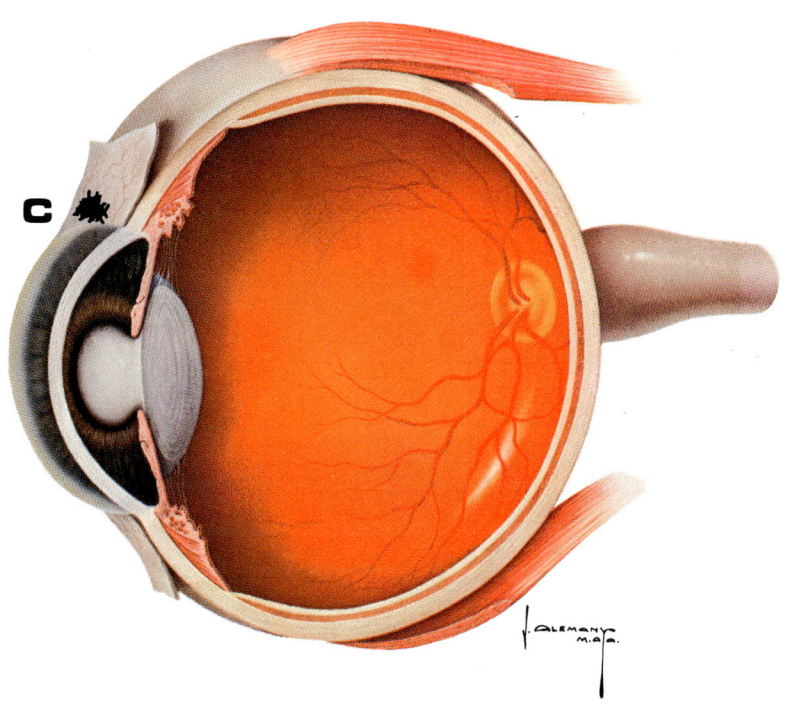

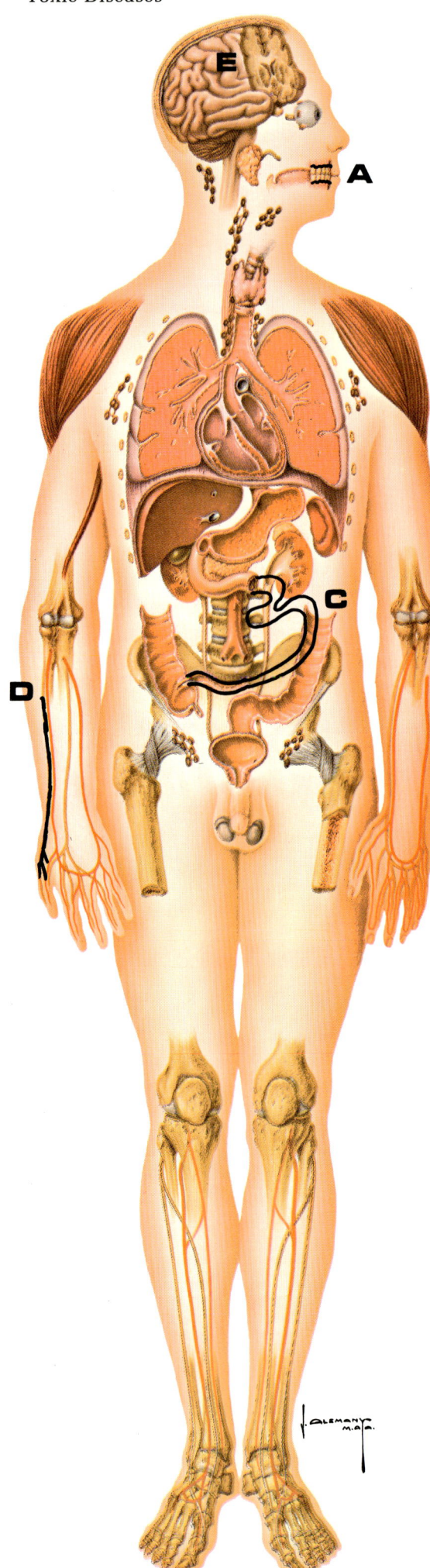

Lead Poisoning

A 36-year-old white male painter complained of colicky abdominal pain, episodic nausea and vomiting, and weakness and stiffness of his upper extremities for 2 weeks prior to admission. On the day of admission he developed a frank wristdrop of his right upper extremity.

Physical examination revealed a pale white male with a blue-black lead line on his gums (A), stippling of the retina adjacent to the optic disk (B), hyperactive bowel sounds, indicating involvement of the intestines (C), and a right wristdrop, indicating involvement of the right radial nerve (D). There was no significant sensory loss.

Laboratory examination revealed a normochromic, microcytic anemia with a basophilic stippling of the red cells, increased coproporphyrin in the urine, and a high blood lead level.

Treatment with calcium disodium edetate was effective.

Differential Diagnosis:
1. Porphyria
2. Periarteritis nodosa
3. Diabetic acidosis
4. Black widow spider bite
5. Arsenic poisoning
6. Serum sickness
7. Sickle cell anemia

8. Hyperthyroidism
9. Pellagra
10. Pernicious anemia
11. Poliomyelitis
12. Syphilis
13. Trichinosis
14. Uremia

Clinical Note. Lead may involve the central or peripheral nervous system, the gastrointestinal tract, or the blood. It is thus extremely similar clinically to porphyria, and there is some similarity to pernicious anemia and pellagra. An acute encephalitis (E) is seen almost exclusively in children, but it may be seen also in workers exposed to tetra-ethyl lead. It may present as coma, convulsions, or psychosis. There may be papilledema, causing confusion, with a brain tumor. When the blood levels of lead are equivocal, urine samples collected after giving calcium disodium edetate may show an increase in excretion of lead. Children may develop lead poisoning by eating white lead paint or from exposure to new water systems in which white lead was used in the joints of pipe. Industrial exposure to lead is rare nowadays because of good standards of environmental control.

Pathology. The lead may be deposited in the bones, liver, kidney, and bone marrow, but there is little cellular reaction. In lead encephalopathy, however, there is perivascular hemorrhage, cell necrosis, and in various parts of the brain the perivascular spaces may be filled with a serous exudate.

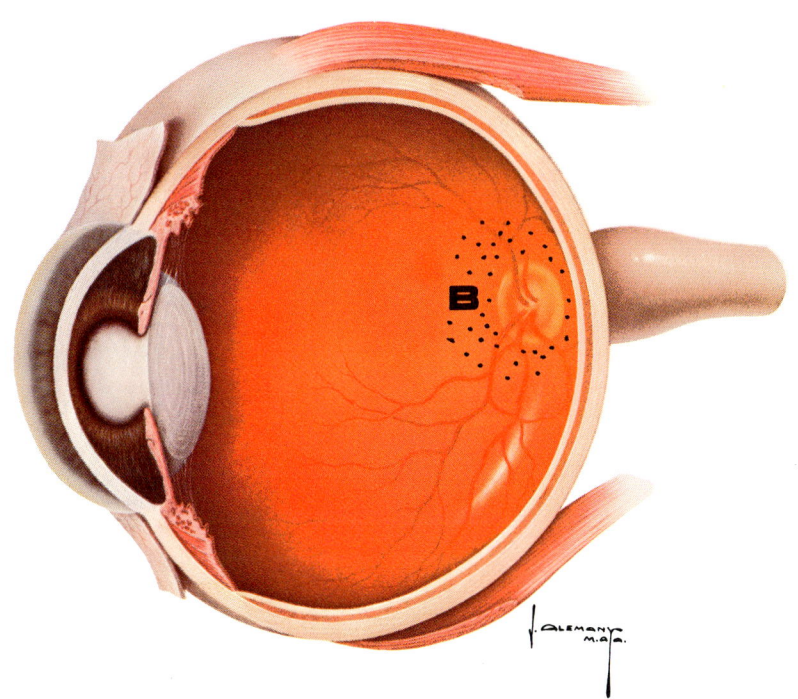

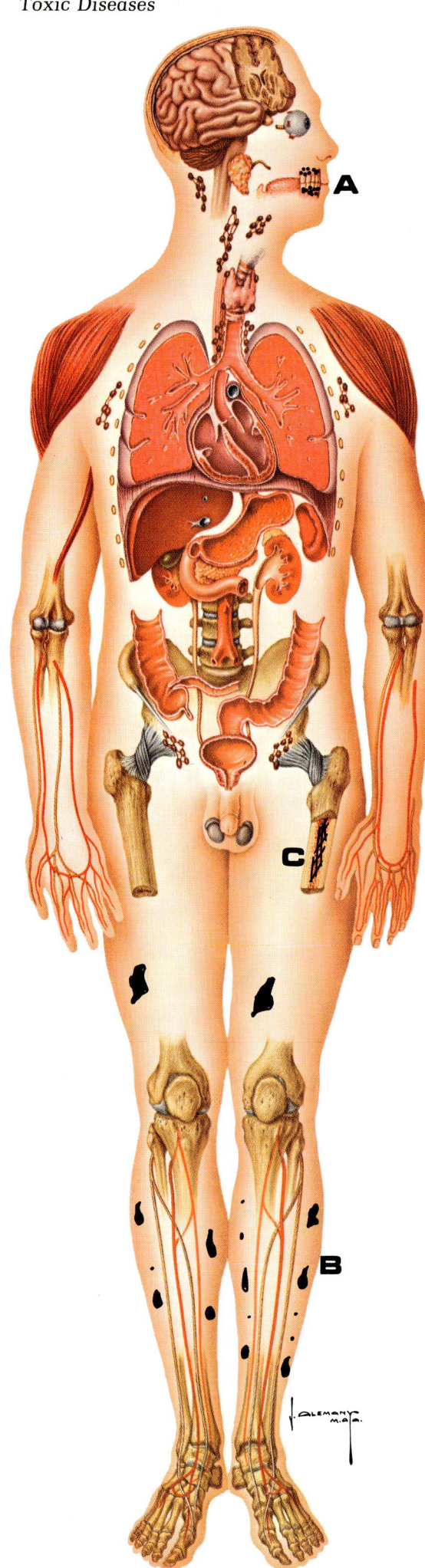

Benzene Poisoning

A 46-year-old white male laborer complained of frequent nosebleeds and bleeding gums.

Physical examination revealed that his gums bled readily (A), and there were a few ecchymoses of the legs and thighs (B).

Laboratory examination revealed a pancytopenia, and bone marrow examination revealed hypoplasia of all elements but an increased number of lymphocytes (C).

Investigation revealed toxic amounts of benzene vapor in the plant where he worked.

Differential Diagnosis:
1. Dicumarol intoxication
2. Hypersplenism
3. Chloromycetin ingestion
4. Idiopathic thrombocytopenic purpura
5. Lupus erythematosus
6. Thrombotic thrombocytopenic purpura
7. Aplastic anemia
8. Myeloid metaplasia
9. Leukemia
10. Osteopetrosis
11. Scurvy

Clinical Note. Although this disease affects only the blood-forming organs, it causes bleeding in various organs, and so it is classified as a systemic disease. Also it is a good example of the growing list of drugs (Chloromycetin, etc.) that are toxic to the bone marrow. Acute exposure, like exposure to many poisons, affects the central nervous system. It is important to get an occupational history on everyone, as occupational disorders are potentially curable.

Pathology. The major lesion is in the bone marrow, as described above; next in importance are hemorrhages in the skin and various organs. Here is one disease of the blood that is rarely associated with splenomegaly.

Chapter 13

Diseases of Unknown Etiology

These diseases have little in common except that the cause is unknown. Yet surprisingly many can be treated at least symptomatically. In diagnosing the disorders listed here, one must be very careful to rule out similar diseases with specific causes. For example, sarcoidosis should not be assumed unless tuberculosis has been definitely excluded—occasionally by even a therapeutic trial. Essential hypertension should not be diagnosed unless renal and adrenal causes of hypertension have been excluded. These diseases require long-term follow-up and observation for complications. In some cases the doctor "lives" with the disease.

Acrodynia

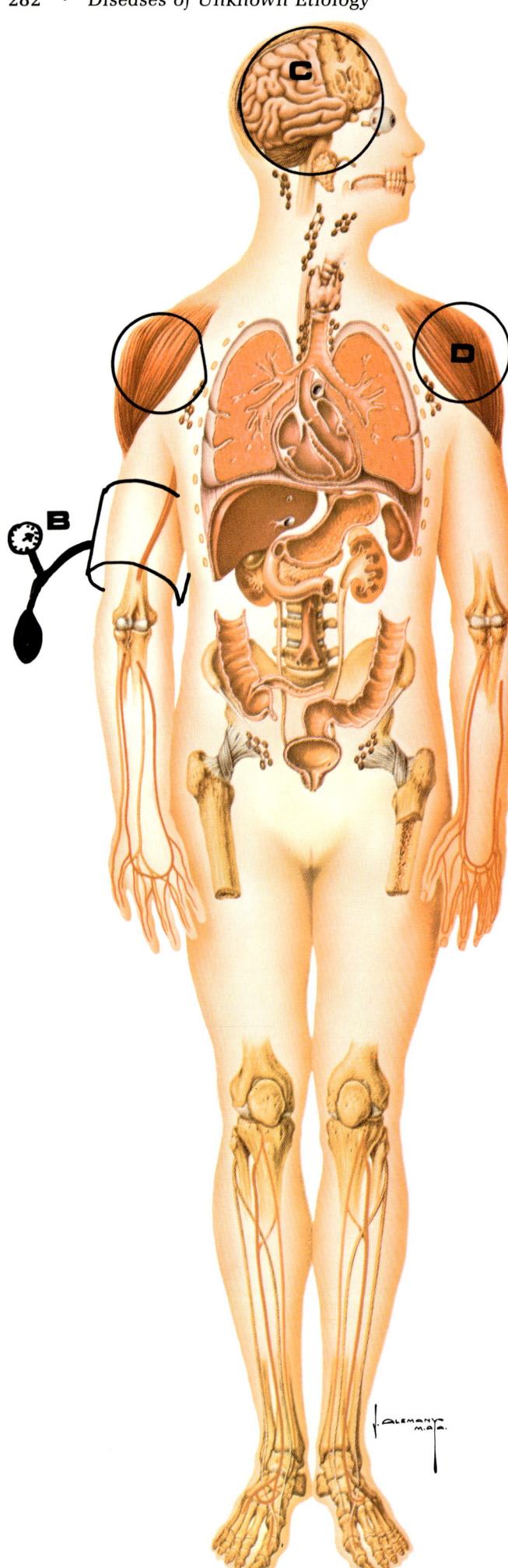

A mother complained that her 2-year-old female child salivated and perspired excessively and was becoming progressively more of an introvert. She also noted breaking of the nails and loss of hair (A).

Physical examination revealed hypertension (B), a shy child who would not communicate well (C), and generalized hypotonia (D).

Laboratory examination was unremarkable. The child improved spontaneously in a few months.

Differential Diagnosis:
1. Lead poisoning
2. Sprue
3. Toxoplasmosis
4. Schilder's disease
5. Pellagra
6. Kwashiorkor
7. Familial dysautonomia
8. Tay-Sachs disease

Clinical Note. This is a rare cause of failure to thrive, but it must be considered if only for the good prognosis. Some of these infants have excessive output of mercury in the urine, but just what role this plays in the etiology is undetermined.

Pathology. Indefinite.

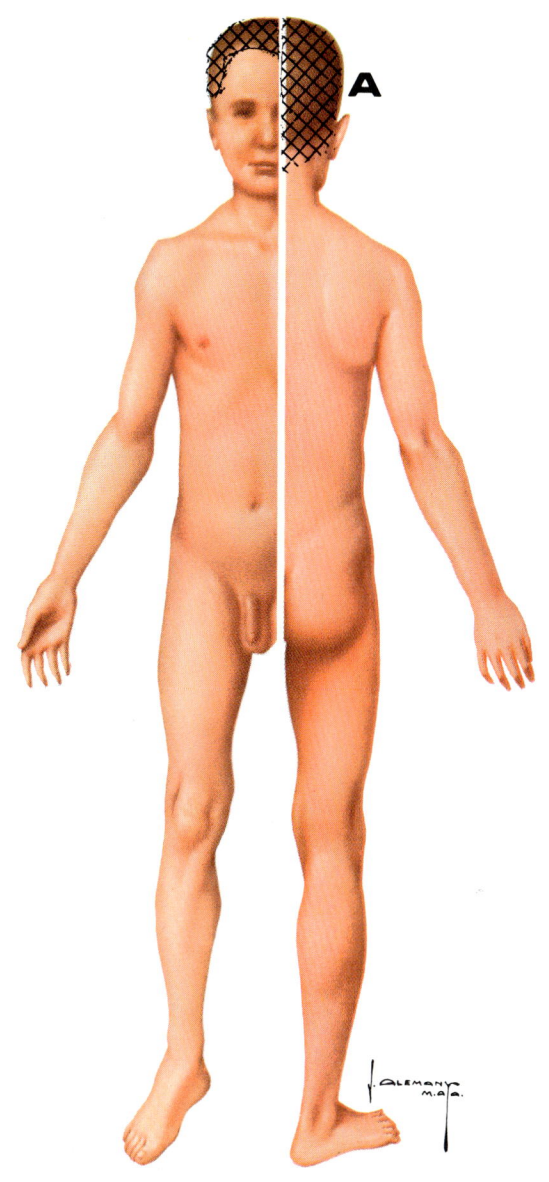

Diseases of Unknown Etiology

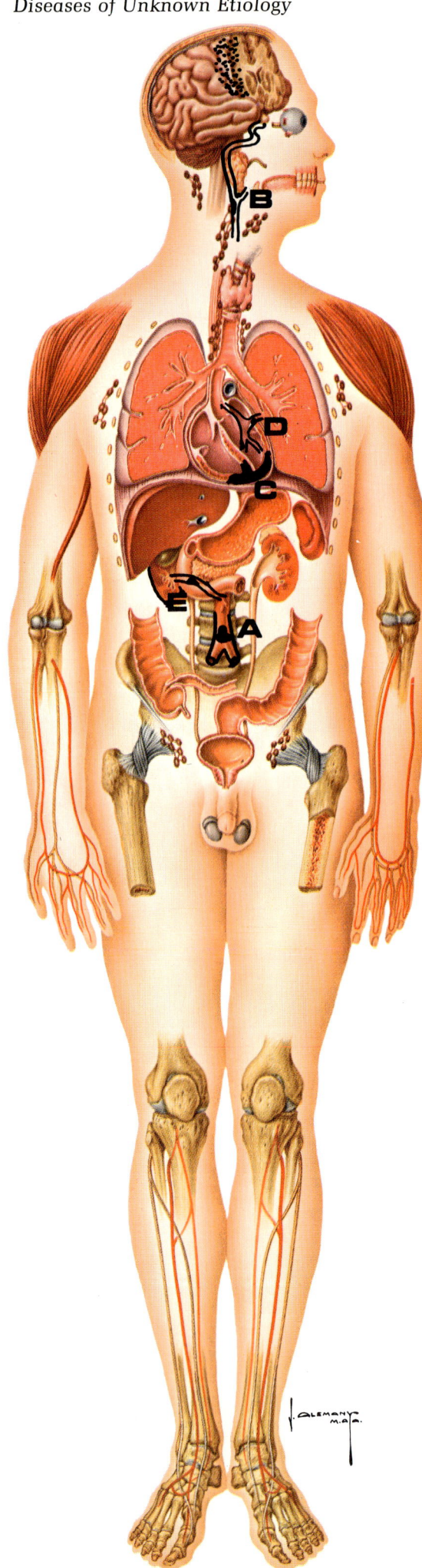

Atherosclerosis

The following cases illustrate a few of the various ways in which this systemic disease may present.

1. A 49-year-old white male gave an 8-month history of numbness in both legs, precipitated invariably by walking 1 or 2 blocks. He also had noted impotence.

Physical examination revealed diminished femoral, popliteal, dorsalis pedis, and tibialis pulses bilaterally and bilateral femoral bruits. An *aortogram* revealed a large atheromatous plaque at the terminal aorta (A).

2. A 63-year-old white female was admitted to the hospital in a comatose state.

Physical examination revealed a right central facial palsy and a right hemiplegia. *Spinal fluid examination* was unremarkable. A *left carotid angiogram* revealed a large atheromatous plaque at the bifurcation of the left carotid artery (B).

3. A 46-year-old Negro male complained of severe left precordial pain.

Physical examination was unremarkable. An *EKG* revealed an inferior wall infarction (C). A *coronary angiogram* revealed a large plaque and thrombosis 1 cm. from the origin of the left circumflex coronary artery (D).

4. A 58-year-old white male complained of severe bitemporal and suboccipital headaches for several months. He had been normotensive 1 year previously.

Physical examination revealed a blood pressure of 220/140 mm. Hg in both arms. A *hypertensive intravenous pyelogram* revealed a delayed nephrogram and filling of the right renal pelvis. A *renal angiogram* revealed an intimal plaque of the right renal artery (E).

Clinical Note. These are the common methods of presentation. Aside from the above methods of presentation, atherosclerosis may manifest as acute popliteal artery thrombosis superimposed on an intimal plaque; a mesenteric infarct, secondary to superior mesenteric artery thrombosis superimposed on an intimal plaque of that vessel; and as plaques and thrombosis of other large vessels. Aortic and basilar artery aneurysms may develop and present characteristic clinical pictures. The unfortunate part is that most cases of atherosclerosis, even severe forms, are asymptomatic and therefore must go undiagnosed until something like this happens.

Pathology. Grossly, there are large and small yellow to white plaques throughout the large arteries. These may be ruptured, contain small and large hemorrhages, or be covered with old or recent thrombotic material. Rarely they may have bacterial vegetations on them. Microscopically the intima shows splitting of the elastic fibrils and destruction of the connective tissue. Lipoid droplets accumulate, and there is associated reaction with proliferation of a dense hyaline tissue on the surface. Calcium may deposit in the atheroma.

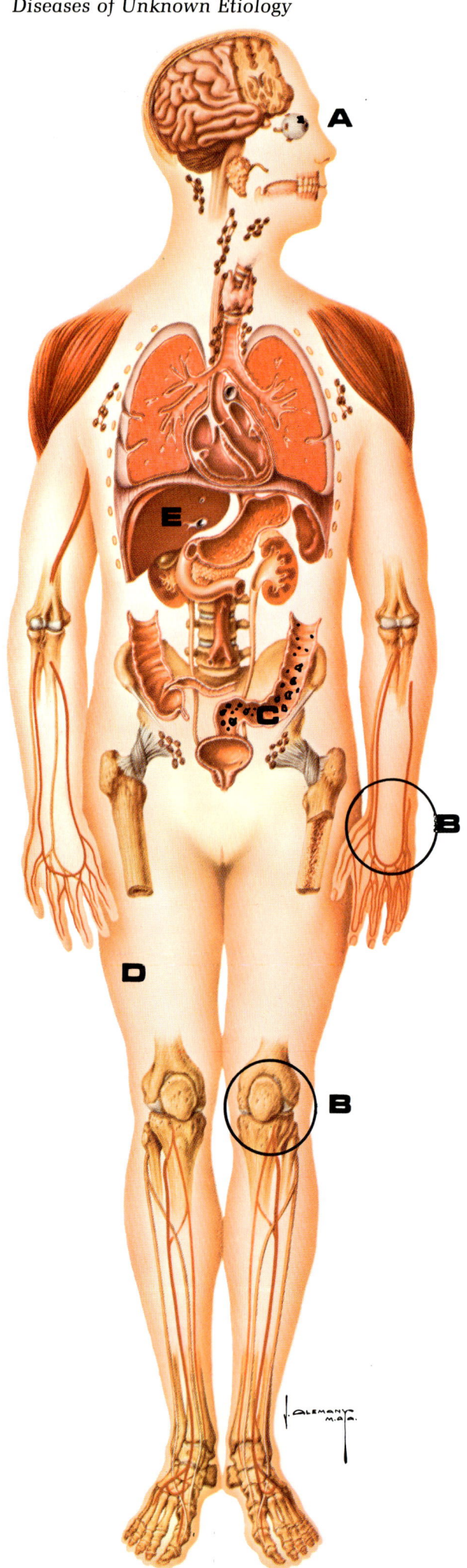

Ulcerative Colitis

A 25-year-old white female developed abdominal pain and diarrhea mixed with blood and mucus 10 days prior to admission. One day prior to admission she noted painful swollen wrists and left knee joint. She had had previous episodes of bloody diarrhea in the past 2 years. Six months prior to admission she had been treated for an episode of episcleritis (A).

Physical examination revealed swollen, tender wrists and left knee joint (B). The abdomen was distended, and there were hyperactive bowel sounds. A rectal examination revealed a loose stool with blood and mucus. At *sigmoidoscopy* petechial hemorrhages and multiple small ulcerations of the rectal mucosa were noted (C).

X-ray examination revealed loss of haustral markings and multiple small ulcerations of the descending colon and sigmoid.

Treatment with bed rest, a low-residue diet, and anticholinergics and Azulfidine was beneficial.

Differential Diagnosis:
1. Amoebic dysentery

2. Irritable colon
3. Diverticulitis
4. Salmonellosis
5. Shigellosis
6. Malabsorption syndrome
7. Carcinoid syndrome
8. Regional ileitis
9. Intestinal tuberculosis
10. Schistosomiasis
11. Lymphogranuloma venereum

Clinical Note. Fifteen per cent of these cases are associated with arthritis. Every patient with arthritis of unknown origin should have a barium enema. There may also be involvement of the skin (D), eye, and liver (E). The skin may be involved with erythema multiforme or pyoderma gangrenosum. In most cases there is fatty infiltration of the liver. To exclude bacillary dysentery and amoebiasis, stool cultures should be done on all cases and stools examined for ova and parasites.

Pathology. Mucosal inflammation and abscess formation at the base of the crypts of Lieberkühn lead to ulceration, perforation, and fistula formation. Later there are pseudopolyps produced by the hypertrophied mucosa between the extensive ulcerations. There may by strictures, and carcinoma of the colon develops in perhaps 10 per cent of these cases.

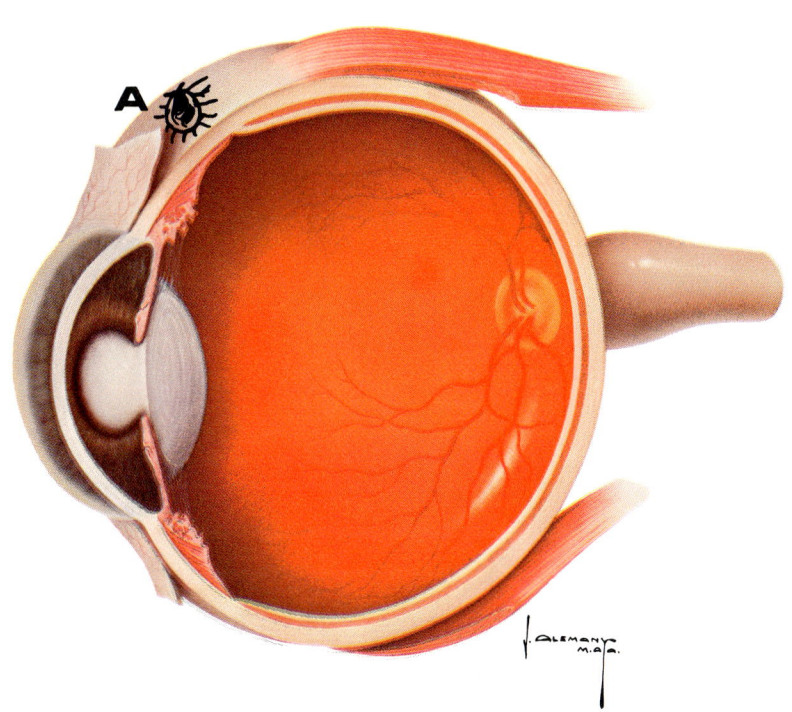

288 · *Diseases of Unknown Etiology*

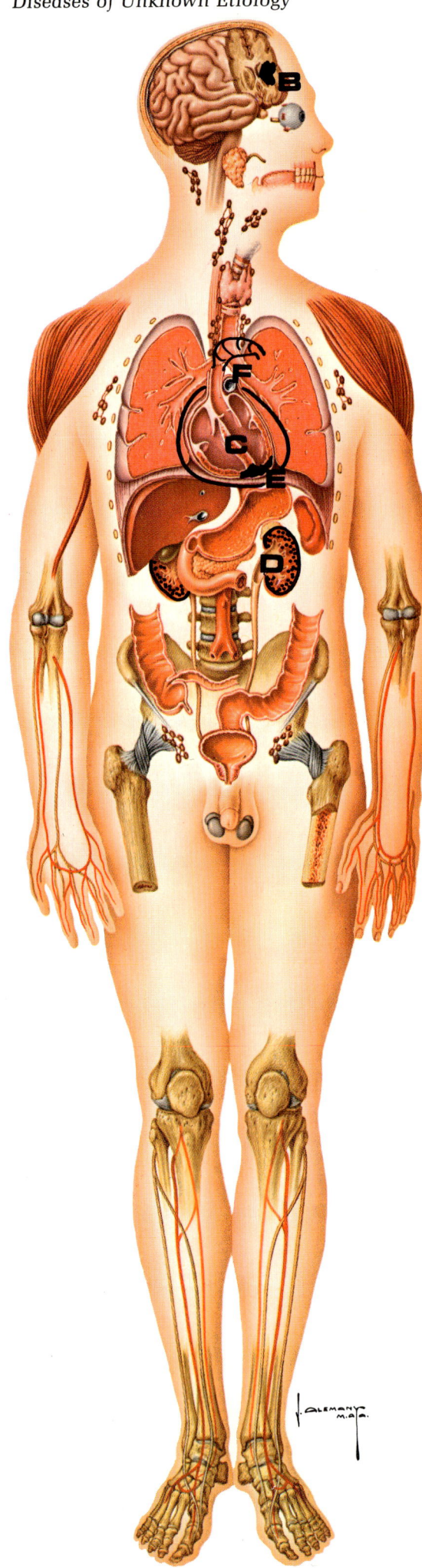

Essential Hypertension

A 56-year-old white male was brought to the emergency room in a semiconscious state. He had wakened the same day with severe headache and difficulty with his speech. He gradually became more lethargic and confused until admission.

Past history revealed that he had had hypertension for 5 years but no previous cardiovascular, renal, or central nervous system diseases. Family history revealed that his mother had hypertension.

Physical examination revealed a blood pressure of 220/110 mm. Hg, flame-shaped retinal hemorrhages, arteriovenous nicking in the eye grounds (A), nuchal rigidity, and left hemiparesis, indicating the cerebral hemorrhage (B) and cardiomegaly (C).

Laboratory examination revealed 3+ albuminuria, and waxy and red cell casts in the urine, indicating renal involvement (D). An EKG revealed left ventricular hypertrophy.

Treatment with reserpine and bed rest was unsuccessful, and the patient died.

Differential Diagnosis:
1. Meningitis
2. Ruptured cerebral aneurysm
3. Brain abscess
4. Pheochromocytoma
5. Cushing's syndrome
6. Aldosteronism, primary
7. Glomerulonephritis
8. Collagen diseases
9. Renal artery stenosis
10. Hypernephroma
11. Subacute bacterial endocarditis with cerebral embolism

Clinical Note. A complete hypertensive work-up, including an IVP, serial serum potassiums, and 24-hour urine catecholamines must be done to rule out most of the above conditions. In most cases of essential hypertension there are no or few symptoms or signs when the patient is first seen in the office. Eventually signs of eye, heart, and kidney involvement appear, as in this case. Headache is not as frequent as was once thought. Cerebral hemorrhages or thromboses develop in 10 per cent. Some present with a myocardial infarction (E). Twenty-five per cent or more eventually develop congestive heart failure. Hypertensive encephalopathy is another mode of presentation, particularly in malignant hypertension. So we see that both atherosclerosis and hypertension may present with several similar clinical pictures.

Pathology. There is arteriolar sclerosis in all the organs of the body, but particularly in the brain, eyes, heart, and kidney (arteriolar nephrosclerosis). In the severe forms there is arteriolar necrosis as well. Atherosclerosis is accelerated and accounts in some cases for the cerebral infarcts, myocardial infarcts, and aortic aneurysms (F). There may be cystic medial necrosis of the aorta, leading to a dissecting aneurysm.

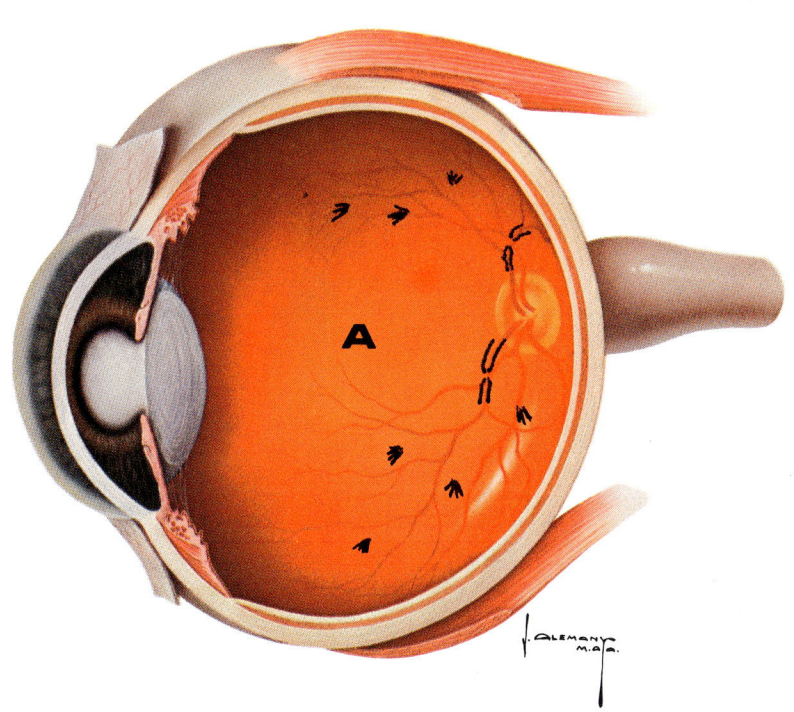

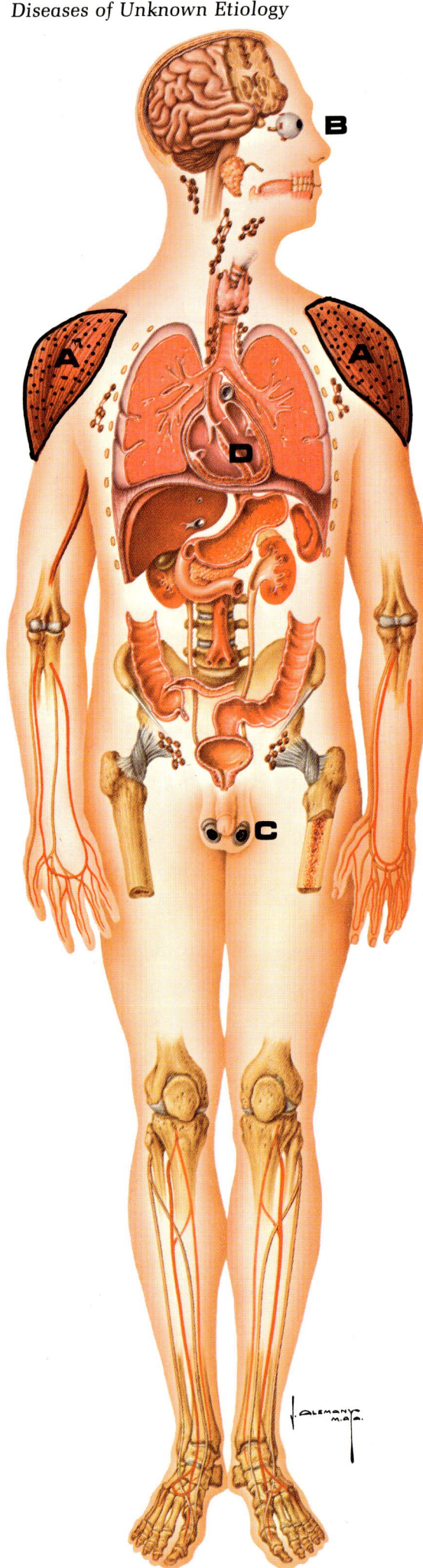

Myotonia Atrophica

A 32-year-old Puerto Rican male complained of increasing diffuse weakness in all 4 extremities for the past 3 years. He noted that his feet slapped and dragged when he walked. His father had been similarly afflicted.

Physical examination revealed atrophy of the facial, sternocleidomastoid, deltoid, and quadriceps femoris muscles bilaterally (A). There were bilateral cataracts (B), testicular atrophy (C), and loss of hair on the scalp. He had difficulty relaxing hand grip promptly (myotonia) and spasm of the tongue muscles on percussion.

Laboratory examination revealed a high urine creatine and low urine creatinine. Serum transaminase and LDH were elevated. *A muscle biopsy and electromyography* were diagnostic.

Differential Diagnosis:
1. Progressive muscular dystrophy
2. Amyotrophic lateral sclerosis
3. Progressive spinal muscular atrophy
4. Myasthenia gravis
5. Myotonia congenita
6. Laurence-Moon-Biedl syndrome

Clinical Note. Since this disorder is transmitted as an autosomal dominant gene, the family history is very important. It is differentiated from the common forms of muscle atrophy and muscular dystrophy by the systemic features (cataracts, etc.). However, both myotonia atrophica and progressive muscular dystrophy may involve heart muscle (D), leading to congestive heart failure; but this is more common in the former.

Pathology. Muscle fibers are of variable size, and there is increase in the numbers of sarcolemmal nuclei. Later the muscle is replaced by fat and fibrous tissue.

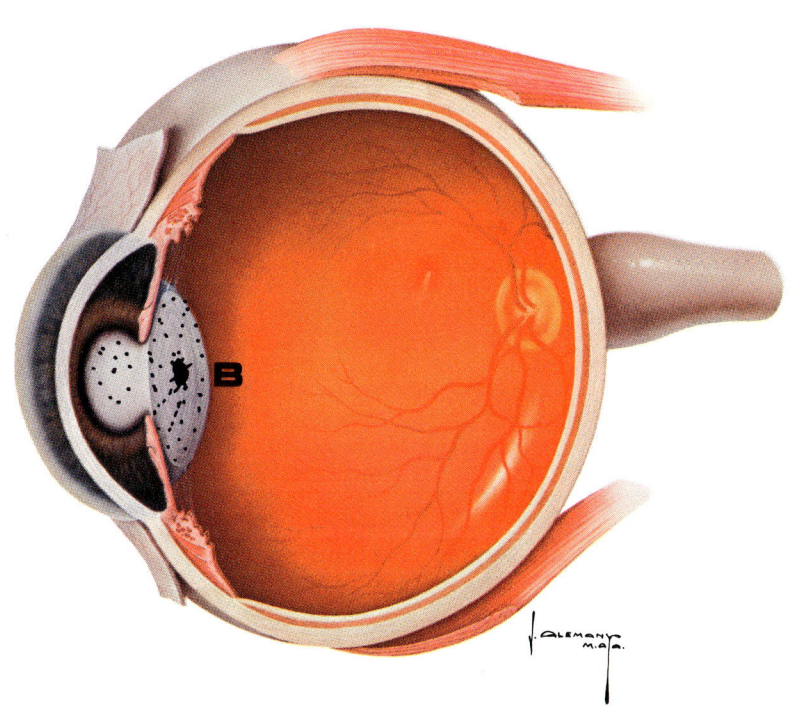

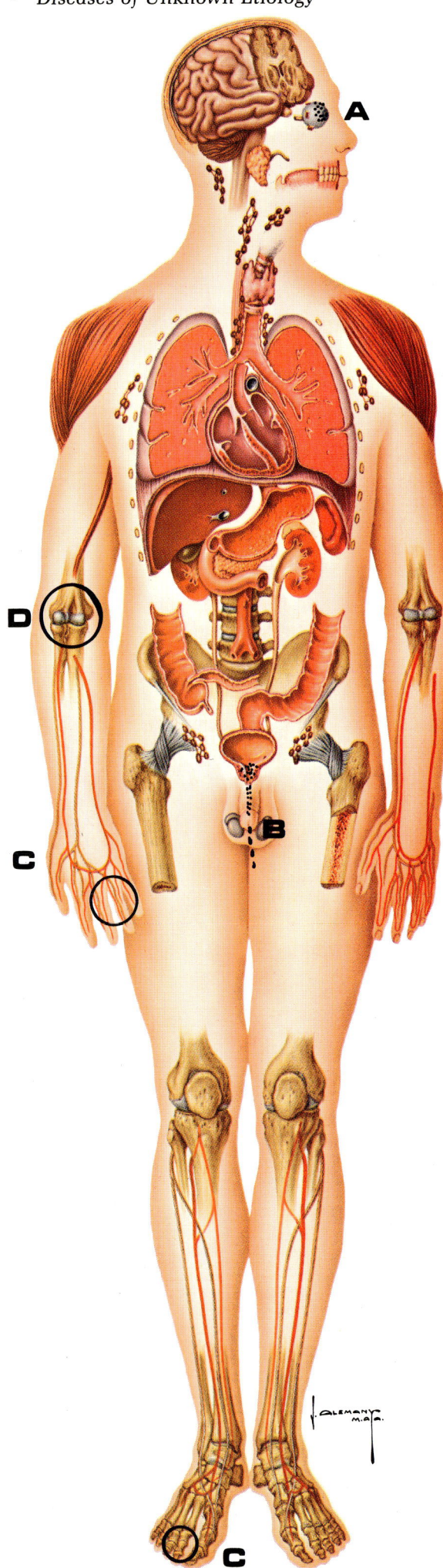

Reiter's Syndrome

A 21-year-old white seaman developed chills, fever, and swelling of the proximal interphalangeal joints of the right hand and the distal interphalangeal joints of the right foot 2 weeks prior to admission. Careful history revealed he had developed a urethral discharge 4 weeks prior to admission and an inflammation of the eyes 3 weeks prior to admission. He had had sexual intercourse 3 weeks prior to the onset of the urethral discharge.

Physical examination revealed bilateral injection of the conjunctiva (A); a serous urethral discharge (B); tender, swollen, and hot proximal interphalangeal joints of the 3rd and 4th fingers of the right hand and tender, swollen distal interphalangeal joints of the right 2nd and 3rd toes (C). The right elbow joint was also involved (D). There were a couple of moist ulcerations of the glans penis (balanitis circinata).

Laboratory examination revealed a rapid sedimentation rate but a negative latex flocculation test and a normal uric acid. Cultures of the urethral, conjunctival, and synovial fluid were negative for gonococcus.

X-rays of the joints were unremarkable.

Treatment with penicillin for 10 days failed to change the clinical picture, but a course of corticosteroids ameliorated all the symptoms.

Differential Diagnosis:
1. Gonorrhea
2. Gout
3. Rheumatoid arthritis
4. Lupus erythematosus
5. Ulcerative colitis
6. Rheumatic fever
7. Brucellosis
8. Haverhill fever
9. Serum sickness

Clinical Note. Since one often obtains a history of sexual exposure in these cases, it has been considered a venereal disease; but no infectious agent has been isolated. This case illustrates that most cases occur in young adult males. The history of urethritis, conjunctivitis, and arthritis is quite typical, and only gonorrhea can duplicate this picture. Since the gonococcus cannot easily be isolated from joints, differentiation can be very difficult at times. Less common manifestations of Reiter's syndrome include keratodermia blennorrhagica and heart block.

Pathology. The synovial membranes are involved with both acute and chronic inflammatory changes, including both neutrophilic and lymphocytic infiltration.

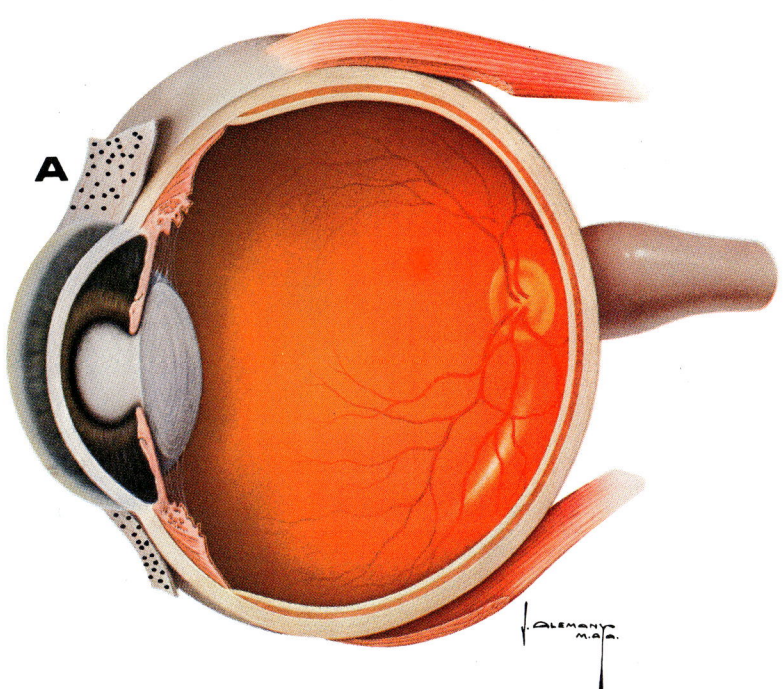

294 · *Diseases of Unknown Etiology*

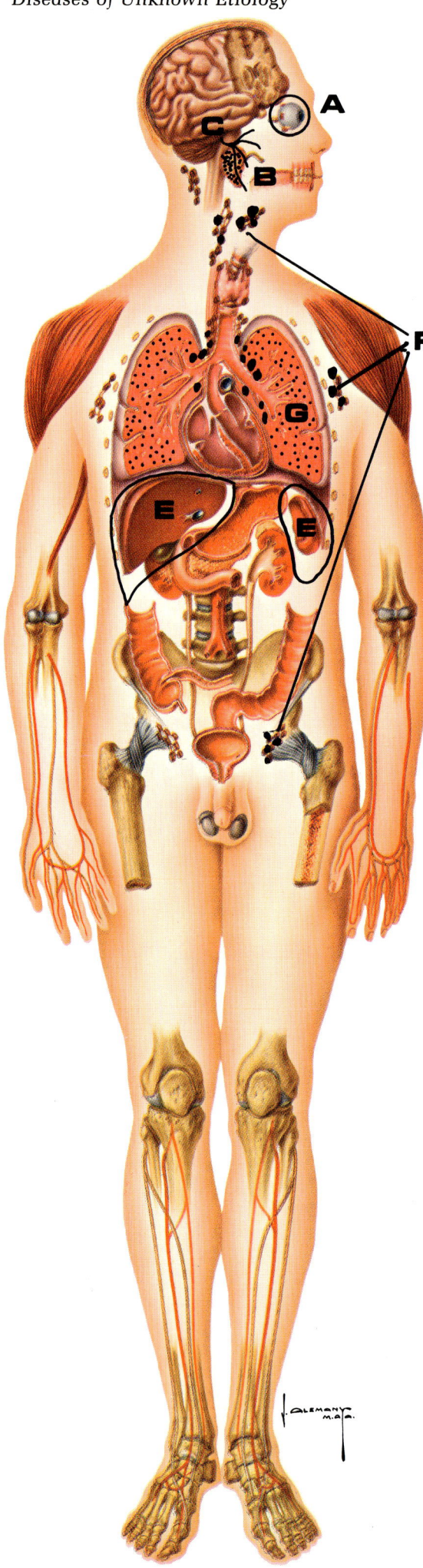

Sarcoidosis

A 37-year-old Negro male was admitted to the hospital because of increasing shortness of breath for 1 month. Two years previously he had had an attack of inflammation of both eyes (A), parotitis (B), and right Bell's palsy (C), which cleared spontaneously.

Physical examination revealed tachycardia, tachypnea, and absence of alveolar breathing throughout the lung fields, but only occasional sibilant rales. There was a polymorphic nodular eruption (D) of the face, shoulders, and extensor surfaces of the extremities. There were mild hepatosplenomegaly (E) and cervical, axillary, and inguinal lymphadenopathy (F).

Laboratory examination revealed a high serum gamma globulin, increased serum alkaline phosphatase, and calcium. Mantoux tests were repeatedly negative, but there was a positive Kveim test. Skin and lymph node biopsy confirmed the diagnosis.

X-ray examination of the chest revealed bilateral hilar adenopathy and diffuse miliary and nodular infiltrates throughout the lung fields (G). X-ray of the hands revealed lace-like and cystic radiolucencies of the phalanges. Corticosteroid therapy failed to produce a lasting remission.

Differential Diagnosis:
1. Tuberculosis
2. Histoplasmosis
3. Lymphoma
4. Hamon-Rich disease
5. Wegener's granulomatosis
6. Collagen disease
7. Berylliosis
8. Leukemia
9. Syphilis

Clinical Note. In few cases are patients as severely ill as this one on presentation. The onset of this disease is frequently asymptomatic; but in some European countries there may be an abrupt onset with fever, polyarthritis, erythema nodosum, and bilateral hilar adenopathy. The contrast of the tremendous involvement of many organs with few clinical symptoms is striking. If skin or lymph node biopsy is inappropriate, a liver biopsy will often be positive. Although Bell's palsy is the most frequent manifestation of nervous system involvement, there may be involvement of the pituitary and hypothalamus or the spinal cord. A variety of ophthalmic lesions, including episcleritis, vitreous opacities, and chorioretinitis, may occur; but iridocyclitis (present in this case) is the most common. The hypercalcemia may lead to nephrocalcinosis. Rarely, the heart and gastrointestinal tract are involved. Is it difficult to differentiate this from tuberculosis? Not if there are skin, salivary gland, small bone, and heart lesions, as these are rarely involved in tuberculosis.

Pathology. Microscopically the tubercles are composed of multinucleated giant cells surrounded by epithelioid histiocytes and only a few lymphocytes. The sparcity of lymphocytes and lack of caseation distinguish these lesions from tuberculosis.

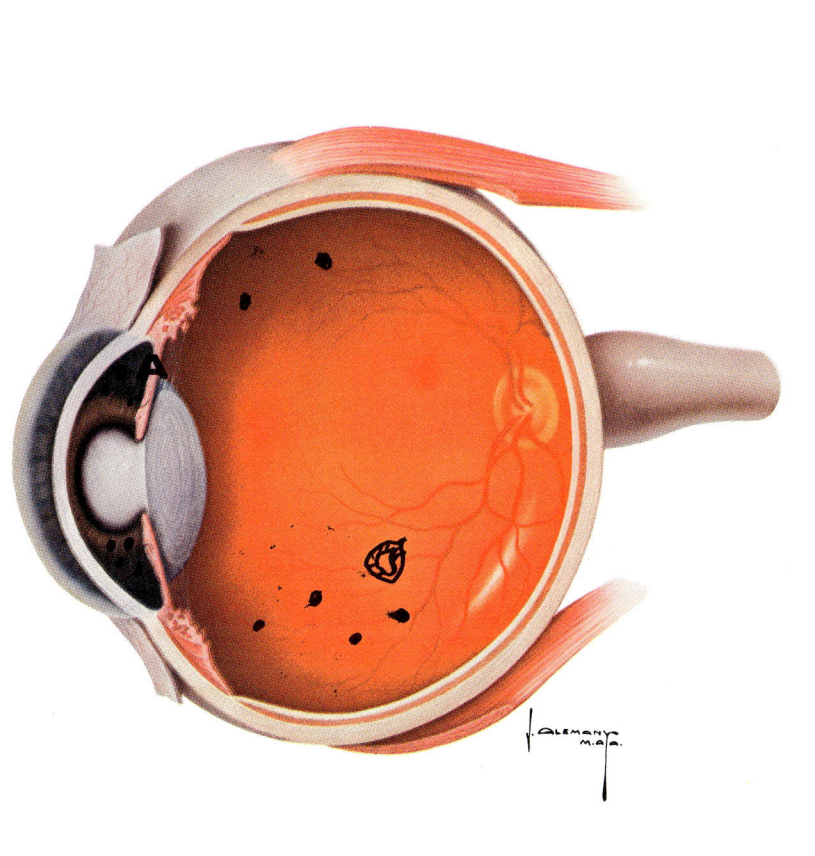

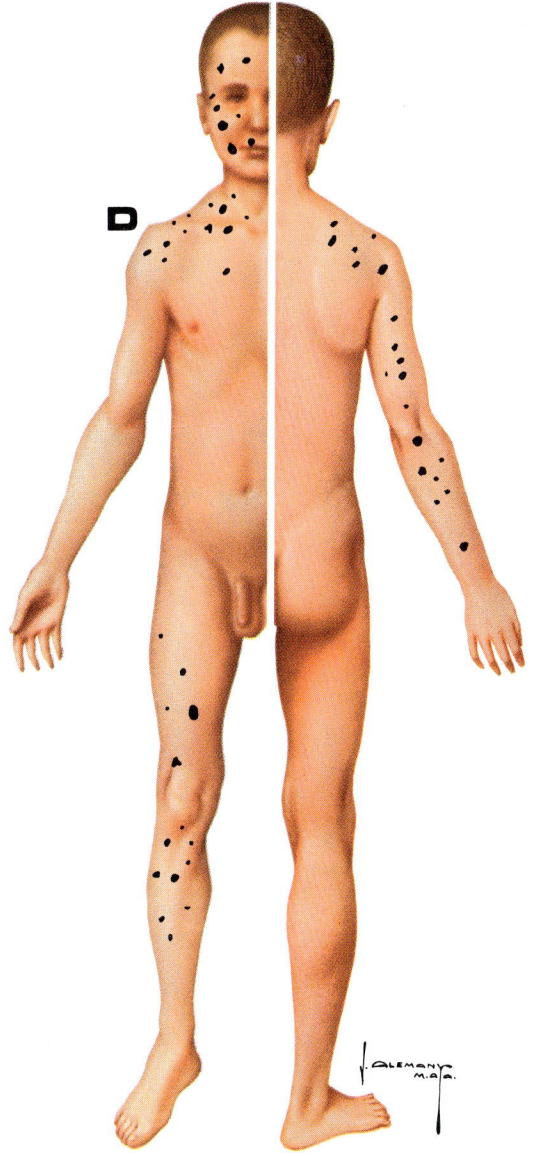

296 · *Diseases of Unknown Etiology*

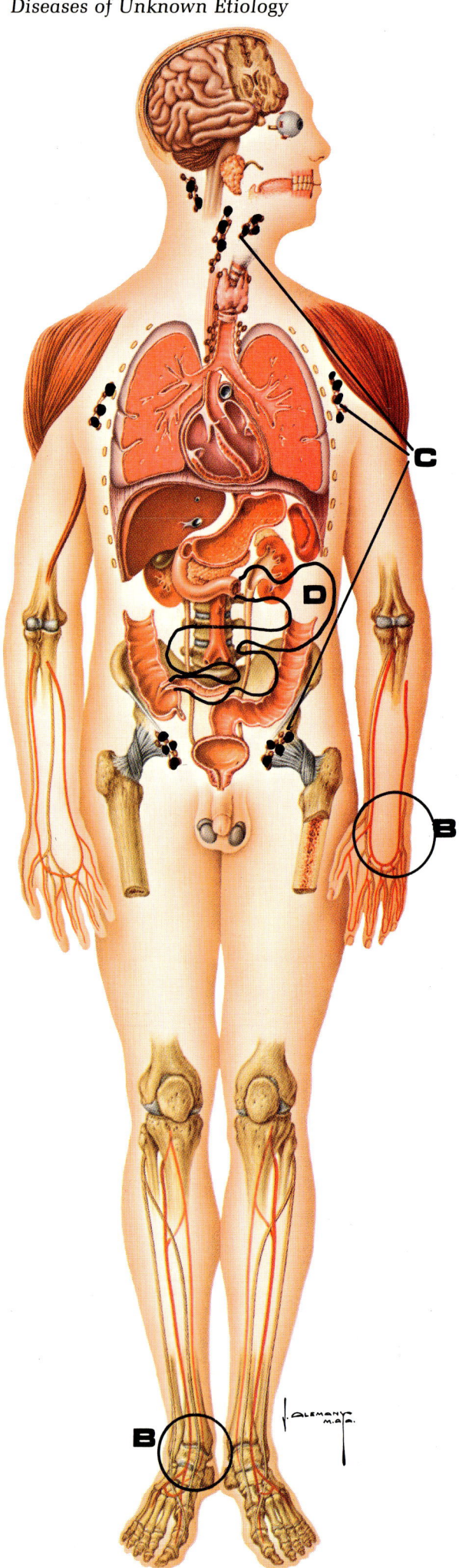

Whipple's Disease

A 48-year-old white male complained of painful left wrist and right ankle joints. He had had intermittent diarrhea for several months and lost several pounds of weight.

Physical examination revealed generalized skin pigmentation (A), swollen, tender, and red left wrist and right ankle joints (B), and generalized lymphadenopathy (C).

Laboratory examination revealed a hypochromic anemia, increased neutral fat in the stool, and decreased uptake of ^{131}I triolein and of ^{131}I oleic acid. The 24-hour urine 5-hydroxyindoleacetic acid was elevated. A transoral suction biopsy was diagnostic.

X-ray examination revealed dilated and thickened loops of small intestine with scattering of barium, indicating involvement of the intestines (D).

Differential Diagnosis:
1. Regional enteritis
2. Ulcerative colitis
3. Rheumatoid arthritis
4. Rheumatic fever

5. Gout
6. Addison's disease
7. Gonorrhea
8. Serum sickness
9. Tuberculosis of the intestines
10. Adult celiac disease
11. Carcinoid syndrome

Clinical Note. Three intestinal conditions, Whipple's disease, regional enteritis, and ulcerative colitis, present with joint symptoms, but the finding of increased stool fat helps to distinguish Whipple's disease from the other two. The other conditions in the differential rarely present with diarrhea as well. Like gout, Whipple's disease is rare in females. There is usually a hypochromic anemia, as in this case, secondary to toxic depression of the bone marrow, as the hypochromic anemia does not respond to folic acid.

Pathology. The most striking finding on both lymph node and intestinal biopsy are macrophages filled with glycoprotein (not cholesterol), which stain with periodic acid-Schiff material. A verrucous endocarditis has been reported. If lymph node and peroral suction biopsy are negative, it may be necessary to perform an exploratory laparotomy to get the diagnosis.

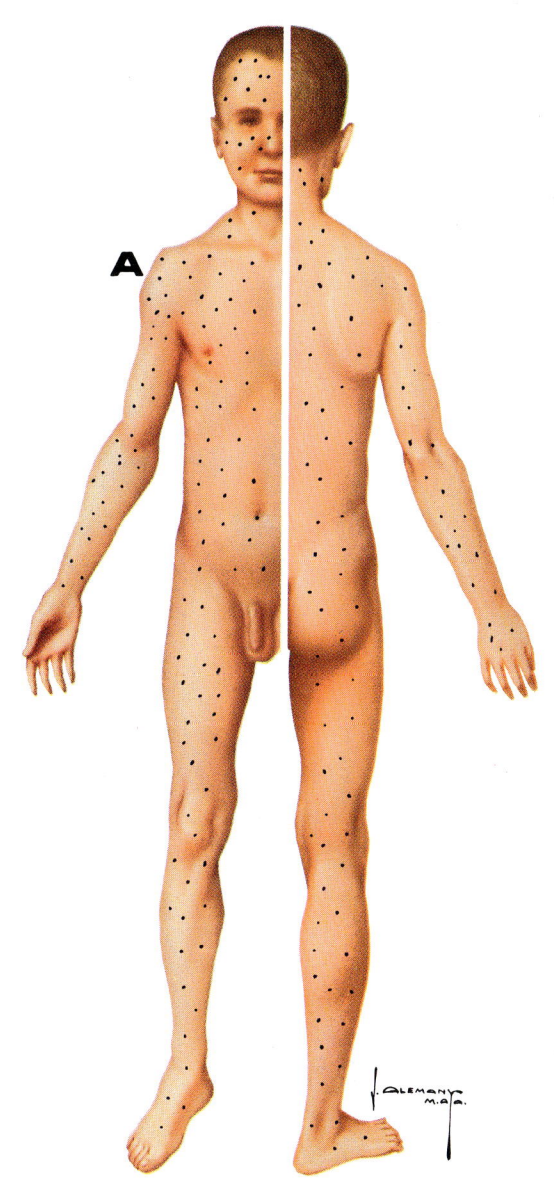

Part Two

Tables

I. Clinical Key to Organ System Involvement

II. Prominent Physical Signs of Systemic Disease

III. Organ Involvement as a Key to the Diagnosis of Systemic Disease

IV. Systemic Disease With the Organs That Show Significant Functional or Pathologic Changes

V. Local Disease as a Symptom of Systemic Disease

VI. Laboratory Work-up of Systemic Diseases

VII. Laboratory Tests of Organ Involvement

Table I.
Clinical Key to Organ System Involvement

	Symptoms	Signs
Adrenal Gland		
Pain:	—	—
Mass:	Rarely (neuroblastoma)	Flank mass rarely (neuroblastoma)
Functional changes:	Shock, chills, pigmentation changes, weakness, fatigue, weight loss, syncope	Low blood pressure, pigmentary changes in skin, hirsutism, change in secondary sex characteristics
Aorta		
Pain:	Occasionally dull chest pain	—
Mass:	Pulsatile mass in neck or abdomen	Bulging of chest or pulsatile mass of neck or abdomen
Functional changes:	Shock	Low blood pressure, loss of pulses in extremities, palpable thrills
	—	Palpable thrill, aortic diastolic murmur, systolic murmur over mass
Auscultatory changes:	—	Systolic and diastolic murmurs over aorta and its branches
Arteries		
Pain:	Chest pain, headache, pain in extremities	Tender temporal artery
Mass:	—	Nodules of arteries
Discharge:	Epistaxis	Epistaxis
Functional changes:	Fainting, cold in extremities, convulsions	Cold extremities, absent pulses, bruits over arteries
Changes in shape:	—	Hardening of arteries, aneurysm, tortuosity
Color changes:	Blue or black extremities	Blue or gangrenous extremities, silver or copper wiring
Bladder, Urinary		
Pain:	Dysuria	Tender suprapubic area
Mass:	Not noted by patient	Suprapubic mass
Discharge:	Bloody or cloudy urine	Bloody or cloudy urine
Functional changes:	Frequency, difficulty voiding, incontinence	Residual urine on catheterization
Blood		
Pain:	Occasional bone pain	Occasional bone tenderness
Mass:	—	Bone hypertrophy, splenomegaly, lymphadenopathy
Discharge:	Bleeding from any body orifice and skin	Bleeding from any body orifice and skin. Retinal hemorrhages
Functional changes:	Fatigue, weight loss, fainting	Drop in blood pressure, tachycardia
Color changes:	Pallor possibly noted by patient	Pallor or plethora
Ulcers:	In the mouth	In the mouth
Auscultation:	—	Heart murmurs
Constitutional changes:	Fever, chills	Fever

Table I. Clinical Key to Organ System Involvement

	Symptoms	Signs
Bone		
Pain:	Pain in back, neck, skull, extremities	Tenderness in back, neck, skull, or extremities
Mass:	Lump on any bone	Focal or diffuse enlargement of bone
Discharge:	Occasionally skin discharge	Fistulous tract from bone to skin
Functional changes:	Limitation of motion	Limitation of motion
Changes in shape:	Occasionally noted by patient	Saber shin, enlarged skull circumference, etc., long fingers
Breast		
Pain:	Focal or diffuse pain in breasts	Focal or diffuse tenderness in the breast
Mass:	Lump in the breast	Mass or diffuse hypertrophy of breasts; axillary adenopathy, supraclavicular adenopathy
Discharge:	Yellow or bloody discharge from nipple	Serous, purulent, or bloody discharge from nipple
Ulcers:	Ulceration of skin of breast	Ulceration of skin of breast
Functional changes:	Inability, overproduction or inappropriate production of milk	Inability, overproduction or inappropriate production of milk
Ear		
Pain:	Otalgia, headache	Tender ear or mastoids
Mass:	Lump or swelling of external ear	Ear swelling, mass on drum, cervical lymphadenopathy
Discharge:	Yellow or bloody aural discharge	Serous, purulent, or bloody aural discharge
Color changes:	None	Red eardrum, scarred eardrum
Changes in shape:	Elf ears, etc.	Elf ears, large ears, perforated drum
Functional changes:	Loss of hearing, tinnitus	Loss of hearing, positive Weber and Rinne test, lack of drum movement
Esophagus		
Pain:	Chest pain, epigastric pain, or heartburn increased by swallowing or breathing	Occasionally tenderness in the neck
Mass:	Rarely a mass in neck (diverticulum)	Rarely a mass in neck (diverticulum)
Discharge:	Hematemesis, regurgitation of food or acid	Hematemesis, regurgitation of food or acid
Functional changes:	Dysphagia	———
Eye		
Pain:	Eye pain, headache	Tender eyeball or eyelid
Mass:	Swollen eye or eyelid; lump on lid, protrusion of eye	Orbital mass, lid mass; exophthalmos, periorbital edema
Discharge:	Watery, yellow, or bloody discharge	Watery, purulent or bloody discharge
Color changes:	Red eye	Infected conjunctiva, circumcorneal injection, scleral injection, blue sclera
		Kayser-Fleischer ring, calcium deposits in cornea; cataracts, corneal opacities, disk pallor

Table I. Clinical Key to Organ System Involvement

	Symptoms	Signs
Functional changes:	Blurred vision, double vision, blindness, color blindness	Refractive error, astigmatism, field defect, strabismus; change in reaction of pupillary reflexes, increase in ocular tension
Gastrointestinal Tract		
Pain:	Focal or diffuse abdominal pain	Focal or diffuse abdominal tenderness
Mass:	Abdominal mass	Virchow's node abdominal mass, distended abdomen, rectal mass
Discharge:	Hematemesis, melena, excess mucus in stool	Hematemesis, melena, excess mucus in stool
Functional changes:	Anorexia, weight loss, vomiting, diarrhea, constipation, obstipation	Hyperactive or hypoactive bowel sounds; visible peristalsis
Genitourinary Tract		
Pain:	Flank pain, lower abdominal pain, testicular pain, back pain, dysmenorrhea, dysuria	Flank tenderness, lower abdominal tenderness, testicular tenderness, tenderness on pelvic or rectal examination
Mass:	Flank mass, lower abdominal mass, testicular mass	Flank mass, lower abdominal mass, testicular mass, adnexal or uterine mass, cystocele, rectocele
Discharge:	Urethral or vaginal discharge, cloudy or bloody urine	Urethral or vaginal discharge, cloudy or bloody urine
Functional changes:	Hypermenorrhea, amenorrhea, metrorrhagia, menorrhagia, infertility, impotence, frequency of urination, difficulty in voiding	Low sperm count, poor maturation of vaginal epithelium, observations during voiding
Gums		
Pain:	Painful gums and teeth	Tender gums
Mass:	Gum mass or hypertrophy	Gum mass or hypertrophy
Discharge:	Yellow or bloody discharge	Purulent or bloody discharge from gums
Color changes:	———	Lead line, etc.
Hair		
Pain:	———	———
Mass:	Thickening of hair	Thickening of hair strands
Discharge:	———	———
Functional changes:	Hypertrichosis, hirsutism, hair loss, thinning of hair strand	Same
Heart		
Pain:	Chest pain at rest or on exercise; midepigastric pain, referred pain to back, neck, arms, etc.	Usually no significant tenderness of precordium
Mass:	———	Precordial bulge, cardiomegaly, hepatomegaly, neck vein distention, ascites and pitting edema

Table I. Clinical Key to Organ System Involvement

	Symptoms	Signs
Discharge:	Cough with foamy or blood-tinged sputum	Foamy or blood-tinged sputum
Color changes:	Cyanosis, plethora	Cyanosis, plethora
Changes in shape:	Stunted growth	Clubbing of fingers and toes
Functional changes:	Palpitations, syncope, dyspnea	Tachycardia, bradycardia, arrhythmias
Auscultatory changes:	———	Heart murmurs, pericardial friction rubs, changes in heart sounds
Islet Cells of Pancreas		
Pain:	———	———
Mass:	———	Occasional midepigastric mass noted
Discharge:	———	Sugar in urine
Functional changes:	Coma, syncope, sweating, fatigue, hunger, polyuria, polydypsia, weight loss, weight gain	Coma, syncope, neuropathy, arteritis
Joints		
Pain:	Joint pain	Joint tenderness
Mass:	Joint swelling	Joint swelling
Discharge:	———	———
Functional changes:	Limitation of motion	Limitation of motion
Auscultatory changes:	Joint crepitus	Joint crepitus
Kidney		
Pain:	Flank pain, lower abdominal pain, testicular pain, dysuria	Murphy's sign
Mass:	Flank mass	Flank mass
Discharge:	Cloudy, dark, or bloody urine	Cloudy, dark, or bloody urine
Functional changes:	Frequency of urination, nocturia, anuria, polyuria, incontinence	Incontinence, anuria
Liver		
Pain:	Right upper quadrant pain radiating to right shoulder or right scapula	Tender right upper quadrant
Mass:	Enlarged liver or spleen occasionally noticed by patient	Hepatomegaly or enlarged gallbladder, splenomegaly, ascites, edema of lower extremities, hemorrhoids, caput medusae
Discharge:	Dark urine, light stool, hematemesis	Dark urine, light stool, hematemesis
Color changes:	Yellow skin and eyes	Jaundice, icteric sclera, orange-yellow to green-yellow, spider angiomata
Functional changes:	Weakness, fatigue, weight loss, nausea and occasional vomiting, coma	Loss of hair, gynecomastia, testicular atrophy, coma, delirium
Lung		
Pain:	Chest pain, back pain, occasional abdominal pain	Rarely tenderness in chest

Table I. Clinical Key to Organ System Involvement

	Symptoms	Signs
Mass:	—	Rarely a lung neoplasm or abscess may bulge to surface; barrel chest, hepatomegaly, neck vein distention, axillary or cervical adenopathy
Discharge:	White, yellow, or bloody sputum	Mucoid, purulent, or bloody sputum; rarely a bronchocutaneous fistula
Color changes:	Cyanosis, plethora	Cyanosis, plethora
Changes in shape:	—	Tracheal deviation, retraction
Functional changes:	Dyspnea, tachypnea, wheezing cough, halitosis, coma	Tachypnea, tachycardia, coma
Percussion:	—	Dullness, flatness, hyperresonance
Auscultatory changes:	—	Crepitant, sibilant, sonorous rales, changes in breath sounds, egophony, bronchophony, etc.

Lymph Nodes

Pain:	Occasional pain noted in lymph glands	Tender lymph glands
Mass:	Enlarged lymph nodes	Enlarged lymph nodes
Discharge:	Occasional skin discharge	Occasionally development of a fistula from lymph nodes to skin
Functional changes:	Enlarged extremity or scrotum	Lymphedema

Mouth

Pain:	Painful mouth	Painful mouth
Mass:	Mass of lip or mucous membranes	Mass of lip or mucous membranes
Discharge:	White or yellow coating	White or yellow coating
Color changes:	—	Brown pigment of mucous membranes
Ulcers:	Ulcers of lips or mucous membranes	Ulcers of lips or mucous membranes

Muscle

Pain:	Painful muscles	Tender muscles
Mass:	Lump or diffuse enlargement	Focal or diffuse hypertrophy
Functional changes:	Weakness, fatigue, loss of power	Loss of power, loss of deep tendon reflexes
Atrophy:	Focal or diffuse atrophy	Focal or diffuse atrophy

Nails

Pain:	Pain under nails	Tender nails
Mass:	Swelling of nail and digit	Swelling or thickening of nail
Discharge:	Splinter hemorrhages, yellow discharge	Splinter hemorrhages, purulent discharge
Functional changes:	Brittle nails	Brittle nails
Changes in shape:	—	Clubbing, longitudinal ridging, loss of the lunula of the nail

Nervous System

Pain:	Headache, earache, ocular pain, neck pain, back pain, face pain	Tenderness in head, neck, back, nerve bundles, nuchal rigidity
Mass:	Enlarged head, mass on head or spine	Enlarged head, mass on head or spine, mass on nerve bundles, nerve hypertrophy, papilledema

Table I. Clinical Key to Organ System Involvement

	Symptoms	Signs
Discharge:	Ear or nose discharge	Aural discharge, rhinorrhea
Functional changes:	Blindness, double vision, deafness, tinnitus	Blindness, field defect, diplopia
	Loss of smell	Perceptive deafness
		Weber and Rurne test
	Loss of taste	Anosmia
		Loss of taste
	Loss of pain	Analgesia
		Anesthesia
	Loss of touch	Loss of vibratory and position sense
	Paresthesias	Loss of muscle power
		Dyskinesia
	Weakness	Dysmetria
		Ataxia
	Paralysis	Spastic gait
		Nystagmus
	Incoordination	Aphasia
		Dysarthria
	Difficulty in walking	Tremor
		Rigidity
	Incontinence	Chorea
		Athetosis
	Aphasia	Hyperactive deep tendon reflexes
		Absent deep tendon reflexes
		Pathologic reflexes
		Absent superficial abdominal reflexes
Ovary		
Pain:	Lower abdominal pain	Tender adnexa
Mass:	Lower abdominal mass	Lower abdominal mass, adnexal mass
Discharge:	———	———
Functional changes:	Amenorrhea, metorrhagia, hypermenorrhea, sterility	———
Parathyroid Gland		
Pain:	Occasional bone pain	Occasional bone tenderness
Mass:	Mass in thyroid gland	Mass in thyroid gland; cystic mass on bone occasionally
Discharge:	———	———
Functional changes:	Weakness, tetany, convulsions, confusion, polyuria, diarrhea	Convulsions, Trousseau's phenomenon, Chvostek's sign
Penis		
Pain:	Painful penis	Tender penis
Mass:	Penile mass or ulcers	Penile mass or ulcers, inguinal adenopathy
Discharge:	Urethral discharge; discharge from ulcer	Urethral discharge; discharge from ulcer
Functional changes:	Priapism; impotence, premature ejaculation	Priapism
Changes in shape:	———	Epispadius, hypospadius
Pituitary Gland		
Pain:	Headache	———
Mass:	Bone hypertrophy; gigantism	Bone hypertrophy; gigantism

Table I. Clinical Key to Organ System Involvement

	Symptoms	Signs
Discharge:	—	—
Functional changes:	Weight loss, fainting spells, blindness, impotence	Hair loss, skin atrophy, hypertrichosis, nail changes, thyroid and testicular atrophy, hypotension
Rectum		
Pain:	Rectal pain, pain on bowel movement	Rectal tenderness
Mass:	Perirectal mass	Rectal and perirectal mass, hemorrhoids, warts, skin tags, condyloma latum, sentinel pile
Discharge:	Blood or mucus in stool or after stool; bloody or yellow discharge	Blood or mucus in stool or after stool; bloody or yellow discharge; fistula
Functional changes:	Constipation, incontinence	Poor sphincter tone and control
Sinuses		
Pain:	Supra-orbital or maxillary pain	Tender frontal or maxillary sinuses
Mass:	—	—
Discharge:	White, yellow, or bloody nasal or postnasal drip	Mucoid, purulent or bloody nasal or postnasal discharge
Functional change:	Blocking of nasal passages	Blocking of nasal passages
Skin		
Pain:	Painful skin; pruritus	Tender skin
Mass:	Lumps in the skin	Papular to nodular lesions; skin masses
Discharge:	Weeping of skin	Clear, purulent, or bloody discharge from lesions
Color changes:	Erythematous rash; pigmentary changes	Erythematous rash, pigmentary changes
Atrophy:	Focal or diffuse atrophy, or thinning of the skin	Focal or diffuse atrophy, or thinning of the skin
Spleen		
Pain:	Right upper quadrant pain	Tenderness in right upper quadrant
Mass:	Occasionally enlarged spleen felt by patient	Splenomegaly
Discharge:	—	—
Functional changes:	Purpura, pallor, hemorrhages from any body orifice	Pallor, anemia, leukopenia, thrombocytopenia, petechiae
Auscultatory changes:	—	Friction rub over spleen
Testicles		
Pain:	Testicular pain	Tender testicles
Mass:	Scrotal mass	Scrotal mass, inguinal adenopathy
Discharge:	—	—
Functional changes:	Sterility	Low sperm count
Throat		
Pain:	Sore throat	Tender peritonsillar nodes
Mass:	Enlarged tonsils and cervical lymph nodes	Enlarged tonsils and cervical lymph nodes
Discharge:	—	Tonsillar exudates or ulcers
Functional changes:	Difficulty in swallowing, anorexia	—

Table I. Clinical Key to Organ System Involvement

	Symptoms	Signs
Thyroid Gland		
Pain:	Pain in thyroid and neck	Tender thyroid gland
Mass:	Mass in neck	Enlarged thyroid gland, cervical lymphadenopathy, exophthalmos
Discharge:	——	——
Functional changes:	Palpitations, weakness, weight loss, polyuria, polyphagia, polydypsia, depression, diarrhea, sweating, intolerance to cold, intolerance to heat, constipation, loss of appetite, amenorrhea, menorrhagia, hung-up deep tendon reflexes	Smooth warm skin, thick cold skin, tremor, tachycardia, bradycardia, nail changes, cardiac arrhythmias, muscle atrophy, hung-up deep tendon reflexes
Auscultatory changes:	——	Thyroid bruit
Tongue		
Pain:	Painful tongue	Tender tongue
Mass:	Mass in tongue	Mass in tongue, hypertrophy
Discharge:	——	——
Atrophy:	——	Atrophy of papillae or muscle

Table II.
Prominent Physical Signs of Systemic Disease

Sign	Disease
Ears, Nose and Throat	
1. Angular stomatitis	Riboflavin deficiency
2. Arched palate	Marfan's syndrome, Turner's syndrome
3. Blue line of gums	Lead poisoning
4. Flushed face	Carcinoid syndrome, polycythemia vera, menopause syndrome
5. Koplik's spots	Measles
6. Moon face	Cushing's syndrome
7. Pigmentation of the buccal mucosa	Peutz-Jegher's disease, Addison's disease
8. Saddle nose	Congenital lues
Extremities	
1. Arterial nodules	Periarteritis nodosa
2. Cubitus valgus	Turner's syndrome
3. Nail hemorrhages	Subacute bacterial endocarditis, trichinosis
4. Polydactylia	Turner's syndrome, Laurence-Moon-Biedl syndrome
5. Raynaud's phenomenon	Scleroderma, macroglobulinemia, periarteritis nodosa
6. Short fingers	Pseudohypoparathyroidism, mongolism
7. Spider hands	Arachnodactyly
8. Spoon nails	Plummer-Vinson syndrome
9. Tendon xanthoma	Essential hypercholesterolemia
10. Tophi	Gout
Eye	
1. Angioid streaks of retina	Pseudoxanthoma elasticum
2. Argyll Robertson pupil	Neurosyphilis
3. Blue sclera	Osteogenesis imperfecta
4. Cataracts	Diabetes mellitus, galactosemia, myotonia atrophica
5. Cherry red macula	Niemann-Pick disease, Tay-Sachs disease
6. Choroidal tubercle	Tuberculosis
7. Chorioretinal scar	Toxoplasmosis
8. Corneal opacities	Hurler's disease, hypercalcemia
9. Exophthalmos	Hyperthyroidism
10. Kayser-Fleischer ring	Wilson's disease
11. Lens dislocation	Arachnodactyly
12. Microaneurysms of retina	Diabetes mellitus
13. Peripapillary arteriovenous anastomosis	Takayasu's syndrome
14. Pinguecula	Gaucher's disease, Hodgkin's disease, ochronosis
15. Retinal exudates and/or hemorrhages	Numerous systemic diseases
16. Retinitis pigmentosa	Laurence-Moon-Biedl syndrome
17. Salt and pepper fundus	Congenital lues
18. Tears, absence of	Sjögren's syndrome, familial dysautonomia
19. Von Graefe's sign	Hyperthyroidism
20. Xanthelasma	Diabetes mellitus, essential hypercholesterolemia, essential hypertriglyceridemia, primary biliary cirrhosis

Table II. Prominent Physical Signs of Systemic Disease

Sign	Disease
Neck	
1. Thyroid bruit	Hyperthyroidism
2. Web neck	Turner's syndrome
Nervous System	
1. Chvostek's sign	Hypoparathyroidism and related diseases
2. Hung-up deep tendon reflexes	Hypothyroidism
3. Trousseau's phenomenon	Hypoparathyroidism and related diseases
Skin	
1. Absent axillary and pubic hair	Hypopituitarism
2. Adenoma sebaceum	Tuberosclerosis
3. "Bronze" skin	Addison's disease, hemochromatosis
4. Butterfly rash	Lupus erythematosus
5. Café au lait spots	Neurofibromatosis
6. Capillary telangiectasis	Rendu-Osler-Weber syndrome
7. Cream or orange papules in neck and axilla	Pseudoxanthoma elasticum
8. Erythema induratum	Tuberculosis
9. Erythema multiforme	Rheumatic fever, Stevens-Johnson syndrome
10. Erythema nodosum	Rheumatic fever, coccidioidomycosis
11. Hirsutism	Adrenogenital syndrome, Cushing's syndrome
12. Janeway spots	Subacute bacterial endocarditis
13. Osler's nodules	Subacute bacterial endocarditis
14. Port-wine stain	Sturge-Weber syndrome
15. Sclerodactyly	Scleroderma, macroglobulinemia, periarteritis nodosa
16. Spider angioma	Cirrhosis of the liver
17. Subcutaneous nodules	Rheumatic fever, rheumatoid arthritis

Table III.

Organ Involvement as a Key to the Diagnosis of Systemic Disease

Note: A list of conditions to be considered in the differential diagnosis of each organ is in the right-hand column under each individual heading. Knowledge of the full scope of organ involvement in each patient will aid in establishing diagnosis from the combinations of organs listed in the left-hand column.

Adrenal Gland:

Arteries, gastrointestinal tract, skin, mouth	Addison's disease
Arteries, heart	Pheochromocytoma
Arteries, muscle, nervous system	Aldosteronism
Arteries, skin, bone	Cushing's syndrome
Blood vessels, nervous system	Meningococcemia
Liver, spleen, kidney, eye	Secondary amyloidosis
Lungs, lymph nodes, kidneys, nervous system	Tuberculosis
Lungs, lymph nodes, spleen, eye	Histoplasmosis
Pituitary gland, testicles, thyroid, skin	Hypopituitarism
Pituitary gland, liver, spleen, bone	Acromegaly
Skin, nervous system, bone	Neurofibromatosis

Aorta:

Arteries, heart, nervous system	Atherosclerosis
Bone, eye	Arachnodactyly
Heart, blood vessels, kidney, nervous system	Subacute bacterial endocarditis
Heart, eyes, kidney, nervous system	Essential hypertension with medionecrosis
Joints, heart, skin, nervous system	Rheumatic fever
Ovaries, bone, skin	Turner's syndrome
Skin, nervous system	Syphilis

Arteries:

Adrenal gland, heart	Pheochromocytoma
Adrenal gland, muscle, nervous system	Aldosteronism
Adrenal gland, nervous system, blood vessels	Meningococcemia
Adrenal gland, skin, bone	Cushing's syndrome
Adrenal gland, skin, gastrointestinal tract	Addison's disease
Blood, lymph nodes, eyes	Macroglobulinemia
Blood, multiple organs	Sickle cell anemia
Heart, kidney, eyes, nervous system	Essential hypertension
Heart, nervous system	Atherosclerosis
Heart, skin, tendons	Essential hypercholesterolemia
Islet cells, kidney, eye, nervous system	Diabetes mellitus
Nervous system, gastrointestinal tract, kidney	Periarteritis nodosa
Pituitary gland, skin, sex glands, thyroid	Hypopituitarism
Skin, aorta, nervous system	Syphilis
Skin, blood, joints, kidney	Lupus erythematosus
Skin, gastrointestinal tract, lung	Scleroderma
Skin, nervous system	Epidemic typhus
Thyroid, eyes, heart, nervous system, skin	Hyperthyroidism

Bladder:

Urinary, liver	Schistosomiasis
Urinary, lung, kidney	Tuberculosis
Urinary, skin, aorta, nervous system	Syphilis

Blood:

Bone	Osteopetrosis
Bone, gastrointestinal tract	Multiple myeloma
Gastrointestinal tract, mucous membranes	Peutz-Jegher's disease
Gastrointestinal tract, nervous system	Porphyria
Gastrointestinal tract, tongue, nails	Plummer-Vinson syndrome
Gastrointestinal tract, tongue, skin	Malabsorption syndrome
Gums, nervous system, gastrointestinal tract	Lead poisoning
Gums, skin, joints	Scurvy
Kidney, heart, nervous system	Renal failure
Liver, lung, nervous system, bone	Metastatic carcinoma
Liver, nervous system	Hepatic failure
Lung, heart, nervous system	Pulmonary emphysema
Lung, spleen, lymph nodes	Histoplasmosis
Lymph nodes, spleen	Lymphatic leukemia
Lymph nodes, spleen	Hodgkin's disease
Lymph nodes, spleen, arteries, eye	Macroglobulinemia
Mucous membranes, skin, spleen	Aplastic anemia
Multiple organs	Sickle cell anemia
Nervous system, eye, spleen, skin	Niemann-Pick disease
Nervous system, gastrointestinal tract	Pernicious anemia
Nervous system, spleen, skin	Thrombotic, thrombocytopenic purpura
Spleen	Chronic myelogenous leukemia
Spleen, bone, liver, skin	Gaucher's disease
Spleen, heart, veins	Polycythemia vera
Spleen, liver	Myeloid metaplasia
Spleen, liver, bone	Mediterranean anemia
Spleen, liver, lymph nodes	Kala-azar
Spleen, liver, nervous system	Malaria
Skin, gastrointestinal tract, spleen	Idiopathic thrombocytopenic purpura
Skin, joints	Hemophilia
Skin, joints, spleen, kidney	Lupus erythematosus

Bone:

Adrenal gland	Cushing's syndrome
Blood	Osteopetrosis
Blood	Osteogenesis imperfecta
Blood, gastrointestinal tract	Multiple myeloma
Blood, gums	Scurvy
Blood, spleen	Mediterranean anemia
Eye, skin	Hand-Schüller-Christian disease

Table III. Organ Involvement as a Key to the Diagnosis of Systemic Disease

Eye, teeth	Congenital syphilis
Kidney, gastrointestinal tract	Primary hyperparathyroidism
Kidney, muscle	Renal tubular acidosis
Kidney, muscle, eye	Lignac-Fanconi syndrome
Liver, lung	Echinococcosis
Liver, lung, nervous system, bone	Metastatic carcinoma
Liver, nervous system	Gargoylism
Lung, eye, skin	Sarcoidosis
Lung, heart, nervous system	Pulmonary emphysema
Lung, lymph nodes, kidney	Tuberculosis
Lung, skin	Coccidioidomycosis
Lung, skin, kidney	North American blastomycosis
Lymph nodes, skin	Sporotrichosis
Muscle	Rickets
Muscle, parathyroid gland	Pseudohypoparathyroidism
Nervous system, eye, testicles	Laurence-Moon-Biedl syndrome
Nervous system, gastrointestinal tract, blood	Lead poisoning
Nervous system, liver, eye	Wilson's disease
Nervous system, spleen, liver	Niemann-Pick disease
Nervous system, skin	Tuberosclerosis
Nervous system, skin, heart	Mongolism
Ovaries, skin, heart	Turner's syndrome
Ovaries, skin, nervous system	Menopause
Pituitary gland, liver, spleen	Acromegaly
Spleen, liver, blood, lymph nodes	Letterer-Siwe disease
Spleen, skin, eye, blood	Gaucher's disease
Skin, nervous system, adrenal gland	Neurofibromatosis
Skin, nervous system, liver	Hypervitaminosis A
Thyroid, skin, nervous system	Cretinism

Breast:

Adrenal gland, skin	Adrenogenital syndrome
Liver, nervous system, skin	Hepatic failure
Lung, lymph nodes, kidney	Tuberculosis
Lung, skin, kidney	Blastomycosis
Ovaries, skin, bone	Turner's syndrome
Skin, aorta, nervous system	Syphilis
Skin, bone, lymph nodes	Actinomycosis
Testicles, nervous system	Klinefelter's syndrome

Ear:

Bone, joints, urine	Ochronosis
Eye, skin, teeth	Congenital syphilis
Joints, kidney, heart	Gout

Esophagus:

Blood, tongue	Plummer-Vinson syndrome
Liver, nervous system, skin	Hepatic failure
Skin, heart, lung, kidney	Scleroderma

Eye:

Arteries, heart	Atherosclerosis
Arteries, heart, kidney, nervous system	Essential hypertension
Arteries, heart, skin	Essential hypercholesterolemia
Blood, blood vessels, lymph nodes	Macroglobulinemia
Blood, blood vessels, spleen, kidney	Lupus erythematosus
Blood, blood vessels, multiple organs	Sickle cell anemia
Bone, aorta, kidney	Arachnodactyly
Bone, kidney	Hyperparathyroidism
Bone, skin, lungs	Hand-Schüller-Christian disease
Gastrointestinal tract, nervous system	Digitalis intoxication
Gastrointestinal tract, joints	Ulcerative colitis
Heart, lymph nodes	Chagas' disease
Islet cells, blood vessels, kidney, skin	Diabetes mellitus
Joints, heart	Ankylosing spondylitis
Joints, skin	Rheumatoid arthritis
Joints, skin, ear, urine	Alcaptonuria
Joints, urethra	Gonorrhea
Joints, urethra	Reiter's syndrome
Kidney, muscle, bone	Lignac-Fanconi syndrome
Liver, spleen, blood	Kala-azar
Liver, spleen, kidney	Secondary amyloidosis
Liver, spleen, nervous system	Galactosemia
Liver, spleen, nervous system, bone	Gargoylism
Liver, spleen, skin	Essential triglyceridemia
Lung, lymph nodes, kidney, nervous system	Tuberculosis
Lung, lymph nodes, nervous system, skin	Sarcoidosis
Lung, lymph nodes, blood, spleen, adrenal gland	Histoplasmosis
Muscle, testicles, skin	Myotonia atrophica
Nervous system, spleen, liver, blood, skin	Niemann-Pick disease
Nervous system, testicles, bone	Laurence-Moon-Biedl syndrome
Nose, lungs, nervous system, kidneys	Mucormycosis
Penis, lymph nodes, rectum	Lymphogranuloma venereum
Skin, lungs, nervous system	Measles
Teeth, ear, skin, bone	Congenital syphilis
Throat, lymph nodes, nervous system	Listeriosis
Thyroid, heart, arteries, nervous system	Hyperthyroidism

Gastrointestinal Tract:

Adrenal gland, arteries, skin	Addison's disease
Arteries, nervous system, kidney	Periarteritis nodosa
Blood, blood vessels, multiple organs	Sickle cell anemia
Blood, nervous system	Pernicious anemia
Blood, skin	Hemophilia
Blood, skin, spleen	Idiopathic thrombocytopenia purpura
Blood, tongue, bone, nervous system	Malabsorption syndrome
Eye, nervous system	Digitalis intoxication
Joints, eye	Ulcerative colitis
Joints, lymph nodes, skin	Whipple's disease
Kidney, bone	Hyperparathyroidism
Liver, kidney	Carbon tetrachloride poisoning
Liver, lungs	Amebiasis
Liver, lungs, skin, heart	Carcinoid syndrome
Liver, nervous system	Alcoholism
Liver, nervous system, skin	Hepatic failure
Liver, spleen	Schistosomiasis
Lung, skin, spleen	Typhoid fever
Mucous membranes	Peutz-Jegher's syndrome
Muscle, nervous system	Cysticercosis
Nervous system	Poliomyelitis

Table III. Organ Involvement as a Key to the Diagnosis of Systemic Disease

Nervous system, blood, liver, skin... Porphyria
Nervous system, blood, gums .... Lead poisoning
Nervous system, muscle, heart ...... Hypokalemia
Nervous system, skin..................... Arsenic poisoning
Nervous system, skin..................... Pellagra
Pancreas, endocrine glands............ Zollinger-Ellison syndrome
Pancreas, islet cells, liver............... Chronic pancreatitis
Pancreas, lungs, skin..................... Fibrocystic disease
Skin, arteries, heart, lungs .... Scleroderma

Genitourinary Tract:

See also Kidney, Penis, Testicle
Eyes, joints .... Gonorrhea
Eyes, joints .... Reiter's syndrome
Lungs, lymph nodes, kidney .... Tuberculosis
Skin, aorta, nervous system........... Syphilis

Gums:

Blood, skin, bone .... Scurvy
Blood, spleen, skin....................... Leukemia
Gastrointestinal tract, nervous system .... Lead poisoning
Liver, heart .... Yellow fever
Nervous system, skin..................... Dilantin intoxication
Skin, mucous membranes .... Smallpox
Spleen, liver, skin, bone .... Letterer-Siwe disease

Hair:

Adrenal gland, arteries, skin bone... Cushing's syndrome
Muscle, eye, testicles..................... Myotonia atrophica
Pituitary gland, adrenal gland, thyroid, testicles........................ Hypopituitarism
Skin, aorta, nervous system........... Syphilis
Skin, nervous system..................... Phenylpyruvic oligophrenia
Skin, nervous system, arteries......... Acrodynia
Skin, sex glands, breasts .... Adrenogenital syndrome
Thyroid, skin, heart, nervous system. Hyperthyroidism
Thyroid, skin, heart, nervous system. Hypothyroidism

Heart:

Adrenal gland, arteries................... Pheochromocytoma
Arteries, kidney, nervous system ... Essential hypertension
Arteries, nervous system .... Atherosclerosis
Arteries, skin, tendons .... Essential hypercholesterolemia
Blood, blood vessels, other organs... Sickle cell anemia
Blood, blood vessels, kidney, spleen. Lupus erythematosus
Blood, spleen .... Polycythemia vera
Blood, blood vessels, spleen, skin ... Subacute bacterial endocarditis
Bone, eye, aorta .... Arachnodactyly
Eye, nervous system, spleen, liver... Gargoylism
Eye, skin, lymph nodes.................. Chagas' disease
Gastrointestinal tract, muscle, nervous system .... Hypokalemia
Gastrointestinal tract, skin, lungs ... Carcinoid syndrome
Gastrointestinal tract, nervous system .... Digitalis intoxication
Gastrointestinal tract, nervous system .... Poliomyelitis
Joints, liver, spleen........................ Still's disease
Joints, skin, nervous system............ Rheumatic fever
Kidney, nervous system, blood ...... Chronic renal failure
Liver, gums, kidney .... Yellow fever
Liver, nervous system, eye .... Glycogen storage disease

Liver, pancreas, testicles .... Hemochromatosis
Lungs, liver .... Q-fever
Lung, liver, nervous system............ Chronic congestive heart failure
Lung, liver, nervous system, blood... Pulmonary emphysema
Nervous system .... Beriberi
Nervous system, skin, bone............ Mongolism
Nose, lungs, kidney .... Mucormycosis
Ovaries, skin, bone........................ Turner's syndrome
Pituitary gland, bone, liver, spleen... Acromegaly
Skin, aorta, nervous system............ Syphilis
Skin, gastrointestinal tract, arteries... Scleroderma
Throat, nervous system.................. Diphtheria
Thyroid, nervous system, skin ...... Hyperthyroidism
Thyroid, skin, nervous system ...... Hypothyroidism
Tongue, muscle, skin..................... Primary amyloidosis

Islet cells:

Blood vessels, eye, kidney .... Diabetes mellitus
Gastrointestinal tract, endocrine glands .... Zollinger-Ellison syndrome
Nervous system .... Islet cell adenoma
Pancreas, liver, gastrointestinal tract .... Chronic pancreatitis

Joints:

Blood, skin .... Hemophilia
Blood, blood vessels, spleen, kidney. Lupus erythematosus
Blood, blood vessels, skin .... Ehlers-Danlos syndrome
Eye, ear, urine.............................. Alcaptonuria
Eye, heart .... Ankylosing spondylitis
Gastrointestinal tract, eye .... Ulcerative colitis
Gastrointestinal tract, lymph nodes. Whipple's disease
Heart, skin, nervous system............ Rheumatic fever
Lungs, kidney, lymph nodes .... Tuberculosis
Penis, lymph nodes, rectum .... Lymphogranuloma venereum
Skin, eye .... Rheumatoid arthritis
Skin, kidney................................. Gout
Skin, lymph nodes........................ Serum sickness
Skin, lymph nodes........................ Streptobacillary fever
Skin, lymph nodes, bone .... Sporotrichosis
Skin, nervous system, aorta............ Syphilis
Throat, skin................................. Scarlet fever
Urethra, eye................................. Gonorrhea
Urethra, eye................................. Reiter's syndrome

Kidney:

Arteries, nervous system .... Glomerulonephritis
Arteries, nervous system .... Toxemia of pregnancy
Arteries, nervous system, gastrointestinal tract .... Periarteritis nodosa
Arteries, nervous system, heart ...... Essential hypertension
Arteries, nose, lung .... Wegener's granulomatosis
Blood, blood vessels, spleen .... Lupus erythematosus
Blood, bone, gastrointestinal tract ... Multiple myeloma
Blood, nervous system, spleen ...... Thrombotic thrombocytopenia purpura
Blood, spleen, skin....................... Leukemia
Blood, spleen, liver, nervous system. Malaria
Bone, eye, aorta .... Arachnodactyly
Bone, gastrointestinal tract .... Hyperparathyroidism
Bone, muscle .... Renal tubular acidosis
Bone, muscle, parathyroid gland ... Pseudohypoparathyroidism

314 · Table III. Organ Involvement as a Key to the Diagnosis of Systemic Disease

Gastrointestinal tract, liver .... Carbon tetrachloride poisoning
Heart, blood vessels, nervous system, skin .... Subacute bacterial endocarditis
Heart, gastrointestinal tract, muscle . Hypokalemia
Heart, lung, liver, nervous system ... Congestive heart failure
Islet cells, blood vessels, skin, eye ... Diabetes mellitus
Joints, skin, heart .... Gout
Liver, bone .... Echinococcosis
Liver, eye, nervous system .... Galactosemia
Liver, gums, heart .... Yellow fever
Liver, muscle, nervous system ...... Glycogen storage disease
Liver, nervous system, eye .... Weil's disease
Liver, spleen, adrenal gland .... Secondary amyloidosis
Lung, lymph nodes, adrenal gland ... Tuberculosis
Muscle, bone, eye .... Lignac-Fanconi syndrome
Nervous system, heart .... Chronic renal failure
Nose, lung .... Mucormycosis
Ovary, skin, bone .... Turner's syndrome
Skin, gastrointestinal tract .... Scleroderma

Large intestine:

Eye, joints .... Ulcerative colitis
Liver, lung .... Amebiasis
Liver, spleen .... Schistosomiasis
Nervous system, skin .... Pellagra

Liver:

Blood, blood vessels, spleen .... Lupus erythematosus
Blood, bone .... Osteopetrosis
Blood, gastrointestinal tract, nervous system .... Pernicious anemia
Blood, lymph nodes, spleen .... Macroglobulinemia
Blood, spleen, bone .... Mediterranean anemia
Blood, spleen, multiple organs ...... Sickle cell anemia
Blood, spleen, nervous system ...... Thrombotic thrombocytopenic purpura
Blood, spleen, skin, mucous membranes .... Aplastic anemia
Blood, spleen .... Myeloid metaplasia
Blood, spleen, nervous system ...... Malaria
Bone, lung .... Echinococcosis
Gastrointestinal tract, bladder, spleen .... Schistosomiasis
Gastrointestinal tract, eye, joints ... Ulcerative colitis
Gastrointestinal tract, heart, kidney . Yellow fever
Gastrointestinal tract, kidney .... Carbon tetrachloride poisoning
Gastrointestinal tract, lung .... Amebiasis
Gastrointestinal tract, nervous system .... Alcoholism
Gastrointestinal tract, skin, lung, heart .... Carcinoid syndrome
Heart, lungs .... Congestive heart failure
Lung, bone, nervous system .... Metastatic carcinoma
Lung, heart .... Q-fever
Lung, heart, nervous system .... Pulmonary emphysema
Lung, spleen, eye, lymph nodes ...... Miliary tuberculosis
Muscle, heart, nervous system .... Glycogen storage disease
Nervous system, arteries .... Phenothiazine intoxication
Nervous system, eye .... Wilson's disease
Nervous system, eye, kidney .... Weil's disease
Nervous system, eye, lymph nodes ... Toxoplasmosis
Nervous system, eye, spleen, blood .... Niemann-Pick disease
Nervous system, eye, spleen, bone ... Gargoylism
Nervous system, eye, spleen, kidney .... Galactosemia
Nervous system, kidney .... Polycystic disease
Pancreas, gastrointestinal tract ...... Chronic pancreatitis
Pancreas, lung .... Fibrocystic disease
Pancreas, thyroid, skin .... Hemochromatosis
Pituitary gland, spleen, endocrine glands .... Acromegaly
Skin, aorta, nervous system .... Syphilis
Skin, pancreas .... Kwashiorkor
Skin, lymph nodes, lungs .... Tularemia
Spleen, blood, lymph nodes .... Kala-azar
Spleen, bone, blood .... Gaucher's disease
Spleen, eye, skin .... Essential hypertriglyceridemia
Spleen, gastrointestinal tract, skin ... Hepatic failure
Spleen, joints .... Still's disease
Spleen, kidney .... Secondary amyloidosis
Spleen, lymph nodes .... Relapsing fever
Spleen, lymph nodes, nervous system .... Brucellosis
Spleen, skin, blood, bone .... Letterer-Siwe disease
Throat, spleen, lymph nodes .... Infectious mononucleosis

Lung:

Arteries, gastrointestinal tract, nervous system .... Periarteritis nodosa
Arteries, nose, kidney .... Wegener's granulomatosis
Bone, eye .... Hand-Schüller-Christian disease
Eye, skin .... Vitamin A deficiency
Gastrointestinal tract, liver .... Amebiasis
Gastrointestinal tract, liver, heart ... Carcinoid syndrome
Gastrointestinal tract, liver, spleen ... Schistosomiasis
Gastrointestinal tract, skin, spleen ... Typhoid fever
Heart, lung, nervous system .... Congestive heart failure
Heart, lung, nervous system, blood ... Pulmonary emphysema
Liver, bone .... Echinococcosis
Liver, bone, nervous system .... Metastatic carcinoma
Liver, heart .... Q-fever
Liver, spleen, skin, bone .... Letterer-Siwe disease
Lymph nodes, nervous system, kidney .... Tuberculosis
Lymph nodes, nervous system, skin, spleen .... Sarcoidosis
Lymph nodes, spleen, blood .... Histoplasmosis
Lymph nodes, spleen, blood .... Hodgkin's disease
Nervous system .... Nocardiosis
Nervous system, liver, spleen, eye ... Niemann-Pick disease
Nose, kidney, eye .... Mucormycosis
Pancreas, gastrointestinal tract ...... Fibrocystic disease
Skin, bone .... Coccidioidomycosis
Skin, gastrointestinal tract .... Scleroderma
Skin, kidney, bone .... Blastomycosis
Skin, lymph nodes .... Plague
Skin, lymph nodes, liver, spleen ... Tularemia
Throat, lymph nodes, liver, spleen ... Infectious mononucleosis

Lymph nodes:

Blood, spleen, liver, eye .... Lymphatic leukemia
Blood, spleen, liver, eye .... Macroglobulinemia
Blood, spleen, nervous system .... Thrombotic thrombocytopenic purpura
Eye, nervous system, liver .... Toxoplasmosis
Gastrointestinal tract, skin, joints ... Whipple's disease

Gastrointestinal tract, skin, spleen	Typhoid fever
Joints, skin	Serum sickness
Joints, skin	Streptobacillary fever
Joints, spleen, liver	Still's disease
Liver, spleen, blood	Kala-azar
Liver, spleen, blood, skin, bone	Letterer-Siwe disease
Liver, spleen, skin, throat	Infectious mononucleosis
Lung, blood, spleen	Histoplasmosis
Lung, eye, nervous system	Sarcoidosis
Lung, kidney, nervous system	Tuberculosis
Lung, liver, nervous system, bone	Metastatic carcinoma
Nervous system, spleen, skin	African trypanosomiasis
Penis, rectum, eye, joints	Lymphogranuloma venereum
Skin	Filariasis
Skin	Rubella
Skin, aorta, nervous system	Syphilis
Skin, joints, bone	Sporotrichosis
Skin, lung	Tularemia
Skin, lung	Plague
Skin, nervous system	Scrub typhus
Skin, nervous system	Chickenpox
Spleen, nervous system	Brucellosis
Spleen, nervous system, skin	Hodgkin's disease
Throat, nervous system	Listeriosis
Throat, nervous system, heart	Diphtheria
Throat, skin, joints	Scarlet fever
Throat, spleen, liver	Infectious mononucleosis

Mouth:

Adrenal gland, arteries, skin	Addison's disease
Blood, skin, spleen	Blood dyscrasias
Gastrointestinal tract	Peutz-Jegher's syndrome
Gastrointestinal tract, nervous system, skin	Pellagra
Liver, spleen, blood, bone	Letterer-Siwe disease
Skin, aorta, nervous system	Syphilis
Skin, gastrointestinal tract	Smallpox

Muscle:

Adrenal gland, arteries	Aldosteronism
Adrenal gland, sex organs, skin	Adrenogenital syndrome
Bone, nervous system	Rickets
Bone, skin, kidney	Pseudohypoparathyroidism
Eye, kidney, bone	Lignac-Fanconi syndrome
Eye, nails, nervous system	Trichinosis
Eye, nervous system, liver	Toxoplasmosis
Eye, nervous system, liver, kidney	Weil's disease
Eye, testicles	Myotonia atrophica
Gastrointestinal tract, nervous system	Cysticercosis
Heart, gastrointestinal tract, nervous system	Hypokalemia
Kidney, bone	Renal tubular acidosis
Kidney, bone, blood, heart, skin	Chronic renal failure
Liver, heart, nervous system	Glycogen storage disease
Parathyroid gland, nervous system	Hypoparathyroidism
Skin	Dermatomyositis
Skin, nervous system, nails, arteries	Acrodynia
Thyroid, nervous system, heart, skin	Hyperthyroidism
Thyroid, nervous system, heart, skin	Hypothyroidism
Thyroid, nervous system, heart, skin, bone	Cretinism
Tongue, heart, skin	Primary amyloidosis

Nails:

Esophagus, blood, tongue	Plummer-Vinson syndrome
Eye, liver, nervous system	Wilson's disease
Eye, skin	Vitamin A deficiency
Heart, blood vessels, kidney, spleen	Subacute bacterial endocarditis
Lung, heart, liver, nervous system	Pulmonary emphysema
Muscle, nervous system	Trichinosis
Parathyroid gland, bone, kidney	Hyperparathyroidism
Parathyroid gland, nervous system, muscle	Hypoparathyroidism
Pituitary gland, endocrine glands, skin	Hypopituitarism
Skin, nervous system, arteries	Acrodynia
Thyroid, nervous system, heart, skin	Hyperthyroidism
Thyroid, nervous system, heart, skin	Hypothyroidism

Nervous system:

Adrenal gland, arteries, muscle	Aldosteronism
Adrenal gland, throat, skin, blood vessels	Meningococcemia
Arteries, heart, eye	Atherosclerosis
Arteries, heart, eye, kidney	Essential hypertension
Arteries, lung, kidney, gastrointestinal tract	Periarteritis nodosa
Blood, blood vessels, many organs	Sickle cell anemia
Blood, blood vessels, spleen, kidney	Lupus erythematosus
Blood, bone	Osteopetrosis
Blood, bone, gastrointestinal tract	Multiple myeloma
Blood, bone, gastrointestinal tract	Lead poisoning
Blood, gastrointestinal tract, liver	Pernicious anemia
Blood, liver, spleen	Malaria
Blood, skin	Hemophilia
Blood, skin, spleen	Thrombotic thrombocytopenic purpura
Blood, spleen	Polycythemia vera
Blood vessel, skin	Rocky Mountain spotted fever
Bone, lung, liver	Metastatic carcinoma
Bone, muscle	Rickets
Bone, skin, heart	Mongolism
Eye, liver	Wilson's disease
Eye, liver, kidney	Galactosemia, Weil's disease
Eye, liver, lymph nodes	Toxoplasmosis
Eye, liver, spleen, bone	Gargoylism
Eye, liver, spleen, bone	Niemann-Pick disease
Eye, teeth, skin, nose	Congenital syphilis
Eye, testicles, bone	Laurence-Moon-Biedl syndrome
Gastrointestinal tract	Poliomyelitis
Gastrointestinal tract, blood, skin	Malabsorption syndrome

Table III. Organ Involvement as a Key to the Diagnosis of Systemic Disease

Gastrointestinal tract, heart	Digitalis intoxication
Gastrointestinal tract, skin	Pellagra
Gastrointestinal tract, skin, liver	Porphyria
Gums, skin	Dilantin intoxication
Heart	Beriberi
Heart, muscle, gastrointestinal tract	Hypokalemia
Heart, skin, kidney, spleen	Subacute bacterial endocarditis
Islet cells	Islet cell adenoma
Islet cells, blood vessels, kidney	Diabetes mellitus
Joints, heart, skin	Rheumatic fever
Joints, skin, lymph nodes	Serum sickness
Kidney, liver	Polycystic disease
Kidney, skin, gastrointestinal tract	Renal failure
Liver, arteries	Phenothiazine intoxication
Liver, gastrointestinal tract	Alcoholism
Liver, gastrointestinal tract	Hepatic failure
Liver, heart, muscle	Glycogen storage disease
Lung	Nocardiosis
Lung	Cryptococcosis
Lung, heart, liver	Chronic pulmonary emphysema
Lung, lymph nodes, kidney	Tuberculosis
Lung, lymph nodes, salivary gland, eye	Sarcoidosis
Lung, skin	Measles
Lymph nodes, spleen, liver	Brucellosis
Muscle, gastrointestinal tract	Cysticercosis
Muscle, nails, eye	Trichinosis
Nose, lung, kidney	Mucormycosis
Ovary, skin, bone	Menopause
Parathyroid gland, muscle, nails	Hypoparathyroidism
Salivary gland, pancreas, testicles	Mumps
Skin	Phenylpyruvic oligophrenia
Skin	Scrub typhus and epidemic typhus
Skin, aorta, nervous system	Syphilis
Skin, bone, adrenal gland	Neurofibromatosis
Skin, eye	Sturge-Weber syndrome
Skin, eye	Tuberosclerosis
Skin, gastrointestinal tract	Arsenic poisoning
Skin, lymph nodes	Chickenpox
Skin, nails, arteries	Acrodynia
Spleen, lymph nodes	African trypanosomiasis
Testicles, skin	Klinefelter's syndrome
Throat, heart	Diphtheria
Throat, lymph nodes	Listeriosis
Throat, lymph nodes, spleen	Infectious mononucleosis
Thyroid, bone, skin	Cretinism
Thyroid, heart, eye, skin	Hyperthyroidism
Thyroid, heart, skin	Hypothyroidism
Tongue, heart, muscle	Primary amyloidosis

Nose:

Nervous system	Leprosy
Nervous system, eye, lung, kidney	Mucormycosis
Nervous system, eye, lung, kidney, arteries	Wegener's midline granulomatosis
Skin, aorta, nervous system	Syphilis

Ovaries

Adrenal gland, skin	Stein-Leventhal syndrome
Adrenal gland, sex organs	Adrenogenital syndrome
Bone, liver, lung, nervous system	Metastatic carcinoma
Bone, skin, heart	Turner's syndrome
Bone, skin, nervous system	Menopause
Pituitary gland, endocrine glands, skin	Hypopituitarism

Pancreas:

Blood vessels, kidney, skin, nervous system	Diabetes mellitus
Gastrointestinal tract	Zollinger-Ellison syndrome
Kidney, liver, nervous system	Polycystic disease
Liver, gastrointestinal tract	Chronic pancreatitis
Liver, skin, testicles	Hemochromatosis
Lung, gastrointestinal tract	Fibrocystic disease
Nervous system	Islet cell adenoma

Parathyroid gland:

Bone, kidney, gastrointestinal tract, nails	Hyperparathyroidism
Muscle, nervous system, nails	Hypoparathyroidism

Parotid gland:

Joints, eye, skin	Sjögren's syndrome
Lung, lymph nodes, eye, skin	Sarcoidosis
Pancreas, testicles, nervous system	Mumps

Penis:

Lymph nodes, joints, rectum	Lymphogranuloma venereum
Lymph nodes, skin	Lymphogranuloma inguinale
Skin, aorta, nervous system	Syphilis
Urethra, eye, joints	Gonorrhea
Urethra, eye, joints	Reiter's syndrome

Pituitary gland:

Adrenal gland, arteries, bone, skin	Cushing's disease
Bone, eye, skin	Hand-Schüller-Christian disease
Bone, eye, skin	Pituitary adenoma
Bone, skin, liver, spleen	Acromegaly
Endocrine glands, skin	Hypopituitarism
Pancreas, gastrointestinal tract	Zollinger-Ellison syndrome

Rectum:

Joints, skin	Regional ileitis
Large intestine, eye, joints	Ulcerative colitis
Liver, gastrointestinal tract	Amebiasis
Penis, lymph nodes, joints	Lymphogranuloma venereum
Skin, aorta, nervous system	Syphilis

Sinuses:

Nose, lung, kidney	Mucormycosis
Nose, lung, kidney, arteries	Wegener's granulomatosis

Skin:

Adrenal gland, arteries, bone	Cushing's syndrome

Adrenal gland, arteries, gastrointestinal tract .... Addison's disease
Adrenal gland, blood vessels, nervous system .... Meningococcemia
Adrenal gland, sex organs, muscle .... Adrenogenital syndrome
Arteries, gastrointestinal tract, kidney, nervous system .... Periarteritis nodosa
Arteries, heart, tendons .... Essential hypercholesterolemia
Blood, blood vessels, spleen .... Sickle cell anemia
Blood, blood vessels, spleen, kidney, nervous system .... Lupus erythematosus
Blood, bone, gums .... Scurvy
Blood, bone, liver, spleen .... Letterer-Siwe disease
Blood, joints .... Hemophilia
Blood, spleen, mucous membranes .... Leukemia
Blood, spleen, mucous membranes .... Aplastic anemia
Blood, spleen, mucous membranes .... Thrombocytopenia purpura
Blood, spleen, mucous membranes, nervous system .... Thrombotic thrombocytopenic purpura
Blood vessels, islet cells, nervous system, kidney .... Diabetes mellitus
Blood vessels, nervous system .... Epidemic typhus
Bone, nervous system, liver .... Hypervitaminosis A
Eye, lung .... Vitamin A deficiency
Eye, spleen, liver, blood, bone .... Gaucher's disease
Gastrointestinal tract, blood, bone .... Malabsorption syndrome
Gastrointestinal tract, eye, joints ... Ulcerative colitis
Gastrointestinal tract, joints, lymph nodes .... Whipple's disease
Gastrointestinal tract, liver, lung, heart .... Carcinoid syndrome
Gastrointestinal tract, lung, heart ... Scleroderma
Gastrointestinal tract, lymph nodes, spleen, lung .... Typhoid fever
Gastrointestinal tract, nervous system .... Arsenic poisoning
Gastrointestinal tract, nervous system .... Pellagra
Gastrointestinal tract, nervous system, liver .... Porphyria
Heart, blood vessels, spleen, kidney, nervous system .... Subacute bacterial endocarditis
Heart, lymph nodes .... Chagas' disease
Joints, eye .... Rheumatoid arthritis
Joints, heart, nervous system .... Rheumatic fever
Joints, kidney, heart .... Gout
Joints, lymph nodes .... Streptobacillary fever
Joints, lymph nodes, heart .... Serum sickness
Joints, urine .... Alkaptonuria
Liver, gastrointestinal tract, nervous system .... Hepatic failure
Liver, pancreas .... Kwashiorkor
Liver, pancreas, testicles .... Hemochromatosis
Liver, spleen, eye .... Essential triglyceridemia
Lung, bone .... Coccidioidomycosis
Lung, bone, kidney .... North American blastomycosis
Lung, mucous membranes, nervous system .... Measles
Lung, lymph nodes, nervous system .... Sarcoidosis
Lymph nodes .... Filariasis
Lymph nodes .... Rubella
Lymph nodes, joints .... Sporotrichosis
Lymph nodes, joints, rectum .... Lymphogranuloma venereum
Lymph nodes, liver, spleen .... Relapsing fever
Lymph nodes, lung .... Plague
Lymph nodes, lung .... Tularemia
Lymph nodes, nervous system ...... Chickenpox
Lymph nodes, spleen .... Hodgkin's disease
Lymph nodes, spleen .... Spirillary rat-bite fever
Lymph nodes, spleen, nervous system .... Scrub typhus
Mucous membranes, gastrointestinal tract .... Smallpox
Muscle .... Dermatomyositis
Nervous system .... Phenylpyruvic oligophrenia
Nervous system, bone .... Tuberosclerosis
Nervous system, bone, adrenal gland .... Neurofibromatosis
Nervous system, bone, heart .... Mongolism
Nervous system, bone, liver, spleen .... Niemann-Pick disease
Nervous system, eye .... Sturge-Weber syndrome
Nervous system, gums .... Dilantin intoxication
Nervous system, lymph nodes ...... African trypanosomiasis
Nervous system, nails, arteries ...... Acrodynia
Ovaries, bone, sex organs .... Menopause
Ovaries, bone, sex organs, heart ... Turner's syndrome
Parathyroid gland, bone, kidney ... Primary hyperparathyroidism
Parathyroid gland, nervous system, muscle .... Hypoparathyroidism
Penis, aorta, nervous system .... Syphilis
Pituitary gland, bone, liver, spleen .... Acromegaly
Pituitary gland, endocrine glands .... Hypopituitarism
Testicle, sex organs, breast .... Klinefelter's syndrome
Throat, joints, kidney .... Scarlet fever
Throat, lymph nodes, spleen, liver .... Infectious mononucleosis
Thyroid, bone, nervous system ...... Cretinism
Thyroid, heart, nervous system ...... Hypothyroidism
Thyroid, heart, nervous system ...... Hyperthyroidism
Tongue, heart, muscle .... Primary amyloidosis

Spleen:

Blood .... Chronic myelogenous leukemia
Blood, blood vessels, kidney, nervous system .... Lupus erythematosus
Blood, blood vessels, liver, nervous system .... Sickle cell anemia
Blood, bone .... Osteopetrosis
Blood, bone, liver .... Mediterranean anemia
Blood, bone, liver, skin .... Letter-Siwe disease
Blood, gastrointestinal tract, nervous system .... Pernicious anemia
Blood, heart, nervous system .... Polycythemia vera
Blood, liver .... Myeloid metaplasia

Blood, liver, mucous membranes, skin .... Aplastic anemia
Blood, liver, nervous system .... Malaria
Blood, liver, skin, other organs .... Acute leukemia
Blood, lymph nodes .... Chronic lymphatic leukemia
Blood, lymph nodes, eye, liver .... Macroglobulinemia
Blood, nervous system .... Thrombotic thrombocytopenic purpura
Blood, nervous system, liver, bone .... Niemann-Pick disease
Blood vessels, skin, nervous system .... Rocky Mountain spotted fever
Eye, liver, bone, nervous system .... Gargoylism
Eye, liver, bone, skin .... Gaucher's disease
Eye, liver, kidney, nervous system .... Galactosemia
Gastrointestinal tract, liver, bladder .... Schistosomiasis
Heart, blood vessels, kidney, nervous system .... Subacute bacterial endocarditis
Joints, liver .... Still's disease
Liver, blood, skin .... Cirrhosis of the liver
Liver, eye, skin .... Hypertriglyceridemia
Liver, eye, skin, kidney .... Secondary amyloidosis
Liver, lymph nodes .... Kala-azar
Liver, lymph nodes .... Relapsing fever
Lung, lymph nodes, blood, eye .... Histoplasmosis
Lung, lymph nodes, kidney, nervous system .... Tuberculosis
Lung, lymph nodes, nervous system, eye .... Sarcoidosis
Lymph nodes, blood, nervous system .... Hodgkin's disease
Lymph nodes, liver, nervous system .... Brucellosis
Lymph nodes, skin .... Spirillary rat-bite fever

Nervous system, lymph nodes .... African trypanosomiasis
Pituitary gland, bone, liver .... Acromegaly
Skin, lymph nodes, lung .... Tularemia
Skin, lymph nodes, lung, gastrointestinal tract .... Typhoid fever
Throat, lymph nodes, liver .... Infectious mononucleosis

Testicles:

Eye, muscle, skin .... Myotonia atrophica
Eye, nervous system, bone .... Laurence-Moon-Biedl syndrome
Liver, pancreas, skin .... Hemochromatosis
Lung, lymph nodes, kidney .... Tuberculosis
Parotid glands, pancreas .... Mumps
Pituitary gland, endocrine gland, skin .... Hypopituitarism
Sex organs, skin, nervous system .... Klinefelter's syndrome

Throat:

Adrenal gland, blood vessels, nervous system .... Meningococcemia
Blood, spleen .... Aplastic anemia
Blood, spleen, other organs .... Leukemia
Heart, nervous system .... Diphtheria
Lymph nodes, liver, spleen .... Infectious mononucleosis
Lymph nodes, nervous system .... Listeriosis
Skin, lymph nodes .... Scarlet fever

Tongue:

Blood, esophagus, nails .... Plummer-Vinson syndrome
Blood, gastrointestinal tract, nervous system .... Pernicious anemia
Gastrointestinal tract, blood, bone .... Malabsorption syndrome
Heart, muscle, skin .... Primary amyloidosis
Heart, nervous system .... Beriberi
Pituitary gland, bone, liver, spleen .... Acromegaly

Table IV.

Systemic Disease With the Organs That Show Significant Functional or Pathologic Changes

Note: Many systemic diseases involve the same organs, but there is often one organ that is usually untouched by one disease or the other, or one organ that is distinctly involved by one disease or the other.

Acrodynia: skin, nails, hair, nervous system, muscle, arteries
Acromegaly: pituitary gland, bones, tongue, skin, liver, spleen, heart, nervous system, adrenal gland
Acute lymphatic leukemia: throat, lymph nodes, blood, spleen, skin, liver
Addison's disease: arteries, adrenal gland, skin, gastrointestinal tract, mouth
Adrenogenital syndrome: skin and hair, breasts, muscle, sex organs
African trypanosomiasis: skin, lymph nodes, nervous system, spleen
Alcaptonuria and ochronosis: eye, ears, skin, bone, joints, urine
Alcoholism: nervous system, liver, gastrointestinal tract, heart
Aldosteronism: adrenal gland, arteries, muscles, nervous system
Amebiasis: gastrointestinal tract, liver, lung
Ankylosing spondylitis: joints, heart, eye
Aplastic anemia: mucous membranes, skin, blood, liver, spleen
Arachnodactyly: bone, eyes, heart, aorta, kidney
Arsenic poisoning: skin, nerves, gastrointestinal tract
Atherosclerosis: arteries, heart, nervous system, eyes
Benzene poisoning: blood, skin
Beriberi: heart, nervous system
Brucellosis: lymph nodes, spleen, liver, nervous system
Carbon tetrachloride poisoning: liver, kidney, gastrointestinal tract
Carcinoid syndrome: skin, gastrointestinal tract, liver, lung, heart
Chagas' disease: eye, skin, lymph nodes, heart
Chickenpox: skin, nervous system, lymph nodes
Chronic congestive heart failure: heart, lungs, veins, liver, kidneys
Chronic hepatic failure: liver, skin, breasts, testes, spleen, blood, nervous system, gastrointestinal tract
Chronic lymphatic leukemia: lymph nodes, blood, spleen
Chronic myelogenous leukemia: spleen, blood
Chronic pancreatitis: pancreas, liver, islet cells, gastrointestinal tract
Chronic pulmonary emphysema: lung, heart, blood, nervous system, liver, bone
Chronic renal failure: kidney, heart, blood, muscle, nervous system, skin, gastrointestinal tract
Coccidioidomycosis: lung, skin, bone.
Congenital syphilis: eye, bone, teeth, ear, nervous system
Cretinism: thyroid, bone, nervous system, skin, muscle
Cryptococcosis: lung, nervous system
Cushing's syndrome: skin, arteries, adrenal gland, bone
Cysticercosis: subcutaneous tissue, muscle, nervous system, gastrointestinal tract
Dermatomyositis: skin, muscles
Diabetes mellitus: pancreas, eye, arteries, nervous system, skin, kidney
Digitalis intoxication: nervous system, heart, gastrointestinal tract, eyes
Dilantin intoxication: skin, gums, nervous system
Diphtheria: throat, lymph nodes, heart, nervous system
Disseminated histoplasmosis: lung, lymph nodes, spleen, blood, adrenal gland, eye
Echinococcosis: liver, lung, bone, kidney
Epidemic typhus: skin, blood vessels, nervous system
Essential hypercholesterolemia: arteries, heart, skin, eye, tendons
Essential hypertension: arteries, heart, nervous system, kidneys, eyes
Essential hypertriglyceridemia: eye, liver, spleen, skin
Fibrocystic disease: pancreas, gastrointestinal tract, lungs, liver
Filariasis: skin, lymph node
Galactosemia: eye, liver, spleen, nervous system, kidney
Gargoylism: nervous system, eye, heart, liver, spleen, bone
Gaucher's disease: eye, spleen, liver, skin, blood, bone
Glycogen storage disease: liver, muscle, heart, brain, kidney
Gonorrhea: urethra, genitourinary tract, joints, eye
Gout: skin, joints, kidney, arteries
Hemophilia: blood, skin, joints, gastrointestinal tract, nervous system
Histiocytosis X (Hand-Schüller-Christian disease): eye, skin, bone, lungs
Histiocytosis X (Letterer-Siwe disease): skin, liver blood, spleen, lymph nodes, lungs, bone, gums, mouth
Hodgkin's disease: lymph nodes, spleen, skin
Hyperparathyroidism: see Primary Hyperparathyroidism
Hyperthyroidism: thyroid, eyes, arteries, heart, nervous system, skin, muscle
Hypervitaminosis A: bone, nervous system, liver, skin
Hypokalemia: nervous system, muscle, gastrointestinal tract, heart, kidneys
Hypoparathyroidism: parathyroid gland, nervous system, skin, eye
Hypopituitarism: pituitary gland, skin, testicles or ovaries, arteries, thyroid, adrenal gland
Hypothyroidism: thyroid, skin, nervous system, muscle, heart
Idiopathic hemochromatosis: liver, spleen, skin, pancreas, testes, heart

Table IV. Systemic Disease With Organs Showing Significant Changes

Idiopathic thrombocytopenic purpura: blood, skin, mucous membranes, gastrointestinal tract
Infectious mononucleosis: throat, lymph nodes, liver, spleen, skin, nervous system
Islet cell adenoma: pancreas, sympathetic nervous system, central nervous system
Kala-azar: spleen, liver, blood, lymph nodes
Klinefelter's syndrome: testicles, breast, skin, nervous system
Kwashiorkor: skin, liver, pancreas
Laurence-Moon-Biedl syndrome: nervous system, testicles or ovaries, eyes, bone
Lead poisoning: nervous system, gums, bone, gastrointestinal tract, blood
Lignac-Fanconi syndrome: muscle, eye, kidney, bone
Listeriosis: throat, eye, nervous system, lymph node
Lupus erythematosus: skin, blood, joints, kidney, spleen, liver, heart, nervous system
Lymphogranuloma venereum: skin, lymph nodes, eye, joints, rectum
Macroglobulinemia: eye, arteries, lymph nodes, blood, spleen, liver
Malabsorption syndrome: gastrointestinal tract, tongue, skin, nervous system, blood, bone
Malaria: spleen, blood, liver, nervous system
Measles: skin, eye, respiratory tract, nervous system
Mediterranean anemia: blood, spleen, liver, bone
Meningococcemia: throat, nervous system, adrenal gland, skin, blood vessels
Menopause: ovaries, skin, mucous membranes, bone, nervous system
Metastatic carcinoma: liver, lung, nervous system, bone
Mongolism: nervous system, skin, bone, heart
Mucormycosis: eye, nose, lung, nervous system, heart, kidneys
Multiple myeloma: blood, bone, kidney, gastrointestinal tract, nervous system
Mumps: parotid glands, testicles, pancreas, nervous system
Myelofibrosis with myeloid metaplasia: blood, liver, spleen
Myotonia atrophica: muscles, eyes, testes, hair
Neurofibromatosis: skin, nervous system, bone, adrenal gland
Niemann-Pick disease: nervous system, eye, skin, liver, spleen, blood, lungs, bone
Nocardiosis: lung, nervous system
North American blastomycosis: skin, lung, kidney, bone
Osteopetrosis: bone, blood, liver, spleen, nervous system
Pellagra: skin, nervous system, gastrointestinal tract
Periarteritis nodosa: arteries, gastrointestinal tract, skin, nerves, lungs, kidneys
Pernicious anemia: blood, gastrointestinal tract, nervous system, liver, spleen, tongue
Peutz-Jegher's syndrome: intestines, blood, mucous membranes
Phenothiazine intoxication: liver, nervous system, arteries
Phenylpyruvic oligophrenia: skin, hair, brain
Pheochromocytoma: adrenal gland, arteries, heart
Plague: skin, lymph node, lungs
Plummer-Vinson syndrome: blood, tongue, esophagus
Poliomyelitis: nervous system, gastrointestinal tract, heart
Polycystic disease: kidneys, brain, liver, pancreas
Polycythemia vera: blood, veins, nervous system, heart, spleen
Porphyria: nervous system, gastrointestinal tract, skin, blood
Primary hyperparathyroidism: parathyroid gland, skin and nails, bone, kidney, gastrointestinal tract, teeth
Primary systemic amyloidosis: tongue, heart, skin, muscle, nervous system
Pseudohypoparathyroidism: bone, muscle, parathyroid gland, kidney
Q-fever: lungs, liver, heart
Reiter's syndrome: urethra, eye, joints
Relapsing fever: skin, liver, spleen, lymph nodes
Renal tubular acidosis: kidney, bone, muscle
Rheumatic fever: joints, skin, heart, nervous system
Rheumatoid arthritis: joints, eye, skin
Rickets: bones, nervous system, muscles
Rocky Mountain spotted fever: skin, blood vessels, spleen, nervous system
Rubella: skin, lymph nodes, fetus
Sarcoidosis: eye, lung, nervous system, skin, lymph nodes, spleen, salivary gland, bone
Scarlet fever: throat, lymph nodes, skin, joints
Schistosomiasis: gastrointestinal tract, liver, bladder, spleen
Scleroderma: skin, gastrointestinal tract, lung, heart, kidney, arteries
Scrub typhus: skin, lymph nodes, spleen, nervous system
scurvy: skin, blood, bone, gums
Secondary amyloidosis: eye, liver, spleen, kidney, adrenal glands
Serum sickness: skin, joints, lymph nodes, nerves
Sickle cell anemia: blood, eye, spleen, liver, skin, heart, nervous system, veins, arteries, intestines
Smallpox: skin, mucous membranes, gastrointestinal tract
Spirillary rat-bite fever: skin, lymph nodes, spleen
Sporotrichosis: skin, lymph nodes, joints, bone
Still's disease: joints, liver, spleen, heart, lymph nodes
Streptobacillary fever: skin, lymph nodes, joints
Sturge-Weber syndrome: skin, nervous system, eye
Subacute bacterial endocarditis: heart, eye, skin, nails, spleen, kidney, nervous system
Syphilis: skin, lymph nodes, aorta, nervous system
Thrombotic thrombocytopenic purpura: blood, central nervous system, liver, spleen, lymph nodes, skin, kidney
Toxoplasmosis: lymph nodes, eye, muscles, liver, brain
Trichinosis: eye, nails, muscle, nervous system
Tuberculosis: lung, lymph node, kidney, adrenal gland, nervous system
Tuberculosis, miliary: lung, liver, spleen, lymph node, eye, nervous system
Tuberosclerosis: skin, nervous system, bone

Table IV. Systemic Disease With Organs Showing Significant Changes

Tularemia: skin, lymph nodes, lungs, liver and spleen

Turner's syndrome: ovaries, bone, skin, breasts, heart, kidney

Typhoid fever: gastrointestinal tract, lymph nodes, skin, spleen, lungs

Ulcerative colitis: gastrointestinal tract, eye, joints, skin, liver

Vitamin A deficiency: eye, skin, lungs

Wegener's granulomatosis: nose, sinuses, lungs, kidney, blood vessels

Weil's disease: eye, liver, nervous system, kidney, muscle

Whipple's disease: gastrointestinal tract, lymph nodes, joints, skin, blood

Wilson's disease: nervous system, eye, liver, bone

Yellow fever: liver, gums, heart, kidney

Zollinger-Ellison syndrome: pancreas, gastrointestinal tract, other endocrine glands

Table V.

Local Disease as a Symptom of Systemic Disease

Abortion
1. Hypothyroidism
2. Adrenal insufficiency
3. Sheehan's syndrome
4. Diabetes mellitus
5. Syphilis

Abscess anywhere
1. Avitaminosis
2. Diabetes mellitus
3. Cushing's syndrome
4. Cirrhosis of liver
5. Multiple myeloma
6. Lupus erythematosus
7. Agranulocytosis
8. Agammaglobulinemia

Acanthosis nigricans
1. Gastrointestinal malignancy

Acne vulgaris
1. Cushing's syndrome

Adenoma of the parathyroid glands
1. Multiple endocrine adenoma

Agranulocytosis
1. Lupus erythematosus
2. Infectious mononucleosis
3. Typhoid fever
4. Brucellosis
5. Tuberculosis
6. Viral infections

Anemia, hypochromic
1. Hypothyroidism
2. Cirrhosis of the liver
3. Malabsorption syndrome
4. Anemia, pernicious

Aneurysm, aortic
1. Syphilis
2. Marfan's syndrome

Aneurysm, berry
1. Polycystic kidney

Aortic insufficiency
1. Syphilis
2. Rheumatic valvulitis
3. Bacterial endocarditis

Appendicitis
1. Carcinoid tumor
2. Tuberculosis
3. Actinomycosis
4. Enterobiasis

Arthritis
1. Gout
2. Gonorrhea
3. Tuberculosis
4. Lupus erythematosus
5. Reiter's disease
6. Drug allergy
7. Rheumatic fever
8. Haverhill fever

Asthma, bronchial
1. Parasitic disease
2. Periarteritis nodosa
3. Tuberculosis
4. Coccidioidomycosis

Atrial fibrillation
1. Rheumatic fever
2. Thyrotoxicosis
3. Essential hypertension
4. Digitalis intoxication

Balanitis
1. Reiter's disease

Basal cell carcinoma
1. Cirrhosis of liver

Bronchitis
1. Wegener's granulomatosis
2. Fibrocystic disease
3. Periarteritis nodosa
4. Typhoid fever

Bursitis
1. Gout
2. Rheumatoid arthritis

Calculus, renal
1. Hyperparathyroidism
2. Vitamin A deficiency
3. Gout
4. Cystinuria
5. Vitamin A intoxication

Cataract
1. Myotonia atrophica
2. Galactosemia
3. Diabetes mellitus
4. Hypoparathyroidism

Cerebellar degeneration
1. Alcoholism
2. Dilantin intoxication
3. Malignancy

Cerebral hemorrhage
1. Mycotic aneurysm
2. Periarteritis nodosa
3. Essential hypertension
4. Macroglobulinemia
5. Syphilitic aneurysm
6. Thrombocytopenia purpura
7. Polycythemia vera
8. Leukemia

Cerebral thrombosis
1. Buerger's disease
2. Polycythemia vera
3. Periarteritis nodosa
4. Sickle cell anemia
5. Macroglobulinemia

  6. Thrombotic thrombocytopenic purpura
  7. Syphilis
  8. Lupus erythematosus
Cholelithiasis
  1. Hereditary spherocytosis
  2. Sickle cell anemia
  3. Diabetes mellitus
  4. Familial hypercholesterolemia
Chorioretinitis
  1. Syphilis
  2. Tuberculosis
  3. Toxoplasmosis
  4. Histoplasmosis
  5. Sarcoidosis
Cirrhosis of the liver
  1. Malaria
  2. Hemochromatosis
  3. Wilson's disease
  4. Schistosomiasis
  5. Kala-azar
Colitis
  1. Carcinoid syndrome
  2. Zollinger-Ellison syndrome
  3. Whipple's disease
  4. Malabsorption syndrome
  5. Amebiasis
  6. Ulcerative colitis
  7. Regional ileitis
Common cold
  1. Agammaglobulinemia
  2. Infectious mononucleosis
  3. Leukemia
  4. Multiple myeloma
  5. Wegener's midline infections
  6. Systemic viral infections
  7. Guillain-Barré syndrome
  8. Fibrocystic disease
Conjunctivitis
  1. Gonorrhea
  2. Reiter's disease
  3. Exanthema (measles, etc.)
  4. Riboflavin deficiency
Cor pulmonale
  1. Carcinoid tumor
  2. Hemochromatosis
Coronary insufficiency
  1. Syphilitic aortitis
  2. Rheumatic valvulitis of aortic valves
Cystitis
  1. Tuberculosis
Dementia
  1. Wilson's disease
  2. Syphilis
  3. Thiamine deficiency
  4. Pellagra
  5. Thrombotic thrombocytopenic purpura
  6. Macroglobulinemia
  7. Porphyria
  8. Bromide intoxication
Diabetes insipidus
  1. Pituitary adenoma
  2. Sarcoidosis
  3. Hand-Schüller-Christian disease
Diabetes mellitus
  1. Cushing's syndrome
  2. Acromegaly
  3. Hemochromatosis
  4. Hyperthyroidism
  5. Pheochromocytoma
Dislocation of joint
  1. Myotonia atrophica
  2. Hyperparathyroidism
Dupuytren's contracture
  1. Cirrhosis of the liver
Encephalitis
  1. Cysticercosis
  2. Cryptococcosis
  3. Rheumatic fever
  4. Trichinosis
Encephalopathy
  1. Thiamine deficiency
  2. Hypokalemia
  3. Porphyria
  4. Thrombotic thrombocytopenia purpura
  5. Pernicious anemia
  6. Hypoparathyroidism
Epididymitis
  1. Mumps
  2. Tuberculosis
  3. Gonorrhea
Erythema nodosum
  1. Iodide and bromide toxicity
  2. Tuberculosis
  3. Rheumatic fever
  4. Coccidioidomycosis
  5. Rheumatoid arthritis
Esophageal stricture
  1. Scleroderma
  2. Hodgkin's disease
Fibroma subcutaneous
  1. Von Recklinghausen's disease
Fistula in ano
  1. Tuberculosis
  2. Ulcerative colitis
  3. Actinomycosis
  4. Regional ileitis
Fracture
  1. Hyperparathyroidism
  2. Rickets
  3. Cushing's syndrome
  4. Osteopetrosis
  5. Multiple myeloma
  6. Osteomalacia
  7. Renal disease
Gastroenteritis
  1. Typhoid fever
  2. Carcinoid tumor
  3. Tuberculosis
  4. Multiple myeloma
  5. Pernicious anemia
  6. Trichinosis
  7. Amebiasis
  8. Sprue, idiopathic
  9. Avitaminosis

Table V. Local Disease as a Symptom of Systemic Disease

10. Poliomyelitis
11. Porphyria
12. Lead poisoning
13. Digitalis intoxication

Gingivitis
1. Dilantin toxicity
2. Monocytic leukemia
3. Hand-Schüller-Christian disease

Glaucoma
1. Diabetes mellitus

Glomerulonephritis
1. Lupus erythematosus
2. Periarteritis nodosa
3. Wegener's granulomatosis
4. Subacute bacterial endocarditis

Glossitis
1. Vitamin deficiency
2. Pernicious anemia
3. Iron-deficiency anemia
4. Sprue, idiopathic

Gout
1. Polycythemia vera
2. Lead intoxication
3. Leukemia
4. Chlorothiazide therapy

Hemorrhoids
1. Cirrhosis of the liver

Hernia, inguinal
1. Mongolism
2. Arachnodactyly

Hydrocephalus
1. Toxoplasmosis
2. Tuberculosis

Hydronephrosis
1. Tuberculosis

Infarction, pulmonary
1. Polycythemia vera
2. Sickle cell anemia
3. Congestive heart failure

Infarction, splenic
1. Polycythemia vera
2. Sickle cell anemia
3. Lymphoma
4. Leukemia
5. Cirrhosis of the liver
6. Subacute bacterial endocarditis

Infectious polyneuritis
1. Infectious mononucleosis
2. Diabetes mellitus
3. Porphyria

Iritis
1. Boeck's sarcoid
2. Histoplasmosis
3. Tuberculosis

Islet cell adenoma
1. Multiple endocrine adenomata

Keratitis
1. Hyperparathyroidism
2. Congenital syphilis

Laryngitis
1. Tuberculosis
2. Syphilis
3. Diphtheria

Lens, dislocation of
1. Arachnodactyly

Loeffler's syndrome
1. Amoebiasis
2. Schistosomiasis

Lymphadenitis, generalized
1. Infectious mononucleosis
2. Brucellosis
3. Hodgkin's disease
4. Lymphatic leukemia
5. Typhoid fever
6. Tuberculosis
7. Histoplasmosis

Lymphadenitis, local
1. Tuberculosis
2. Syphilis
3. Lymphogranuloma venereum
4. Tularemia
5. Actinomycosis
6. Hodgkin's disease

Malunion of fracture
1. Osteomalacia
2. Hyperparathyroidism
3. Idiopathic sprue
4. Cushing's syndrome
5. Scurvy
6. Tuberculous osteomyelitis
7. Ovarian insufficiency

Manic-depressive psychosis
1. Hyperparathyroidism
2. Hypoparathyroidism
3. Hyperthyroidism
4. Cushing's syndrome
5. Carcinoid tumor
6. Brucellosis
7. Islet cell tumor
8. Ovarian insufficiency
9. Porphyria

Mastitis
1. Cirrhosis of the liver
2. Thorazine intoxication

Mitral stenosis
1. Rheumatic fever
2. Subacute or acute bacterial endocarditis
3. Lupus erythematosus

Myasthenia gravis
1. Metastatic carcinoma
2. Thymoma
3. Hyperthyroidism

Myositis
1. Trichinosis
2. Dermatomyositis
3. Periarteritis nodosa

Nephritis
1. Lupus erythematosus
2. Amyloidosis
3. Malaria
4. Multiple myeloma
5. Diabetes mellitus

Table V. Local Disease as a Symptom of Systemic Disease

6. Subacute bacterial endocarditis
7. Leptospirosis hemorrhagica
8. Yellow fever

Obesity, exogenous
1. Cushing's disease
2. Pituitary dystrophy
3. Myxedema
4. Laurence-Moon-Biedl syndrome

Optic neuritis
1. Diabetes mellitus
2. Syphilis

Orchitis
1. Mumps
2. Brucellosis
3. Tuberculosis
4. Leprosy
5. Gonorrhea
6. Syphilis

Osteomalacia
1. Vitamin D deficiency
2. Celiac disease
3. Fibrocystic disease

Osteomyelitis
1. Tuberculosis
2. Syphilis
3. Amyloidosis
4. Multiple myeloma
5. Metastatic carcinoma

Pancreatitis
1. Periarteritis nodosa
2. Mumps

Paralysis agitans
1. Thorazine intoxication
2. Wilson's disease
3. Rheumatic fever

Paralytic ileus
1. Hypokalemia
2. Diabetic acidosis
3. Subacute bacterial endocarditis with embolism

Peptic ulcer
1. Islet cell adenoma (Zollinger-Ellison syndrome)
2. Cushing's syndrome
3. Uremia

Pericarditis
1. Tuberculosis
2. Uremia
3. Rheumatic fever

Peritonitis
1. Tuberculosis
2. Cirrhosis of the liver
3. Meig's syndrome
4. Lupus erythematosus

Pharyngitis
1. Leukemia
2. Agammaglobulinemia
3. Infectious mononucleosis
4. Diphtheria
5. Herpangina
6. Guillain-Barré syndrome

Pinguecula
1. Hodgkin's disease
2. Gaucher's disease
3. Ochronosis

Platybasia
1. Osteomalacia
2. Rickets
3. Paget's disease

Pleurisy
1. Tuberculosis
2. Lupus erythematosus
3. Rheumatic fever
4. Congestive heart failure
5. Nocardiosis

Pneumonia
1. Tuberculosis
2. Histoplasmosis
3. Coccidioidomycosis
4. Infectious mononucleosis
5. Typhoid fever
6. Tularemia
7. Sarcoidosis
8. Periarteritis nodosa
9. Cystic fibrosis

Pneumothorax, spontaneous
1. Arachnodactyly
2. Tuberculosis

Polycythemia vera
1. Cushing's syndrome
2. Congestive heart failure
3. Congenital heart disease
4. Hypernephroma
5. Lindau-von Hippel disease

Porphyria
1. Lead intoxication
2. Hodgkin's disease
3. Alcoholism

Priapism
1. Leukemia
2. Sickle cell anemia

Psoriasis
1. Rheumatoid arthritis
2. Hyperparathyroidism

Pyelonephritis
1. Tuberculosis
2. Diabetes mellitus
3. Multiple myeloma
4. Arachnodactyly
5. Hypernephroma

Raynaud's disease
1. Periarteritis nodosa
2. Macroglobulinemia
3. Paroxysmal cold hemoglobinuria
4. Scleroderma
5. Lupus erythematosus

Retinal detachment
1. Diabetes mellitus
2. Cysticercosis

Rhinitis
1. Wegener's granulomatosis

Scleritis
1. Ulcerative colitis
2. Rheumatoid arthritis

Table V. Local Disease as a Symptom of Systemic Disease

   3. Syphilis
   4. Tuberculosis
   5. Sarcoidosis
Stomatitis
   1. Diabetes mellitus
   2. Riboflavin deficiency
   3. Plummer-Vinson syndrome
Thrombophlebitis
   1. Ulcerative colitis
   2. Macroglobulinemia
   3. Pancreatic carcinoma
   4. Polycythemia vera
   5. Sickle cell anemia
Urethritis
   1. Reiter's disease
   2. Gonorrhea
Vaginitis
   1. Diabetes mellitus
Xanthelasma
   1. Diabetes mellitus
   2. Myxedema
   3. Biliary cirrhosis
   4. Familial xanthomatosis

Table VI.
Laboratory Work-up of Systemic Diseases

Acromegaly: skull x-ray, x-ray of hands, serum phosphorus, FBS

Actinomycosis: smear for sulfur granules, culture of skin lesions

Addison's disease: urinary 17-hydroxycorticosteroids and 17-ketosteroids before and after ACTH

Adrenogenital syndrome: urinary 17-ketosteroids and 17-hydroxycorticosteroids, ACTH test, dexamethasone suppression test

Albright's syndrome: x-ray of long bones

Alcaptonuria: urinary homogentisic acid, x-ray of spine

Aldosteronism: serum electrolytes, 24-hour urine potassium, 24-hour urine aldosterone

Amebiasis: stool for ova and parasites, rectal biopsy

Amyloidosis (secondary and primary): Congo red test, rectal biopsy, liver biopsy, gingival biopsy

Anthrax: smear and culture, skin biopsy

Aplastic anemia: bone marrow, lymph node biopsy

Banti's syndrome: liver functions, bone marrow examination, spleen-liver ratio, epinephrine test

Beriberi: serum pyruvic acid, urine thiamine after load

Bilharziasis: stool or urine sediment for eggs

Blastomycosis: culture of pus from skin lesions (or other tissue), skin test

Boeck's sarcoid: Kveim test, x-ray of hands, scalene node biopsy, tuberculin test

Botulism: clinical diagnosis, culture of stool and food

Brucellosis: serologic tests, skin tests, blood cultures

Bubonic plague: culture of bubo, blood or sputum; animal inoculation, serologic tests

Carbon tetrachloride poisoning: liver function tests, infrared spectrometry, liver biopsy

Carcinoid syndrome: urine 5-HIAA, exploratory laparotomy

Celiac disease: D-xylose absorption, urine 5-HIAA, mucosal biopsy, small bowel series

Chagas' disease: blood smear and culture, smear or culture of CSF, bone marrow or tissue biopsy, animal inoculation, serologic tests

Cirrhosis of the liver: liver function tests, liver biopsy

Craniopharyngioma: skull x-ray, PBI, urine 17-ketosteroids and 17-hydroxysteroids, FBS, urine HPG (human pituitary gonadotropin)

Cretinism: x-ray for bone age, PBI

Cryptococcosis: spinal fluid examination, smear and culture, sputum or blood culture

Cushing's syndrome: urinary 17-ketosteroids and 17-hydroxysteroids before and after ACTH, dexamethasone suppression test

Cystic fibrosis of the pancreas: quantitative sweat test, duodenal drainage, chest x-ray, stool for fat and trypsin

Cysticercosis: biopsy of subcutaneous cysticerci

Cystinosis: slit-lamp examination for crystals, urine for cystine

Cytomegalic inclusion disease: clinical diagnosis, urine for intraepithelial inclusion bodies

Dengue: viral isolation from blood or serum, serologic test

Dermatomyositis: muscle biopsy, electromyography, sedimentation rate, serum transaminase, LDH and aldolase, *Trichinella* skin test

Diabetes mellitus: FBS, 2-hour postprandial blood sugar, fractional urines, cortisone glucose tolerance test

Digitalis intoxication: ECG, observe effect of infusion of potassium on heart rate, atropine test

Di Guglielmo's disease: bone marrow, peripheral blood study

Diphtheria: nose and throat culture on Loeffler's slant

Diphyllobothrium latum: stool for eggs of the worm, x-ray following a barium meal

Echinococcosis: x-ray of long bones, Casoni intracutaneous test, serologic tests, liver biopsy of cyst wall

Eclampsia: uric acid, renal function tests, renal biopsy, urinalysis

Emphysema: pulmonary function tests, arterial oxygen saturation, CO_2

Erythroblastosis fetalis: bilirubin, CBC, agglutination of red cells by antiglobulin serum in human or bovine serum albumin, Coombs' test

Fanconi syndrome: x-ray (pelvis, scapula, femur, humerus, ribs); urinary amino acid and glucose, calcium, potassium, phosphates, urates; serum alkaline phosphatase, uric acid

Filariasis: blood smears for microfilariae, *Dirofilaria* antigen intradermal test, complement-fixation test

Galactosemia: urinary galactose, galactose tolerance test, erythrocyte assay of the enzyme uridyl-diphosphogalactose transferase

Gaucher's disease: bone marrow, x-ray of femur

General paresis: spinal fluid examination, Wassermann test of blood and cerebrospinal fluid, TPI, FTA

Gigantism: skull x-ray, FBS, serum phosphorus, x-ray of long bones

Glycogen-storage disease: liver biopsy, glucose tolerance test, galactose tolerance test, epinephrine test

Gonorrhea: urethral or vaginal smear and culture

Gout: serum or urinary uric acid, synovialysis for urate crystals, x-ray of bones

Graves' disease: see Hyperthyroidism, this table

Hand-Schüller-Christian disease: x-ray of skull, bone biopsy, bone marrow examination

Hansen's disease: Wade's scraped incision procedure, x-ray of hands and feet, biopsy of skin, nerves

Hartnup disease: urinary amino acid, indican and indoleacetic acid

Hashimoto's thyroiditis: PBI, RAI, serum antibodies

Haverhill fever: agglutination titer, fluid aspiration from affected joint or abscess for *Streptobacillus moniliformis*

Heart failure: vital capacity, venous pressure and circulation time, chest x-ray, ECG

Hemochromatosis: serum iron and iron-binding capacity, liver or skin biopsy, glucose tolerance test, bone marrow biopsy

Hemolytic anemia: radioactive-chromium-tagged red cell survival, measurement of fecal urobilinogen excretion, Coombs' test, blood smears

Hemophilia: blood coagulation time, thromboplastin generation test

Hepatolenticular degeneration: urine amino acid and copper, serum ceruloplasmin, liver function tests, liver biopsy with histochemical staining of copper by rubeanic acid, slit-lamp examination of the cornea

Histoplasmosis: sputum culture, bone marrow smear and culture and animal inoculation, spinal tap, skin test, serologic tests, liver biopsy

Hodgkin's disease: lymph node biopsy, bone marrow examination, lymphangiogram

Hookworm disease: stool for ova and parasites, eosinophil count

Hurler's syndrome: urinary acid mucopolysaccharides, tissue biopsy

Hyperaldosteronism: serum potassium, sodium, bicarbonate, pH, urine potassium, 24-hour urine aldosterone, plasma renin, exploratory surgery

Hypernephroma: urinalysis, intravenous or retrograde pyelogram, renal angiogram, exploratory laparotomy

Hyperparathyroidism: serum calcium, phosphorus alkaline phosphatase, x-ray of mandible and long bones, urinary calcium, exploratory surgery

Hypersplenism: CBC, red cell survival, spleen-liver ratio, spleen scan, bone marrow, epinephrine test

Hypertension, essential: ECG, renal functions, renal biopsy, clinical observations, tests to exclude secondary hypertension

Hyperthyroidism: PBI, RAI uptake, T_3 uptake, BMR

Hypoparathyroidism: serum calcium, phosphorus, 24-hour urine calcium, alkaline phosphatase, skull x-ray

Hypopituitarism: PBI, 17-ketosteroids, 17-hydroxycorticosteroids, skull x-ray, visual fields, Hickey-Hare test, glucose tolerance test, urine HPG

Hypothyroidism: BMR, PBI, ECG, serum cholesterol, RAI uptake

Hypovitaminosis: see specific vitamin deficiency

Infectious mononucleosis: heterophil antibody titer, smear for atypical lymphocytes, liver function tests

Insulinoma (see Islet cell tumor, this table): Blood sugar, glucose tolerance test, plasma insulin concentration, 36-hour fast, tolbutamide tolerance test, exploratory laparotomy

Iron deficiency anemia: serum iron and iron-binding capacity, CBC, bone marrow for hemosiderin content

Islet cell tumor: FBS, glucose tolerance test, 36-hour fast, tolbutamide tolerance test, exploratory laparotomy

Kala-azar: blood smear, bone marrow or splenic aspirate for parasites, serologic test

Klinefelter's syndrome: sex chromatin pattern, testicular biopsy, urine HPG (human pituitary gonadotropin)

Kwashiorkor: serum albumin, CBC

Laennec's cirrhosis: Bromsulfalein, cephalin-flocculation test, serum protein and albumin/globulin ratio, bilirubin, liver biopsy

Larva migrans, visceral: eosinophil count and serum globulin, skin testing, serologic tests, liver biopsy

Lead intoxication: serum and urine lead content; urine for ALA, coproporphyrin, FEPP; test dose of EDTA

Leishmaniasis: CBC, serum protein, cephalin-flocculation, thymol turbidity, blood and bone marrow smears for parasites

Leprosy: Wade's scraped incision procedure, culture of lesion, biopsy of skin nerves, x-ray of hands and feet, histamine test, lepromin test

Leptospirosis: animal inoculation, blood and urine culture, agglutinin titer, complement-fixation test, spinal tap, muscle biopsy

Letterer-Siwe disease: x-ray of bones, bone marrow or lymph node biopsy

Leukemia: hematologic examination of peripheral blood and bone marrow, total leukocyte count, BMR, uric acid, serum vitamin B_{12} concentration and iron-binding capacity

Listeriosis: culture (blood or sputum) for microorganism, serum agglutinin titer, bone marrow biopsy

Lupus erythematosus: serologic tests, Coombs' test, clotting time, L.E. cell preparations; skin, tissue, muscle, lymph node, or kidney biopsy

Lymphogranuloma inguinale: Lygranum test, serologic tests, tissue or node biopsy

Lymphogranuloma venereum: serum electrophoresis, Frei test, serologic tests

Lymphoma (see Hodgkin's disease): lymph node biopsy; x-ray of chest, G.I. tract, G.U. system, bones; differential count, bone marrow; alkaline phosphatase, spinal tap

Lymphosarcoma: lymph node biopsy; x-ray of chest, G.I. tract, skeletal system; spinal tap; thoracocentesis; paracentesis; bone marrow

McArdle's syndrome: liver biopsy, FBS, enzyme assay of muscle phosphorylase

Macroglobulinemia: serum electrophoresis and ultracentrifugation, Sia water test

Malabsorption syndrome: mucosal biopsy; serum protein, carotene, calcium, cholesterol, potassium, magnesium; prothrombin time, D-xylose and glucose tolerance test, stool for fat and trypsin, ^{131}I triolein and ^{131}I oleic acid, urinary 5-HIAA; small bowel series

Malaria: blood smear for parasites, bone marrow examination

Marfan's syndrome: x-ray long bones and ribs, slit-lamp examination of eyes, IVP, urinary hydroxyproline

Marie-Strümpell spondylitis: x-ray of lumbosacral spine, sedimentation rate, latex flocculation
Measles: smear of nasal secretions for giant cells, serologic tests
Megaloblastic anemia: see Pernicious anemia, this table
Meig's syndrome: thoracocentesis, culdoscopy, exploratory laparotomy
Meningococcemia: blood cultures, spinal fluid examination, smear and culture, Gram stain of punctured petechiae
Menopause syndrome: urinary gonadotrophins; vaginal smear for estrogenic effects, therapeutic trial
Mikulicz's disease: CBC, bone marrow, tuberculin test, biopsy of lesion
Mongolism: clinical diagnosis, psychometric tests, chromosome study
Moniliasis: tissue smear or biopsy; culture
Mononucleosis, infectious: smear for atypical lymphocytes, heterophil agglutination test
Mucormycosis: nose and throat culture, biopsy
Mucoviscoidosis (see Cystic fibrosis of pancreas): quantitative sweat test, duodenal assay of pancreatic enzymes and bicarbonate, chest x-ray
Multiple myeloma: serum protein electrophoresis, urine for Bence-Jones protein, bone marrow biopsy, serum calcium levels, skeletal survey
Mumps: skin test, serologic tests
Myeloid metaplasia, agnogenic: red cell morphology, CBC, bone marrow examination, splenic aspirate, hepatic function tests, skeletal survey, leukocyte alkaline phosphatase
Myelophthisic anemia: CBC, bone marrow examination, skeletal survey, lymph node biopsy
Myotonia atrophica: BMR, electromyography, urine creatinine, muscle biopsy

Nematodes: gastric analysis, muscle biopsy, eosinophil count, intradermal skin test; precipitin, complement-fixation, and flocculation techniques; ECG; Stoll's egg count in stool, stool cultures and smears; duodenal aspiration, G.I. series; rectal swab with Scotch tape
Neurofibromatosis: biopsy, x-ray of spinal column and long bones, spinal fluid examination, myelogram
Neurosyphilis: spinal tap, serologic tests (Wassermann, TPI, FTA)
Niacin deficiency (see Pellagra): Urine N-methylnicotinamide
Niemann-Pick disease: demonstration of sphingomyelin in reticuloendothelial cells, bone marrow biopsy, tissue biopsy, x-ray of skull and long bones
Nocardiosis: sputum smear and culture
Nutritional neuropathy: serum pyruvic acid, blood pentose concentration, urine niacin or thiamine after loading dose

Ochronosis: urinalysis (Benedict's solution, isolation of homogentisic acid), x-ray of spine
Osteomalacia: serum calcium, phosphorus, alkaline phosphatase, x-ray of long bones, response to vitamin D and calcium

Pancreatitis, chronic: serum and urine amylase and lipase, glucose tolerance test, pancreatic juice volume, bicarbonate and enzyme concentration; G.I. series, cholecystogram, exploratory laparotomy
Pellagra: urinary N-methylnicotinamide
Periarteritis nodosa: muscle, skin, and subcutaneous tissue biopsy; CBC, eosinophil count, urinary sediment
Pernicious anemia: CBC, blood smear, bone marrow, gastric analysis, Schilling test
Peutz-Jeghers syndrome: small bowel series, exploratory laparotomy
Phenylpyruvic oligophrenia: urinalysis for phenylpyruvic acid and phenylalanine
Pheochromocytoma: histamine provocative or Regitine blocking test, plasma and urine for epinephrine and norepinephrine, 24-hour urine test for VMA or catecholamines, IVP, presacral air insufflation, exploratory surgery
Phlebotomus fever: serologic tests
Pituitary adenoma: skull x-ray, PBI, urinary 17-ketosteroids and 17-hydroxycorticosteroids, urine HPG (human pituitary gonadotropin)
Plague: see Bubonic plague, this table
Polycystic ovary (see Stein-Leventhal syndrome, this table): culdoscopy, exploratory laparotomy
Polycythemia vera: CBC, platelet count, blood volume, BMR, serum uric acid, arterial oxygen saturation, pulmonary function tests
Polymyositis: see Dermatomyositis, this table
Porphyria: urine porphyrins and porphobilinogen
Portal cirrhosis: see Laennec's cirrhosis, this table
Pott's disease: x-ray of spine, aspiration and culture of synovial fluid, synovial or bone biopsy, PPD, intermediate
Preeclampsia: see Eclampsia, this table
Pseudohypoparathyroidism: serum calcium, phosphorus, urine calcium, Ellsworth-Howard test, parathyroid tissue biopsy
Pyridoxine deficiency: serum iron concentration, urine concentration of xanthurenic acid, and trial of isoniazid, tryptophan tolerance test

Q-fever: serologic tests

Rat-bite fever: culture of lesion, aspiration and culture of regional lymph node, animal inoculation, serologic tests
Raynaud's disease: L.E. preparations, skin biopsy, muscle biopsy, serum protein electrophoresis
Regional enteritis: small bowel series, surgical exploration
Reiter's disease: clinical diagnosis, laboratory exclusion of other cause of joint pathology
Relapsing fever: peripheral blood for *Borrelia*, inoculation of rats and mice, serologic tests, total leukocytes, spinal tap
Reticuloendotheliosis: x-ray, erythrocyte count, tissue cholesterol content, biopsy skeletal lesion and of bone marrow or lymph nodes
Rheumatic fever: ASO titer, CRP, sedimentation rate, ECG
Rheumatoid arthritis: agglutination test using rheu-

matoid sera, x-ray of affected joints, serum iron, examination of synovial fluid; latex, flocculation test, erythrocyte sedimentation rate
Riboflavin deficiency: clinical diagnosis, therapeutic trial
Rickets: x-ray of bones, serum calcium, phosphorus, alkaline phosphatase, urine calcium
Rocky Mountain spotted fever: specific serologic tests, Weil-Felix test
Rubella: none
Rubeola: see Measles, this table

Sarcoidosis: see Boeck's sarcoid, this table
Scarlet fever: nose and throat culture, ASO titer, Schultz-Charlton reaction
Schistosomiasis: stool for ova or urine for ova, rectal biopsy, liver biopsy
Schönlein-Henoch purpura: urinalysis, platelet count, coagulation studies to exclude other causes of purpura
Schüller-Christian disease: see Hand-Schüller-Christian disease, this table
Scleroderma: skin biopsy, esophagram
Scurvy: x-rays of bones, capillary fragility test, serum ascorbic acid, therapeutic trial
Septicemia: blood cultures
Sexual precocity: skull x-ray, urine 17-ketosteroids and 17-hydroxysteroids, exploratory surgery
Sickle cell anemia: CBC, Wright's stain of peripheral blood, serum bilirubin, sickle cell preparation, x-ray of skull and long bones, hemoglobin electrophoresis
Simmonds' disease: see Hypopituitarism, this table
Sjögren's syndrome: Schirmer test for tear production, latex flocculation, thyroglobulin antibody titer, and other auto-immune antibody titers
Smallpox: smear of vesicular fluid for virus particles, viral isolation, serologic tests
Sporotrichosis: culture of exudate from ulcer, serologic tests
Sprue: see Celiac disease, this table
Steatorrhea: see Celiac disease, this table
Stein-Leventhal syndrome: culdoscopy, urine 17-ketosteroids, exploratory surgery
Stevens-Johnson syndrome: clinical diagnosis
Still's disease: latex flocculation, CRP, ASO titer, synovianalysis
Sturge-Weber syndrome: skull x-ray, clinical observation, EEG
Subacute bacterial endocarditis: blood cultures, urine cultures, bone marrow cultures, smear of petechiae
Syphilis: blood and spinal fluid Wassermann, etc., TPI, FTA, dark-field microscopy

Tabes dorsalis: blood Wassermann, etc., x-ray of spine, spinal fluid for colloidal gold and Wassermann or TPI
Takayasu disease: aortography, clinical observation
Tetanus: clinical diagnosis; positive cultures do not establish diagnosis
Torulosis: see Cryptococcosis, this table
Toxemias of pregnancy: see Preeclampsia, this table

Toxoplasmosis: Sabin-Feldman dye test for *Toxoplasma* antibodies, complement-fixation test, skin test
Trichinosis: WBC and differential, muscle biopsy, *Trichinella* skin test
Trypanosomiasis: smears of blood, CSF, lymph node aspirate for parasites
Tuberculosis: smear and culture of sputum or gastric washings, guinea pig inoculation, skin test, chest x-ray
Tularemia: culture of material from ulcer, lymph nodes, or nasopharynx; Foshay's skin test, serologic tests
Turner's syndrome: urine for human pituitary gonadotropin, buccal smear for chromatins, chromosomal studies
Typhoid fever: culture of blood, bone marrow, urine, or stool; febrile agglutinins (Widal reaction)
Typhus epidemic: serologic tests, Weil-Felix test
Typhus scrub: Isolation from blood and Weil-Felix reaction, serologic tests

Ulcerative colitis: barium enema, sigmoidoscopy

Varicella: serologic tests (although clinical diagnosis is usually sufficient)
Variola: see Smallpox, this table
Vitamin A deficiency: serum vitamin A or carotene, dark-adaptation test, skin biopsy
Vitamin B deficiency: see Beriberi, this table
Vitamin C deficiency: see Scurvy, this table
Vitamin D deficiency: x-ray of skull, chest, and long bones; serum calcium, phosphorus and alkaline phosphatase, urine calcium
von Gierke's disease: see Glycogen-storage disease, this table
von Willebrand's disease: bleeding time, coagulation time, thromboplastin-generation test

Waterhouse-Friderichsen syndrome: blood cultures, spinal fluid examination, nose and throat culture, urine 17-ketosteroids and 17-hydroxysteroids
Wegener's granulomatosis: x-ray of nose, sinuses, and chest; urinalysis, renal biopsy, lung biopsy
Weil's disease: dark-field examination of blood for spirochetes, guinea pig inoculation, serologic tests, spinal fluid examination
Wernicke's encephalopathy: serum pyruvic acid, response to thiamine
Whipple's disease: small bowel series, lymph node biopsy, jejunal mucosa biopsy
Wilson's disease: urine copper and amino acids, serum ceruloplasmin, liver biopsy, slit-lamp examination of cornea

Yellow fever: viral isolation, neutralization tests

Zollinger-Ellison syndrome: 12-hour quantitative gastric analysis, G.I. series, gastroscopy, exploratory laparotomy

Table VII.
Laboratory Tests of Organ Involvement

Adrenal cortex:
    Serum electrolytes
    Glucose tolerance test
    24-hour urine 17-ketosteroids before and after ACTH
    24-hour urine 17-hydroxysteroids before and after ACTH
    24-hour urine aldosterone test
    Plasma renin
    Eosinophil count before and after ACTH
    Robinson-Power-Kepler water test
    Flat plate of abdomen

Adrenal medulla:
    Histamine test
    Regitine test
    24-hour urine catecholamines or VMA
    Perirenal air insufflation
    Aortography

Ear:
    Audiogram
    Caloric tests
    Spinal tap
    X-rays of mastoids and petrous bones

Esophagus:
    Barium swallow
    Esophageal perfusion test
    Esophagoscopy
    Esophageal motility

Eye:
    Tonometry
    Visual activity
    Visual fields

Heart:
    Chest x-ray with barium swallow
    ECG
    Venous pressure and circulation time
    Vital capacity
    Fluoroscopy
    Serum lactic dehydrogenase
    Serum transaminase
    Angiography
    Blood volume
    Arterial gas analysis

Joints:
    Synovialysis
    Arthrogram
    Joint biopsy

Kidney:
    BUN and creatinine
    Serum electrolytes
    Urinalysis
    Addis count
    Creatinine clearance
    Fishberg concentration test
    PSP dye test
    Intravenous pyelogram, retrograde pyelography
    Cystoscopy
    Urine culture, renal biopsy

Large bowel:
    Stool for occult blood
    Barium enema
    Sigmoidoscopy
    Stool for occult blood
    Stool for ova and parasites

Liver:
    BSP dye test
    Serum bilirubin
    Thymol turbidity
    Serum transaminase
    Alkaline phosphatase
    Serum protein and albumin/globulin ratio
    Prothrombin time
    Urine bile and urobilinogen
    Duodenal drainage
    Cholecystogram or I.V. cholangiogram
    Rose bengol ^{131}I uptake
    Liver biopsy

Lung:
    Pulmonary function tests
    Chest x-ray
    Fluoroscopy
    Blood carbon dioxide
    Arterial oxygen saturation
    Serum lactic dehydrogenase
    Bronchoscopy
    Bronchogram

Muscle:
    Serum creatine phosphokinase
    Serum transaminase
    Serum lactic dehydrogenase
    24-hour urine creatinine and creatine
    Electromyography
    Muscle biopsy

Nervous system:
    Spinal tap
    X-rays of the skull or spine
    Electroencephalography
    Visual fields
    Audiogram
    Caloric tests
    Brain scan
    Echoencephalogram
    Electromyography

Ovary:
    24-hour urine gonadotropin
    Vaginal smear for estrogen effects

Temperature chart
Hysterosalpingography
Cervical biopsy
Endometrial biopsy
Culdoscopy

Pancreas:
1. Acinar cells
   Serum amylase
   Serum lipase
   Duodenal drainage
   Stool for fat and trypsin
   Flat plate of abdomen
   G.I. series
   Radioactive trioleic acid uptake
2. Islet cells
   Fasting blood sugar
   Glucose tolerance test
   Fractional urines
   36-hour fast
   Insulin tolerance test
   Tolbutamide tolerance test
   Cortisone glucose tolerance test

Parathyroid:
Serum calcium
Serum phosphorus
Alkaline phosphatase
24-hour urine calcium
X-rays of skull, long bones, and teeth

Pituitary:
See Adrenal cortex, Thyroid, Ovary, and Testicles, this table
Skull x-ray
Hickey-Hare test
Pitressin test
Intake and output

Reticuloendothelial system:
CBC and smear of peripheral blood
Platelet count
Bone marrow aspiration
Serum bilirubin
Flat plate of abdomen for spleen size
X-rays of long bones
Stool for stercobilinogen
Urine urobilinogen
Chromium-tagged red cell survival
Schilling test
Gastric analysis
Serum iron and iron-binding capacity
Coombs' test

Serum protein electrophoresis
Coagulation time
Prothrombin time

Skeleton:
Serum calcium
Serum phosphorus
Alkaline phosphatase
X-rays of skull and long bones
Bone biopsy

Skin:
KOH preparation
Wood's lamp exam
Skin biopsy
Culture

Small bowel:
D-Xylose absorption test
Glucose tolerance test
Serum carotene test
Urine 5-HIAA
Stool for fat content
Radioactive triolein and olein uptake
Small bowel series
Stool for occult blood
Stool culture
Stool for ova and parasites
Peritoneal tap
Peritoneoscopy
Mucosal biopsy

Stomach:
Gastric analysis
Upper G.I. series
Gastroscopy
Stool for occult blood

Testicles:
24-hour urine gonadotropin
24-hour urine 17-ketosteroids
Semen analysis
Acid phosphatase
Testicular biopsy
Buccal smear

Thyroid:
BMR
Serum cholesterol
PBI, free thyroxine
RAI uptake
T_3 uptake, T_4 uptake
Photomotogram

Index

Abdomen, distension of, in porphyria, 62
Abortion, as symptom, 322
Abscess, as symptom, 322
Acanthosis nigricans, as symptom, 322
Achalasia, in Chagas' disease, 183
Acidosis, renal tubular, 202
Acne vulgaris, as symptom, 322
Acrodynia, 282
Acromegaly, 82
Addison's disease, 80
  vs. hypopituitarism, 95
Adenoma, in primary hyperparathyroidism, 90
  islet cell, 100, 105
    as symptom, 324
  of adrenal cortex, in aldosteronism, 85
  of parathyroid, as symptom, 322
  pancreatic, in Zollinger-Ellison syndrome, 105
  pituitary, in acromegaly, 82
Adrenal cortex. See *Cortex, adrenal.*
Adrenal cortical hyperplasia, in Cushing's syndrome, 89
Adrenal gland(s), as clinical key, 301, 311
  atrophy of, in hypopituitarism, 95
  infiltration of, in histoplasmosis, 177
  metastases to, in meningococcemia, 153
Adrenal medulla, tests of, 331
Adrenal tumors, in pheochromocytoma, 104
Adrenocortical atrophy, in Addison's disease, 81
Adrenogenital syndrome, 83
African trypanosomiasis, 194
Agranulocytosis, as symptom, 322
Alcoholism, 268
Aldosteronism, 84
Alkaptonuria, 198
Allergic diseases, 5. See also specific diseases.
Amebiasis, 184
Amino aciduria, in rickets, 78
Amyloidosis, primary systemic, 200
  secondary, 203
Anemia. See also *Blood.*
  aplastic, 10
  hemolytic, in thrombotic thrombocytopenic purpura, 20
  hypochromic, as symptom, 322
  Mediterranean, 12
  microcytic, in osteopetrosis, 50
  of lymphatic leukemia, 236
  pernicious, 63, 64
    vs. lead poisoning, 279
  sickle cell, 14

Aneurysm(s), aortic, as symptom, 322
  arterial, in periarteritis nodosa, 29
  berry, as symptom, 322
  cerebral, in polycystic disease, 51
Angiitis, in epidemic typhus, 131
  thrombosis following, in Rocky Mountain spotted fever, 129
Angiomas, retinal, in Sturge-Weber syndrome, 55
Ankylosing spondylitis, 32
Aorta, as clinical key, 301
  systemic medionecrosis of, in arachnodactyly, 43
  valve of, bacterial endocarditis affecting, 139
Aortic insufficiency, as symptom, 322
  in syphilis, 170
Aortic valvulitis, in ankylosing spondylitis, 32
Appendicitis, as symptom, 322
Arachnodactyly, 40
Arsenic poisoning, 274
Artery(ies). See also specific arteries.
  as clinical key, 301, 311
  in epidemic typhus, 131
  involvement of, in granulomatosis, 35
  necrosis of, in periarteritis nodosa, 29
Arthritis, as symptom, 322
  in rheumatic fever, 141
  in ulcerative colitis, 287
  nonmigratory, in streptobacillary fever, 145
  rheumatoid, 24
    juvenile, 34
    vs. gonorrhea, 149
  septic, with bacteremia, in scarlet fever, 143
Aschoff body, in acute rheumatic fever, 141
Asthma, as symptom, 322
Atherosclerosis, 284
  and beriberi, 66
Atrial fibrillation, as symptom, 322

Bacteremia, with septic arthritis, in scarlet fever, 143
Bacteria, diseases involving, 135. See also specific diseases.
Bacterial endocarditis, subacute, 138
Balanitis, as symptom, 322
Bancroftian filariasis, 187
Benzene poisoning, 280
Beriberi, 66
Bilirubin gallstones, in sickle cell anemia, 15

Bitot's spots, in vitamin A deficiency, 74
Black-water fever, 165, 189
Bladder, as clinical key, 301, 311
  vasculitis of, in periarteritis nodosa, 29
Blastomycosis, North American, 172
Blindness, in osteopetrosis, 50
Blood. See also *Anemia.*
  as clinical key, 301, 311
Blood cultures, in bacterial endocarditis, 139
Blood diseases, 9. See also specific diseases.
Blood-urea-nitrogen, in rickets, 78
Bone(s), as clinical key, 302, 311
  bowing of, in rickets, 78
  changes in, in pseudohypoparathyroidism, 107
  enlargement of, in acromegaly, 82
  fracture of, in rickets, 78
  involvement of, in arachnodactyly, 43
  increased density of, in osteopetrosis, 50
Bone marrow, drugs toxic to, 280
  fatty infiltration of, in aplastic anemia, 10
  invasion of, in kala-azar, 188
  involvement of, in pernicious anemia, 65
  megaloblastic, in pellagra, 71
Bowel. See *Intestine(s).*
Bowel sounds, in Peutz-Jegher's syndrome, 53
Bowel tumors, in Peutz-Jegher's syndrome, 53
Brain, infection of, in nocardiosis, 179
  involvement of, in mongolism, 47
  in toxoplasmosis, 193
Brain damage, in galactosemia, 214
Breast(s), as clinical key, 302, 312
  atrophy of, in adrenogenital syndrome, 83
Bronchi, inflammation of, in typhoid fever, 147
Bronchitis, as symptom, 322
Brucellosis, 148
Bursitis, as symptom, 322

Café au lait spots, in neurofibromatosis, 49
Calculus, renal, as symptom, 322
Capillaries, hyaline thrombi in, in thrombotic thrombocytopenic purpura, 20
Carcinoid syndrome, 228
Carbon tetrachloride, poisoning by, 276

Carcinoma, and dermatomyositis, 26
  basal cell, as symptom, 322
  metastatic, 230, 231, 232
  prostatic, 230
Cardiomegaly, in sickle cell anemia, 14
Carpal tunnel, neurologic involvement of, in rheumatoid arthritis, 25
Cataract(s), as symptom, 322
  in galactosemia, 215
Cerebellar degeneration, as symptom, 322
Cerebral aneurysms, in polycystic disease, 51
Cerebral cortex. See *Cortex.*
Cerebral hemorrhage, as symptom, 322
Cerebral thrombosis, as symptom, 322
Chagas' disease, 182
Chickenpox, 114
  vs. smallpox, 125
Cholelithiasis, as symptom, 323
Cholesterol, and hypercholesterolemia, 210
Chorea, Synderham's, 183
Chorioretinitis, as symptom, 323
Chvostek's sign, in hypoparathyroidism, 92
Cirrhosis, of liver, as symptom, 323
Clitoris, enlargement of, in adrenogenital syndrome, 83
Coccidioidomycosis, 174
Colitis, as symptom, 323
Cold, common, as symptom, 323
Collagen diseases, 23. See also specific diseases.
Condylomata lata, in syphilis, 169
Congenital diseases. See specific diseases.
Conjunctivitis, as symptom, 323
  in Listeriosis, 151
Convulsions, in islet cell adenoma, 100
  in rickets, 78
Cor pulmonale, as symptom, 323
Cornea, bacteria in, in vitamin A deficiency, 75
Corneal opacities, in diagnosis, 1
Coronary insufficiency, as symptom, 323
Cortex, adrenal, adenoma of, in adrenogenital syndrome, 83
  in aldosteronism, 85
  tests of, 331
  angiomas of, in Sturge-Weber syndrome, 55
  calcification of, in Sturge-Weber syndrome, 55
  sclerosis in, in tuberosclerosis, 57

Councilman bodies, in yellow fever, 116
Cretinism, 86
 vs. mongolism, 87
Cryptococcosis, 175
Cushing's syndrome, 88
Cutaneous. See also Skin.
Cutaneous lesions, in tularemia, 158
Cutaneous porphyria, 58
 porphyria erythropoietica as form of, 60
Cystic fibrosis, and vitamin A deficiency, 75
Cysticercosis, 185
Cystinosis, 220
Cystitis, as symptom, 323
Cysts, in echinococcosis, 186
 in polycystic disease, 51

Deafness, in osteopetrosis, 50
Deer fly, and tularemia, 158
Deficiency diseases, 63. See also specific diseases.
Dementia, as symptom, 323
Depression, as factor in diagnosis, 1
 in hypoparathyroidism, 92
Dermatomyositis, 26
Dermatomyositis, vs. trichinosis, 196
Diabetes, cryptococcosis in, 175
 early, and hemochromatosis, 219
Diabetes insipidus, as symptom, 323
 in Hand-Schuller-Christian disease, 261
Diabetes mellitus, 204, 205, 206, 208
 as symptom, 323
Diagnosis, of systemic disease, 1
Diarrhea, and pain, in Zollinger-Ellison syndrome, 105
Digitalis intoxication, 270
Dilantin intoxication, 272
Diphtheria, 136
Diseases, of unknown etiology, 281
Drugs, toxic to bone marrow, 280
Dupuytren's contracture, as symptom, 323
Dwarfism, in Laurence-Moon-Biedl syndrome, 101
Dysgenesis, seminiferous tubule, 98

Ear(s), as clinical key, 302, 312
 diseases in, 309
 tests of, 331
Ecchymoses, in aplastic anemia, 10
 in hemophilia, 22
Echinococcosis, 186
Eczema, in oligophrenia, 223
Electrophoresis, hemoglobin, 13
Elephantiasis, in filariasis, 187
Ellsworth-Howard test, in pseudohypoparathyroidism, 107
Emphysema, chronic pulmonary, 246

Encephalitis, acute, in lead poisoning, 279
 as symptom, 323
 complicating measles, 121
Encephalopathy, as symptom, 323
 Wernicke's in beriberi, 66
Endocarditis, in Q-fever, 134
 subacute bacterial, 138
Endocrine diseases, 79. See also specific diseases.
Enteritis, regional, vs. Whipple's disease, 297
Epidemic typhus, 130
Epididymitis, as symptom, 323
Epilepsy, vs. islet cell adenoma, 100
Epiphyseal growth, in cretinism, 87
Episcleritis, in rheumatoid arthritis, 24
Epistaxis, in idiopathic thrombocytopenic purpura, 18
Erythema multiforme, in ulcerative colitis, 287
Erythema nodosum, as symptom, 323
Erythropoiesis, in anemia, 13
Eschar, in scrub typhus, 133
Esophageal mucosa, involvement of, in Plummer-Vinson syndrome, 67
Esophageal stricture, as symptom, 323
Esophagus, as clinical key, 302, 312
 involvement of, in Chagas' disease, 183
 in scleroderma, 30
 lesions of, in smallpox, 125
 tests of, 331
Exophthalmos, in Hand-Schuller-Christian disease, 261
 in hyperthyroidism, 91
Extrapyramidal symptoms, in phenothiazine intoxication, 271
Extremities, diseases in, 309
Eye(s), as clinical key, 302, 312
 cataracts of, in galactosemia, 215
 diseases in, 309
 examination of, 1
 involvement of, in arachnodactyly, 43
 in syphilis, 167
 in tularemia, 158
 tests of, 331

Fanconi syndrome, vs. rickets, 78
Fatigue, and hyperpigmentation, in Addison's disease, 81
 in hypothyroidism, 96
 in menopause, 103
 in renal tubular acidosis, 202
Felty's syndrome, 34
Fever. See specific types.
 prolonged, in bacterial endocarditis, 139
 rheumatic. See Rheumatic fever.
Fibroma subcutaneous, as symptom, 323
Fibromas, in neurofibromatosis, 49

Filariasis, 187
Fingernails, brittle, in hypoparathyroidism, 92
Fistula in ano, as symptom, 323
Fracture(s), as symptom, 323
 malunion of, as symptom, 324

Galactosemia, 214
 vs. glycogen storage disease, 209
Gallstones, in sickle cell anemia, 15
Gangrene, in epidemic typhus, 131
 in Rocky Mountain spotted fever, 129
 in scleroderma, 30
Gargoylism, vs. congenital syphilis, 167
Gastric mucosa, atrophy of, in pellagra, 71
Gastroenteritis, as symptom, 323
 in poliomyelitis, 126
Gastrointestinal involvement, in pellagra, 71
Gastrointestinal tract, as clinical key, 303, 312
 hemorrhage of, in idiopathic thrombocytopenic purpura, 19
Gaucher's disease, 258
Genitalia, lesions of, in syphilis, 169
Genitourinary tract, as clinical key, 303, 313
Gingivitis, as symptom, 324
Glaucoma, as symptom, 324
 in diabetes, 204
Glomerulonephritis, as symptom, 324
 complicating scarlet fever, 143
Glossitis, as symptom, 324
Glycogen storage disease, 209
 and systemic amyloidosis, 201
Glycogenosis, 209
Goiter, in cretinism, 87
Gonadal dysgenesis, 108
Gonococcal endocarditis, in gonorrhea, 149
Gonorrhea, 149
 vs. sporotrichosis, 180
Gout, 216
 as symptom, 324
Granulomas, of pulmonary tuberculosis, 157
 of tularemia, 158
Granulomatosis, Wegener's, 35
 vs. mucormycosis, 178
Growth, retardation of, in Laurence-Moon-Biedl syndrome, 101
Gums, as clinical key, 303, 313
 swelling of, in scurvy, 72

Hair, absence of, in Turner's syndrome, 108
 as clinical key, 303, 313
 coarseness of, in hypothyroidism, 96
 loss of, in hypothyroidism, 96
Hand-Schuller-Christian disease, 260

Headache, and joint pain, in acromegaly, 82
Heart, as clinical key, 303, 313
 tests of, 331
Heart failure, chronic congestive, 247
 in diphtheria, 137
Heart murmur, in syphilis, 170
Hematuria, in primary hyperparathyroidism, 90
 in purpura, 16
Hemiplegia, in bacterial endocarditis, 139
Hemochromatosis, idiopathic, 218
Hemoglobin electrophoresis, in anemia, 13
Hemoglobinuria, 189
Hemophilia, 22
Hemoptysis, in pulmonary tuberculosis, 157
Hemorrhage, cerebral, as symptom, 322
 in hemophilia, 22
 nasal, in idiopathic thrombocytopenic purpura, 18
 renal, in idiopathic thrombocytopenic purpura, 19
 subarachnoid, in polycystic disease, 51
Hemorrhoids, as symptom, 324
Henoch-Schonlein's purpura, 16
Hepatic failure, chronic, 248
Hepatomegaly, in sickle cell anemia, 14
Hepatorenal syndrome, 165
Hepatosplenomegaly, in amyloidosis, 203
 in myelofibrosis, 240
 in osteopetrosis, 50
 in Still's disease, 34
 in thrombotic thrombocytopenic purpura, 20
Hereditary diseases. See specific diseases.
Hernia, inguinal, as symptom, 324
Herpes zoster, and chickenpox, 115
Hirsutism, in adrenogenital syndrome, 83
 in Cushing's syndrome, 88
 in menopause, 102
Histiocytosis X, 260, 262
Histoplasmosis, disseminated, 176
History, taking of, 1
Homogentisic acid, in alkaptonuria, 198
Hyaline thrombi, in capillaries, in thrombotic thrombocytopenic purpura, 20
Hydrocephalus, as symptom, 324
Hydronephrosis, as symptom, 324
Hypercholesterolemia, essential, 210
 vs. hypertriglyceridemia, 213
Hyperglycemia, in pheochromocytoma, 104
Hyperparathyroidism, primary, 90
 vs. gout, 217
 vs. renal tubular acidosis, 202
Hyperpigmentation, in scleroderma, 30
Hypersplenism, in lupus erythematosus, 37

Hypertension, and adrenal adenoma, 85
   essential, 288
   labile, in pheochromocytoma, 104
Hyperthyroidism, 91
Hypertriglyceridemia, essential, 212
Hyperthyroidism, vs. diabetes, 205
Hypervitaminosis A, 76
Hypogonadism, in hypopituitarism, 95
Hypokalemia, 269
Hypoparathyroidism, 92
Hypopituitarism, 94
   vs. Laurence-Moon-Biedl syndrome, 101
Hypopotassemia, in hypokalemia, 269
Hypothyroidism, 96

Icteric sclera, in anemia, 13, 14
Ilium, Peyer's patch of, hyperplasia in, in typhoid fever, 147
Impotence, in hypopituitarism, 94
Infarction, pulmonary, as symptom, 324
   splenic, as symptom, 324
Infectious diseases, 111. See also specific diseases.
Inguinal node adenopathy, in syphilis, 168
Intestine(s), borborygmi of, in Peutz-Jegher's syndrome, 52
   large, as clinical key, 314
     tests of, 331
     tumors of, metastases of, 231
   musculature of, fibrosis of, in pellagra, 71
   small, tests of, 332
   tumors of, in Peutz-Jegher's syndrome, 53
Intoxication, digitalis, 270
   Dilantin, 272
   phenothiazine, 271
Iritis, as symptom, 324
   in ankylosing spondylitis, 33
Iron, excessive, and hemochromatosis, 219
Iron deficiency, and Plummer-Vinson Syndrome, 67
Islet cell adenoma, 100
   as symptom, 324
Islet cells, as clinical key, 304, 313

Jaundice, in Weil's disease, 165
Joints, as clinical key, 304, 313
   dislocation of, as symptom, 323
   involvement of, in gonorrhea, 149
     in Lupus erythematosus, 37, 40
     in Still's disease, 34
   pain in, in acromegaly, 82
   swelling of, in hemophilia, 22
     in periarteritis nodosa, 28
     in rheumatoid arthritis, 24
   tenderness of, in lymphogranuloma venereum, 118
   tests of, 331

Kala-azar, 188
Keratitis, as symptom, 324
Kidney, as clinical key, 304, 313
   horseshoe, in Turner's syndrome, 108
   involvement of, in pulmonary tuberculosis, 157
   polycystic, 51
   tests of, 331
Kimmelstiel-Wilson's disease, 207
   with diabetes, 208
Klinefelter's syndrome, 98
Koplik's spots, in measles, 120
Kwashiorkor, 68

Laboratory procedures, in diagnosis, 1
   in infectious diseases, 111
   in systemic diseases, 327
Laryngitis, as symptom, 324
Laurence-Moon-Biedl syndrome, 101
Lead poisoning, 278
Lens, dislocation of, as symptom, 324
Leptospirosis, and Weil's disease, 165
   vs. carbon tetrachloride poisoning, 277
Letterer-Siwe disease, 262
Leukemia, acute lymphatic, 234
   chronic myelogenous, 237
   cryptococcosis in, 175
   lymphatic, chronic, 236
     vs. myelogenous leukemia, 237
Leydig cells, in Klinefelter's syndrome, 99
Lice, and relapsing fever, 161
Lignac-Fanconi syndrome, 220
   vs. renal tubular acidosis, 202
Listeriosis, 150
Liver, as clinical key, 304, 314
   cirrhosis of, as symptom, 323
     in galactosemia, 215
   cysts in, of echinococcosis, 186
     in polycystic disease, 51
   enlarged, in anemia, 12
   involvement of, with meningitis, in Weil's disease, 165
   lobules of, necrosis of, in yellow fever, 116
   metastases to, 231
   necrosis of, in pellagra, 71
   tests of, 331
Liver-spleen involvement, in aplastic anemia, 11
Loeffler's syndrome, as symptom, 324
Lungs, as clinical key, 304, 314
   involvement of, in granulomatosis, 35
   in Q-fever, 134
   metastases to, 231
   tests of, 331
   vascular nodular densities in, in periarteritis nodosa, 28
Lupus erythematosus, 36, 38, 40
Lymph node(s), as clinical key, 305, 314
   inquinal, involvement of, in plague, 154
   involvement of, in syphilis, 168

regional, involvement of, in tuberculosis, 157
Lymphadenitis, generalized, as symptom, 324
   local, as symptom, 324
Lymphadenopathy, in Hodgkin's disease, 233
   in rubella, 123
   in serum sickness, 6
   in Still's disease, 34
   in syphilis, 169
   in thrombotic thrombocytopenic purpura, 20
Lymphatic leukemia, acute, 234
   chronic, 236
Lymphogranuloma venereum, 118
Lymphoid hyperplasia, in typhoid fever, 147
Lymphoma, cryptococcosis in, 175

Macroglobulinemia, 238
Malabsorption syndrome, 252
Malaria, 165, 189
   vs. yellow fever, 116
Manic-depressive psychosis, as symptom, 324
Mastitis, as symptom, 324
McArdle's disease, 209
Measles, 120
Meningeal involvement, in mumps, 119
Meningitis, aseptic, in leptospirosis, 165
   in Weil's disease, 165
   chest x-ray in diagnosis of, 175
Meningococcemia, 152
Meningoencephalitis, Chagas', 183
   in mononucleosis, 117
   in mumps, 119
Menopause, 102
Mental disorientation, in pellagra, 71
Mental retardation, in cretinism, 86
   in Laurence-Moon-Biedl syndrome, 101
   in mongolism, 46
   in oligophrenia, 223
   in toxoplasmosis, 192
   in tuberosclerosis, 56
Mercury, in urine, in acrodynia, 283
Mesenteric artery, thrombosis of, in periarteritis nodosa, 29
Metabolic diseases, 197. See also specific diseases.
Mitral stenosis, as symptom, 324
Mitral valve, involvement of, in bacterial endocarditis, 139
Mongolism, 46
   vs. cretinism, 87
Mongoloid features, in anemia, 12
Mononucleosis, infectious, 117
   infectious, vs. listeriosis, 150
   vs. toxoplasmosis, 193
   vs. Weil's disease, 165
Mouth, as clinical key, 305, 315
Mucormycosis, 178
Mucosa, oral. See also Gums.
   atrophy of, in Plummer-Vinson syndrome, 67
   involvement of, in smallpox, 125

swelling of, in scurvy, 72
ulceration of, in aplastic anemia, 11
Mumps, 119
Muscle(s), as clinical key, 305, 315
   increase of mass of, in adrenogenital syndrome, 83
   involvement of, in dermatomyositis, 26
   tests of, 331
   wasting of, in hyperthyroidism, 91
Myasthenia gravis, as symptom, 324
Mycoses, 171
Myelofibrosis, with myeloid metaplasia, 240
Myelogenous leukemia, chronic, 237
Myeloid metaplasia, vs. myelogenous leukemia, 237
   with myelofibrosis, 240
Myeloma, multiple, 241
   vs. macroglobulinemia, 239
Myocarditis, in diphtheria, 137
   in poliomyelitis, 126
Mycordium, involvement of, in Chagas' disease, 183
Myositis, as symptom, 324
Myotonia atrophica, 290
Myxedema, vs. hypopituitarism, 95

Nails, as clinical key, 305, 315
   ridging of, in hyperthyroidism, 91
Nasal septum, involvement of, in granulomatosis, 35
Neck, diseases in, 310
Necrobiosis lipoidica, 207
Neoplasms, 227. See also specific neoplasms.
Nephritis, as symptom, 324
   chronic, vs. rickets, 78
Nephrocalcinosis, in renal tubular acidosis, 202
Nephrolithiasis, in gout, 217
Nephrotic syndrome, and amyloidosis, 203
Nerves, cranial, involvement of, in diphtheria, 137
Nervous system, as clinical key, 305, 315
   examination of, 1
   central, involvement of, in periarteritis nodosa, 29
   involvement of, in diphtheria, 137
   in herpes zoster, 115
   in phenothiazine intoxication, 271
   in Rocky Mountain spotted fever, 129
   in serum sickness, 7
   in trichinosis, 196
   peripheral, in beriberi, 66
   involvement of, in porphyria, 62
   tests of, 331
Neuritis, optic, as symptom, 325
   in serum sickness, 7
Neurofibromatosis, 48

Niemann-Pick disease, 264
  vs. Letterer-Siwe disease, 263
Nocardiosis, 179
  vs. cryptococcosis, 175
North American blastomycosis, 172
Nose, as clinical key, 316
  diseases in, 309
  hemorrhage from, in idiopathic thrombocytopenic purpura, 18

Obesity, as symptom, 325
  in Cushing's syndrome, 88
Ochronosis, 198
Oligophrenia, phenylpyruvic, 222
Optic neuritis, as symptom, 325
Orchitis, as symptom, 325
Organ failure, 245
Organ involvement, clinical key to, 301-308
  laboratory tests of, 331
"Oriental sores," 188
Osteomalacia, as symptom, 325
Osteomyelitis, as symptom, 325
Osteopetrosis, 50
Osteoporosis, in menopause, 102
  of spine, in sickle cell anemia, 14
Ovary(ies), as clinical key, 306, 316
  nonpalpable, in Turner's syndrome, 108
  polycystic, vs. adrenogenital syndrome, 83
  tests of, 331

Pancarditis, in lupus erythematosus, 40
Pancreas, adenoma of, in Zollinger-Ellison syndrome, 105
  as clinical key, 316
  islet cells of, as clinical key, 304, 313
    degeneration of, in diabetes, 205
  tests of, 332
  tumors of, 231
Pancreatic insufficiency, in kwashiorkor, 69
Pancreatitis, as symptom, 325
  chronic, 254
  in mumps, 119
Pancytopenia, in kala-azar, 188
  in lupus erythematosus, 37
Paralysis agitans, as symptom, 325
Paralysis ileus, as symptom, 325
Paraplegia, in hemophilia, 22
Parasites, 181
Parathyroid, adenoma of, as symptom, 322
Parathyroid, tests of, 332
Parathyroid gland, as clinical key, 306, 316
  hyperplasia of, in pseudohypoparathyroidism, 107
Parkinsonism, vs. Wilson's disease, 225
Parotid gland, as clinical key, 316
  infiltration of, in mumps, 119
Pellagra, 70
  vs. lead poisoning, 279
"Pellagra" syndrome, 229

Penis, as clinical key, 306, 316
  lesions of, in syphilis, 168
  ulcer of, in lymphogranuloma venereum, 118
Peptic ulcer, as symptom, 325
Periarteritis nodosa, 28
Pericarditis, as symptom, 325
  in Still's disease, 34
Peritonitis, as symptom, 325
Petechiae, in purpura, 16
  in renal failure, 251
  lower extremity, in idiopathic thrombocytopenic purpura, 18
  in thrombotic thrombocytopenic purpura, 20
Peutz-Jegher's syndrome, 52
Pharyngitis, as symptom, 325
  in poliomyelitis, 126
  streptococcal, 143
Pharynx, mucosa of, atrophy of, in Plummer-Vinson syndrome, 67
Phenothiazine intoxication, 271
Phenylpyruvic oligophrenia, 222
Pheochromocyloma, 104
Physical examination, 1
Pigmentation, hyper-, in Addison's disease, 81
  in kwashiorkor, 68
  in scleroderma, 30
Pinguecula, as symptom, 325
Pituitary, tests of, 332
Pituitary adenoma, in acromegaly, 82
Pituitary gland, as clinical key, 306, 316
Plague, 154
Platybasia, as symptom, 325
Pleura, involvement of, in lupus erythematosus, 40
  in nocardiosis, 179
Pleurisy, as symptom, 325
Plummer-Vinson syndrome, 67
Pneumonia, as symptom, 325
  in plague, 154
  viral, vs. Q-fever, 134
Pneumothorax, spontaneous, as symptom, 325
Poisoning, arsenic, 274
  benzene, 280
  carbon tetrachloride, 276
  lead, 278
Poliomyelitis, 126
Polycystic disease, 51
Polycythemia, secondary, vs. polycythemia vera, 243
Polycythemia vera, 242
  as symptom, 325
Polyneuritis, infectious, 324
Polyps, in Peutz-Jegher's syndrome, 53
Polyarthritis, in lupus erythematosus, 37
Polydypsia, in hyperthyroidism, 91
Polyneuritis, in mononucleosis, 117
Polyserositis, in lupus erythematosus, 40
Polyuria, in hyperparathyroidism, 91
Porphyria, as symptom, 325
  intermittent abdominal, 62

vs. lead poisoning, 279
Porphyria cutanea tarda, 58
Porphyria erythropoietica, 60
Pretibial fever, in leptospirosis, 165
Pretibial ulceration, in sickle cell anemia, 14
Priapism, as symptom, 325
Prostate, carcinoma of, 230
Pseudohypoparathyroidism, 106
Psoriasis, as symptom, 325
Psychoneurotic behavior, in brucellosis, 148
  in carcinoid, 229
  in islet cell adenoma, 100
  in thrombotic thrombocytopenic purpura, 20
Pulmonary disease, in nocardiosis, 179
Pulmonary emphysema, chronic, 246
Pulmonary lesions, and skin lesions, in blastomycosis, 173
Pulmonary tuberculosis, 156
Purpura, anaphylactoid, 17
  Henoch-Schonlein's, 16
  idiopathic thrombocytopenic, 18
  thrombotic thrombocytopenic, 20
Pyelonephritis, as symptom, 325
  in diabetes, 208
Pyoderma gangrenosum, in ulcerative colitis, 287

Q-Fever, 134

Raynaud's disease, 325
Rash, in animal bites, 163
  in chickenpox, vs. smallpox, 125
  in Letterer-Siwe disease, 263
  in lupus erythematosus, 38
  in scarlet fever, 143
  in scrub typhus, 133
  in smallpox, vs. chickenpox, 125
  in tuberosclerosis, 56
  maculopapular, in syphilis, 168
  pattern of, in epidemic typhus, vs. Rocky Mountain spotted fever, 131
  pattern of, in Rocky Mountain spotted fever, vs. epidemic typhus, 131
  purpuric, in meningococcemia, 153
Rat-bite fever, spirillary, 162
  spirillary, vs. streptobacillary fever, 145
  vs. sporotrichosis, 180
Rectal stricture, in lymphogranuloma venereum, 118
Rectum, as clinical key, 307, 316
Reiter's syndrome, 292
  lymphogranuloma venereum, 118
Relapsing fever, 160
Renal calculus, as symptom, 322
Renal failure, chronic, 250
Renal tubular acidosis, 202
Renal tubular degeneration, in hypokalemia, 269

Respiratory infection, history of, in meningococcemia, 153
Respiratory tract, infections of, and lymphatic leukemia, 234
  involvement of, in granulomatosis, 35
  in measles, 121
Reticuloendothelial system, involvement of, in kala-azar, 188
  in mononucleosis, 117
  tests of, 332
Reticuloendothelioses, 257
Retina, hemorrhage of, in polycystic disease, 51
  in sickle cell anemia, 14
Retinal detachment, as symptom, 325
Retinal perivasculitis, in periarteritis nodosa, 29
Retinopathy, hypertensive, in periarteritis nodosa, 28
Rheumatic fever, acute, 140
  as complication of scarlet fever, 143
  vs. Chagas' disease, 183
  vs. sickle cell anemia, 15
Rhinitis, as symptom, 325
Rickets, 78
Rickettsiae, 127
Rocky Mountain spotted fever, 128
  vs. tularemia, 158
Rubella, 122
Rubeola, 120

Sarcoid, Boeck's, vs. Niemann-Pick disease, 265
Sarcoidosis, 294
  vs. histoplasmosis, 177
Scarlet fever, 142
Schistosomiasis, 190
Sclera, icteric, in anemia, 13, 14
Scleritis, as symptom, 325
Scleroderma, 30
Scrub typhus, 132
Scurvy, 72
Seminiferous tubule dysgenesis, 98
Serotonin, secretion of, in carcinoid, 229
Serum sickness, 6
Sheehan's syndrome, vs. hypopituitarism, 95
Sinuses, as clinical key, 307, 316
Sinusitis, resistant, and diagnosis of mucormycosis, 178
Skeletal anomalies, in Klinefelter's syndrome, 98
Skeletal system, involvement of, in arachnodactyly, 43
Skeleton, tests of, 332
Skin. See also Cutaneous and Pigmentation.
  as clinical key, 307, 316
  diseases in, 310
  eschar of, in scrub typhus, 133
  examination of, 1
  hairless, in hypopituitarism, 94
  hemorrhage of, in scurvy, 72
  hyperkeratosis of, in vitamin A deficiency, 74
  involvement of, and bowel tu-

mors, in Peutz-Jegher's syndrome, 53
and oral mucosa, in smallpox, 125
in Chagas' disease, 183
in chickenpox, 114
in hyperthyroidism, 91
in kwashiorkor, 68
in lupus erythematosus, 37, 38, 39
in mongolism, 47
in pellagra, 71
in porphyria cutanea tarda, 58
in porphyria erythropoietica, 60
in Rocky Mountain spotted fever, 129
in tuberosclerosis, 56
in ulcerative colitis, 287
lesions of osteolytic, in Hand-Schuller-Christian disease, 261
in periarteritis nodosa, 29
pulmonary, in blastomycosis, 173
in syphilis, 169
puffiness of, in hypothyroidism, 96
scaly, in hypoparathyroidism, 92
tests of, 332
thinning of, in menopause, 102
Skull, appearance of, in sickle cell anemia, 14
Smallpox, 124
Sodium levels, in Addison's disease, 81
Spinal cord, degeneration of, in pellagra, 71
involvement of, in pernicious anemia, 65
in poliomyelitis, 126
Spinal cord compression, in rheumatoid arthritis, 25
Spine, cervical, in Still's disease, 34
osteoporosis of, in sickle cell anemia, 14
Spirillary rat-bite fever, 162
Spirochetes, 159
Spleen, as clinical key, 307, 317
enlarged, in anemia, 12
in aplastic anemia, 11
infarction of, in sickle cell anemia, 15
Splenectomy, in aplastic anemia, 11
Splenic infarction, as symptom, 324
Splenomegaly, and lymphadenopathy, in Hodgkin's disease, 233
with high temperature, in malaria, 189
without lymphadenopathy, in Gaucher's disease, 259
Spondylitis, ankylosing, 32
Sporotrichosis, 180
Stein-Leventhal syndrome, vs. adrenogenital syndrome, 83
Still's disease, 34
Stomach, tests of, 332
ulceration of, in Zollinger-Ellison syndrome, 105
Stomatitis, as symptom, 326
Stool, fatty, in Whipple's disease, 297
Streptobacillary fever, 144
Sturge-Weber syndrome, 54
Subacute bacterial endocarditis, 138
Subperiosteal hemorrhage, in scurvy, 73
Sulkowitch test, in hypoparathyroidism, 92
Synderham's chorea, 183
Syphilis, 168, 170
congenital, 166
hematogenous, 157
primary, 169
secondary, 169
stages of, vs. tuberculosis, 157
vs. miliary tuberculosis, 155
Systemic disease, diagnosis of, 1
laboratory work-up of, 327
local disease as symptom of, 322
with organs showing clinical change, 319

Tachycardia, in rheumatic fever, 141
Temperature, and splenomegaly, in malaria, 189
spiking, in amebiasis, 184
Testicles, as clinical key, 307, 318
atrophy of, in hypopituitarism, 94
in Klinefelter's syndrome, 99
swelling of, in mumps, 119
tests of, 332
Tetany, in rickets, 78
Throat, as clinical key, 307, 318
diseases in, 309
Thrombophlebitis, as symptom, 326
Thyroid, absence of, in cretinism, 87
atrophy of, in hypopituitarism, 95
enlargement of, 91
tests of, 332
Thyroid gland, as clinical key, 308
Ticks, and relapsing fever, 161
and tularemia, 158
Tongue, as clinical key, 308, 318
Toxic diseases, 267
Toxoplasmosis, 192
Trachea, lesions of, in smallpox, 125
Trichinosis, 196
Trousseau's sign, in hypoparathyroidism, 92
Trypanosomiasis, African, 194
vs. kala-azar, 188
Tuberosclerosis, 56
hematogenous, 157
miliary, 155
vs. histoplasmosis, 177
vs. Niemann-Pick disease, 265
pulmonary, 156
vs. histoplasmosis, 177
vs. cryptococcosis, 175
Tularemia, 158
vs. plague, 154
vs. sporotrichosis, 180
Turner's syndrome, 108
vs. Klinefelter's syndrome, 99
Typhoid fever, 146
Typhus, epidemic, 130
scrub, 132

Ulcer, peptic, as symptom, 325
Ulcerations, mucosal, in aplastic anemia, 11
Ulcerative colitis, 286
vs. Whipple's disease, 297
"Uremic frost," in renal failure, 250
Uremic lung, in renal failure, 251
Urethral inflammation, in gonorrhea, 149
Urethritis, as symptom, 326
Urine, amino-aciduria, in cystinosis, 221
dark, in alkaptonuria, 198
mercury in, in acrodynia, 282
screening of, in oligophrenia, 223
Urticaria, in serum sickness, 6
Uveitis, granulomatous, in histoplasmosis, 177
in ankylosing spondylitis, 33

Vaginal mucosa, atrophy of, in menopause, 102
Vaginitis, as symptom, 326
Varicella, 114
Vasculitis, necrotizing, in granulomatosis, 35
Valvulitis, aortic, in ankylosing spondylitis, 32
Veins, involvement of, in granulomatosis, 35
Viral diseases, 113. See also specific diseases.
Vision, changes in, in acromegaly, 82
peripheral, loss of, in hypopituitarism, 94
Vitamin A, deficiency of, 74
in hypervitaminosis, 76
Von Gierke's disease, 209
vs. Niemann-Pick disease, 265

Waterhouse-Friderichsen syndrome, 153
Wegener's granulomatosis, 35
vs. mucormycosis, 178
Weil's disease, 164
vs. yellow fever, 116
Wernicke's encephalopathy, in beriberi, 66
Whipple's disease, 296
Wilson's disease, 224

Xanthelasma, as symptom, 326
X-ray, in diagnosis, 1

Yellow fever, 116

Zollinger-Ellison syndrome, 105